ASPECTS OF PRAEMATURITY AND DYSMATURITY

Nutricia Symposium

# ASPECTS OF PRAEMATURITY AND DYSMATURITY

*Groningen 10—12 May 1967*

EDITORS:

J. H. P. JONXIS, M.D., H. K. A. VISSER, M.D. AND
J. A. TROELSTRA, M.D.

1968

H. E. STENFERT KROESE N.V. — LEIDEN

# CONTENTS

VI CONTENTS

CLOSING SESSION

SUMMING-UP AND GENERAL DISCUSSION

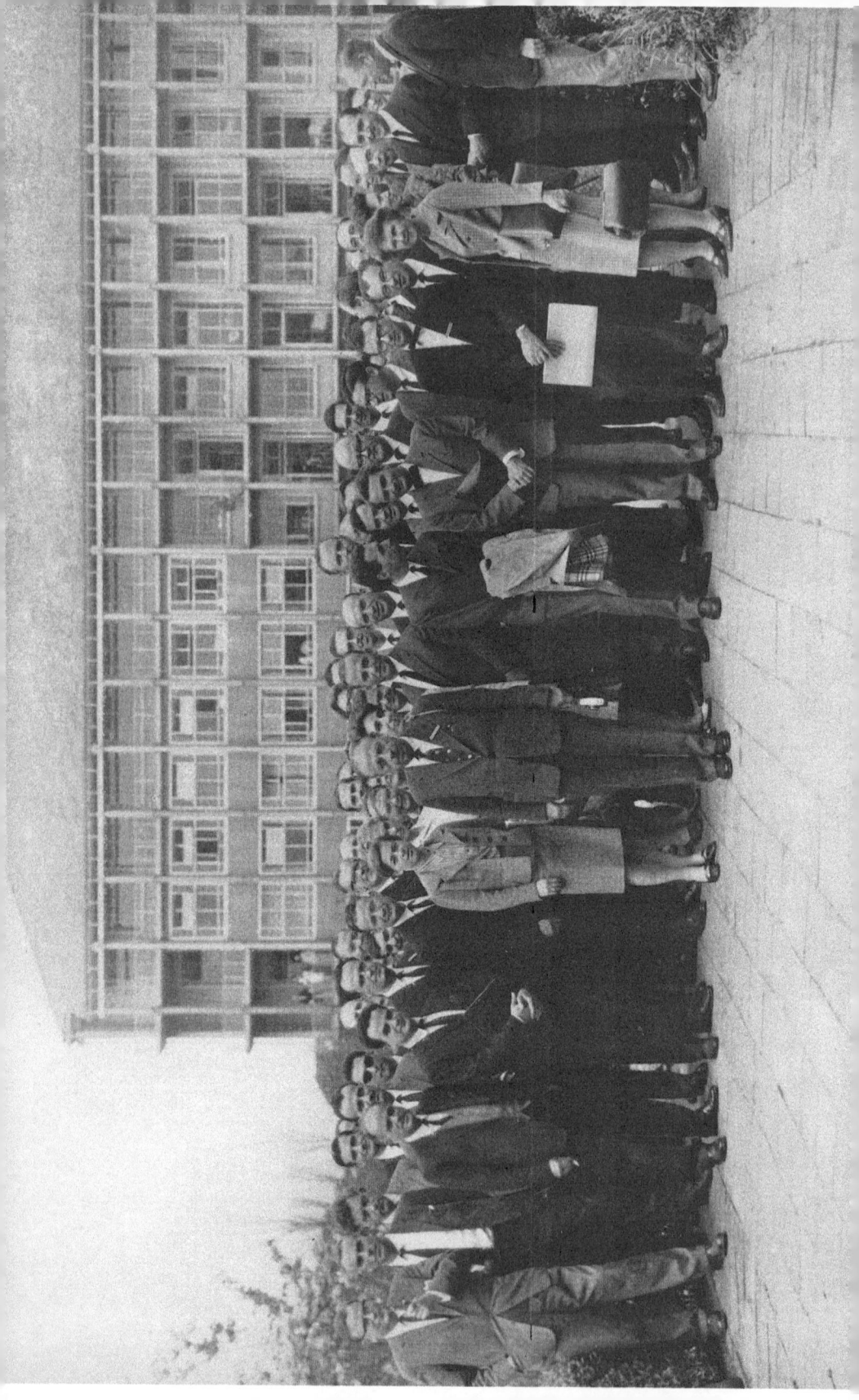

# LIST OF PARTICIPANTS

Mme. D. BLUM-BRACHET, Clinique de Médecine Infantile, Hôpital Universitaire St. Pierre, Bruxelles.

J. H. VAN BOLHUIS, Dept. of Paediatrics, St. Joseph's Hospital, Deventer

J. I. DE BRUIJNE, Dept. of Physiology and Pathology of the Newborn, University of Amsterdam

C. B. F. DAAMEN, Laboratory of Pathology, Dijkzigt Hospital, Rotterdam

N. J. DELBEKE, Dept. of Paediatrics, State University, Gent

M. DIWANY, Children's Hospital, Mounira, Cairo

J. DODION-FRANSEN, Clinique de Médecine Infantile, Hôpital Universitaire St. Pierre, Bruxelles

C. DREYFUS-BRISAC, Centre de Recherches Biologiques Néonatales, Hôpital de Port-Royal, Paris

C. DRILLIEN, Dept. of Child Life and Health, University of Edinburgh

A. C. DROGENDIJK, Dept. of Obstetrics, Vrije Universiteit, Amsterdam

E. EGGERMONT, Lab. de Chimie Physiologique, Université de Louvain

J. ENGELHARDT, Dept. of Paediatrics, Zuiderziekenhuis, Rotterdam

R. FRANÇOIS, Clinique de Pédiatrie, Hôpital Edouard Herriot, Lyon

P. GRUENWALD, Dept. of Pathology, Sinai Hospital of Baltimore

R. GRÜTTNER, Dept. of Paediatrics, State University, Hamburg

P. HADDAD, Maternité Alexandre Khoury, Beirut

P. G. HART, Dept. of Obstetrics, State University, Utrecht

R. HEFFINCK, Paediatrician, Aalst, Belgium

J. JANSSENS, Dept. of Obstetrics, Vrije Universiteit, Amsterdam

J. H. P. JONXIS, Dept. of Paediatrics, State University, Groningen

L. A. JOOSSE, Dept. of Obstetrics, State University, Groningen

B. E. KINGMA, Wilhelmina Children's Hospital, Utrecht

G. J. KLOOSTERMAN, Dept. of Obstetrics, University of Amsterdam

O. KOLDOVSKY, Laboratory of Developmental Nutrition, Prague

F. KUIPERS, Emma Children's Hospital, Amsterdam

A. LAMBRECHTS, Clinique et Policlinique des Maladies d'Enfance, Hôpital de Bavière, Liège

R. DE LEEUW, Dept. of Paediatrics, University of Amsterdam

H. LOEB, Clinique de Médecine Infantile, Hôpital Universitaire St. Pierre, Bruxelles

L. O. Lubchenco, Dept. of Paediatrics, Medical Center, University of Colorado, Denver

B. Luppis, Dept. of Paediatrics, University of Milano

A. S. Majaj, Augusta Victoria Hospital, Jerusalem

J. L. Mastboom, Dept. of Obstetrics, Catholic University, Nijmegen

N. Matsaniotis, Dept. of Paediatrics, University of Athens

A. Minkowski, Centre de Recherches Biologiques Néonatales, Hôpital de Port-Royal, Paris

N. Nicolopoulos, Children's Hospital Aghia Sophia, Athens

M. Ounsted, Nuffield Dept. of Obstetrics and Gynaecology, Radcliffe Infirmy, Oxford

C. Papadatos, Dept. of Paediatrics, University of Athens

H. F. R. Prechtl, Dept. of Developmental Neurology, State University, Groningen

N. C. R. Räihä, Dept. of Paediatrics, University of Helsinki

R. Rappaport, Hôpital des Enfants Malades, Paris

J. W. Reynolds, c/o Hormonlaboratoriet, Karolinska Sjukhuset, Stockholm

J. H. Ruys, Dept. of Paediatrics, State University, Leiden

A. L. C. Schmidt, Dept. of Obstetrics, Dijkzigt Ziekenhuis, Rotterdam

E. D. A. M. Schretlen, Dept. of Paediatrics, Catholic University, Nijmegen

H. Schwartz, Dept. of Pediatrics, Stanford Medical School, Palo Alto

R. Schwartz, Dept. of Pediatrics, Cleveland Metropolitan General Hospital, Cleveland

F. Sereni, Dept. of Paediatrics, University of Milano

A. Sikkel, Dept. of Obstetrics, State University, Leiden

T. D. Stahlie, Dept. of Paediatrics, Vrije Universiteit, Amsterdam

H. Stolley, Institute of Research for Children's Nutrition, Dortmund

S. J. Strich, Institute of Psychiatry, Dept. of Neurology, London

W. Swoboda, Children's Hospital, Vienna

J. A. Troelstra, Dept. of Paediatrics, State University, Groningen

T. Valaes, The Anne-Marie Institute of Child Health, Athens

G. H. M. Veeneklaas, Dept. Paediatrics, State University, Leiden

W. Verhoeven, Nutricia Co., Zoetermeer

H. K. A. Visser, Dept. of Paediatrics, Medical School, Rotterdam

E. M. Widdowson, Medical Research Council, Infant Nutrition Research Division, University of Cambridge

J. S. Wigglesworth, Dept. of Child Health, Hammersmith Hospital, London

J. C. H. N. Wijffels, Dept. of Paediatrics, University of Amsterdam

W. van Zeben, Juliana Children's Hospital, The Hague

# OPENING

PROF. DR. J. H. P. JONXIS

I am happy to welcome you at this second Nutricia Symposium and I am glad that you all arrived safely here in Groningen. The first Nutricia Symposium dealt with a related subject. I see some faces belonging to participants of that meeting and many new ones. I hope that we shall have as good a time as we had three years ago here.

When I look around I see a group of very quiet people in front of me. Yet we are interested in revolutions, for we are studying the most revolutionary moment in mammalian life: birth. In all forms of mammals, whether small or large litters are concerned, or animals born more or less maturely or praematurely, each time birth is a very dangerous moment in the surviving of the species. In the human being, especially in recent years, birth has become a rather safe event thanks to our neighbours, the obstetricians. Still many of us doubt whether always the nervous central system ends up completely undamaged whereas that very system is the most precious possession of man. So there are also in man still many problems about birth we might discuss. I hope that this meeting will not only be one where we enjoy ourselves and that opens possibilities to exchange scientific views, but also one of some practical results.

# ROLE OF THE PLACENTA

# ASPECTS OF STEROID METABOLISM IN THE FOETO-PLACENTAL UNIT AND THE NEWBORN INFANT

JOHN W. REYNOLDS*

One of the striking features of steroid metabolism during human pregnancy is the marked rise in urinary oestrogen excretion. The urinary concentrations of all oestrogens are increased, compared to the non-pregnant levels, but the increase of the 16α-hydroxylated oestrogens is particularly great. The critical role of the foetus in the increased oestrogen production of pregnancy was first shown by CASSMER (1) who found that after inducing foetal death *in utero*, the maternal pregnanediol** excretion fell slightly but the oestrogen excretion showed a marked decrease. FRANDSEN and STAKEMAN (2) reported the first evidence, based on studies of oestrogen excretion by women bearing anencephalic foetuses, that the foetal adrenal gland may produce essential oestrogen precursors. They found that these women, bearing infants with the adrenal hypoplasia characteristic of the anencephalic anomaly, excreted greatly reduced amounts of oestrogens, particularly the 16α-hydroxylated oestrogen, oestriol.

With these beginnings, and with the data derived from many detailed *in vivo* studies to be discussed later in this paper, the concept of the foeto-placental unit as an integrated endocrine organ developed (3, 4). The essence of the concept is that the placenta and foetus acting together are necessary for most of the increased oestrogen production of pregnancy and for the provision of glucocorticoids and aldosterone to the foetus. Neither the foetus nor the placenta alone have the enzyme systems necessary for the production of these various steroids. However, when the foetus and placenta function as a unit,

* Department of Pediatrics, University of Minnesota, Minneapolis, Minn. (Temporarily at the Hormone Laboratory, Karolinska sjukhuset, Stockholm, Sweden).
** See page 18.

1*

all of the enzymes are present for the synthesis of these steroids from circulating cholesterol.

Before discussing the biogenesis of specific steroids in the foeto-placental unit, it may be helpful to review the essential enzyme reactions controlling the synthesis of steroids in endocrine glands. Cholesterol is synthesized from acetate and the cholesterol is converted to the 21-carbon steroid, pregnenolone. Pregnenolone has the same 3β-OH-Δ 5 structure as cholesterol. Pregnenolone is converted to the 19-carbon steroid dehydroepiandrosterone (DHA) through the intermediate 17α-OH-pregnenolone (fig. 1). Hydroxy-

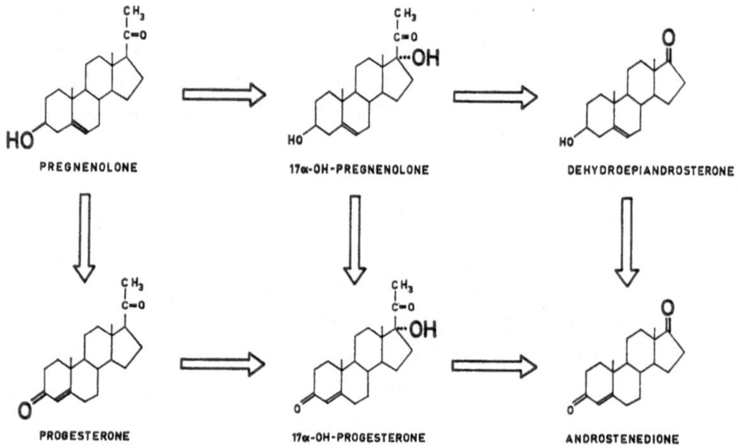

*Fig.* 1. Steps in the conversion of pregnenolone to C-19 steroids.

lation at C-17 is necessary before the side chain can be removed. Pregnenolone can be converted to the biologically active Δ 4-3-keto steroid, progesterone, by two enzymes, 3β-hydroxysteroid dehydrogenase and Δ 4-Δ 5-isomerase (fig. 2). These two enzymes will be called the 3β-hydroxysteroid dehydrogenase system (3β-HSD system) for the sake of simplicity. Progesterone can undergo 17α-hydroxylation and side-chain loss to form androstenedione, and 17α-OH-pregnenolone and DHA can be converted to 17α-OH-progesterone and androstenedione, respectively, by the 3β-HSD system. Oestrogens are formed by the process of aromatisation with 19-carbon, Δ 4-3-keto steroids as substrates (fig. 3). Δ 5-3β-OH steroids are not suitable substrates for aromatisation, but must first be converted to Δ 4-3-keto steroids

CONVERSION OF PREGNENOLONE INTO PROGESTERONE

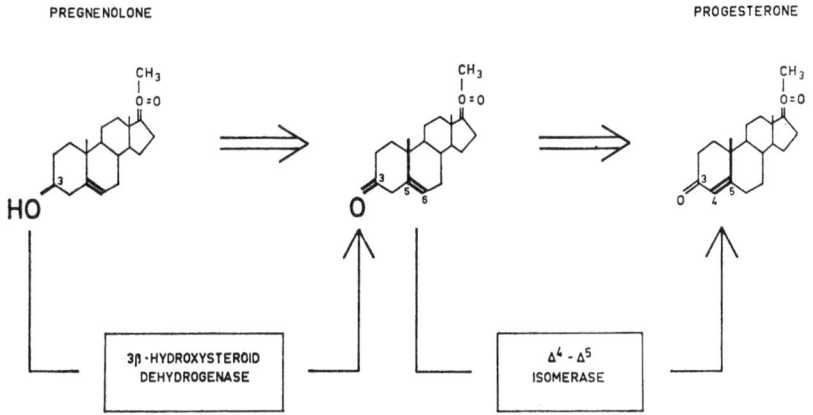

*Fig.* 2. The two enzyme reactions involved in the conversion of pregnenolone into progesterone.

AROMATISATION

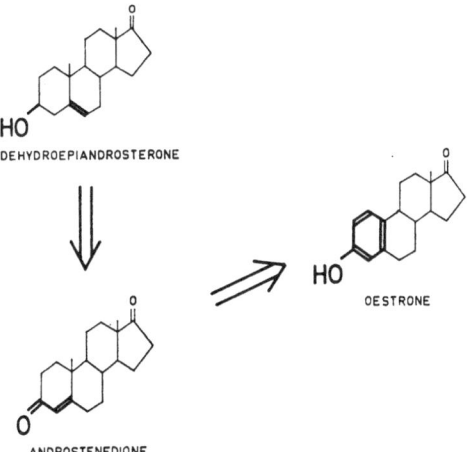

*Fig.* 3. Simplified representation of the conversion of a Δ 5-3β-OH steroid into an oestrogen.

by the 3β-HSD system. Formation of the sulfate-conjugate is mediated by a sulfokinase enzyme and hydrolysis of the conjugate by a sulfatase enzyme. There are separate sulfokinase and sulfatase enzymes for Δ 5-3β-hydroxysteroids (neutral steroids) and oestrogenic steroids.

Further metabolism of steroid hormones can involve one or more hydroxylation reactions, each governed by a specific hydroxylase enzyme (fig. 4). Hydroxylation at C-11 and C-21 are necessary for

PROGESTERONE       DESOXYCORTICOSTERONE       CORTICOSTERONE

17α-OH-PROGESTERONE       DESOXYCORTISONE       CORTISOL

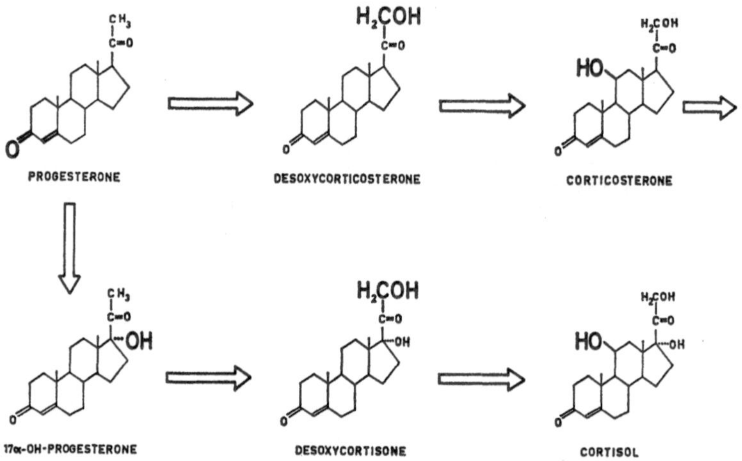

*Fig.* 4. Hydroxylation reactions required for the conversion of progesterone into corticosteroids.

the conversion of 17α-OH-progesterone to the basic glucocorticoid, cortisol, and hydroxylation at C-11 and C-21 are necessary for the synthesis of corticosterone from progesterone. Corticosterone is converted to aldosterone by hydroxylation then dehydrogenation at C-18. Hydroxylation at C-16 is an important foetal reaction in the biogenesis of oestriol in the foeto-placental unit.

The concept of the foeto-placental unit is based on the results of many *in vivo* experiments, using labeled steroids, carried out at the 17th—20th week of gestation in human volunteers undergoing therapeutic abortion. Several different approaches have been used in these experiments, including: perfusion of the placenta *in situ*, perfusion of the foetus after removal from the uterus, study of the foeto-placental unit by injection of labeled steroid into the umbilical circulation *in situ*, and intraamniotic injection of labeled steroid many hours before termination of the pregnancy. Foetal and placental tissues exposed to the labeled steroid are extracted and analyzed for their content of labeled steroid and, in the *in situ* experiments, the maternal urine is analyzed.

In contrast to other endocrine organs, there is only very limited synthesis of cholesterol from acetate by the placenta (5, 6). However, *in situ* perfusion of placentas with labeled cholesterol has shown that at midpregnancy (7) and at term (8), significant amounts are converted to pregnenolone (fig. 5). Midterm foetuses perfused with labeled acetate and cholesterol demonstrated a conversion of acetate into cholesterol but only a minute conversion of the cholesterol into pregneolone or 17α-OH-pregnenolone (9). The same workers perfused labeled cholesterol sulfate in a mid-term foetus and likewise found no conversion to steroids. Thus neither the foetus nor the placenta are able to carry out all steps in the synthesis of pregnenolone from acetate but the placenta, in contrast to the foetus, can form significant amounts of pregnenolone from the abundantly available precursor, circulating cholesterol. This placenta-derived pregnenolone serves as the precursor for all steroid biogenesis in the foeto-placental unit.

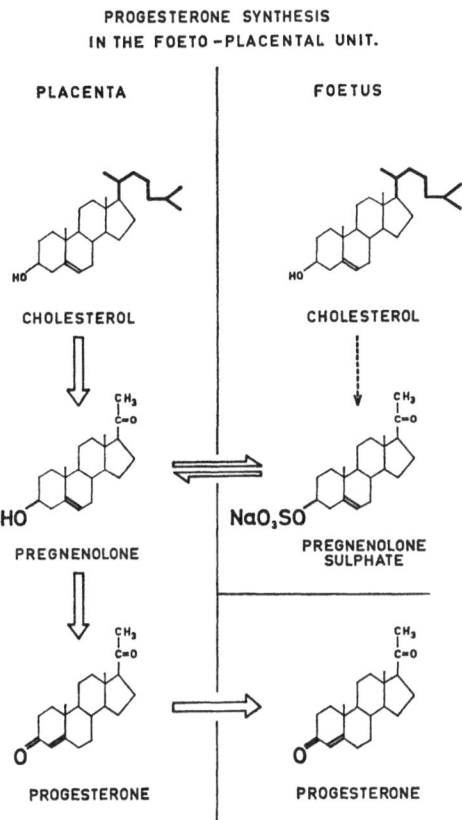

*Fig.* 5. Simplified representation of the origins of pregnenolone and progesterone in the foeto-placental unit.

Pregnenolone entering the foetus from the placenta undergoes 17α-hydroxylation and sulfurylation in the adrenals, being transformed into 17α-OH-pregnenolone sulfate (9). 17α-OH-pregnenolone is converted by the foetal adrenal to dehydroepiandrosterone sulfate (DHAS) which is then released into the foetal circulation (10). DHAS entering the placenta is rapidly hydrolysed by a neutral steroid sulfatase and free DHA is liberated. The DHA is converted to androstenedione by the 3β-HSD system and the androstenedione is then converted to oestrone and oestradiol-17β by the aromatising enzyme (11, 12) (fig. 6). The bulk of these oestrogens are rapidly transferred across the placenta into the maternal circulation but some are released into the umbilical circulation and are transported to the foetus. No oestriol and no 16α-hydroxylated intermediates were found in these studies of DHA and DHAS metabolism by the placenta perfused *in situ*, indicating the lack of placental 16α-hydroxylase activity under these *in situ* conditions. DHAS is present in high concentration in the umbilical arterial blood (13, 14) and thus is considered to serve as the foetal precursor for oestrone and oestradiol-17β synthesis by the placenta. Pregnenolone and 17α-OH-pregnenolone cannot serve as direct precursors to oestrogen production by the placenta. On perfusion of placentas with these two steroids, only progesterone was found as a product of pregnenolone and only 17α-OH-progesterone as a

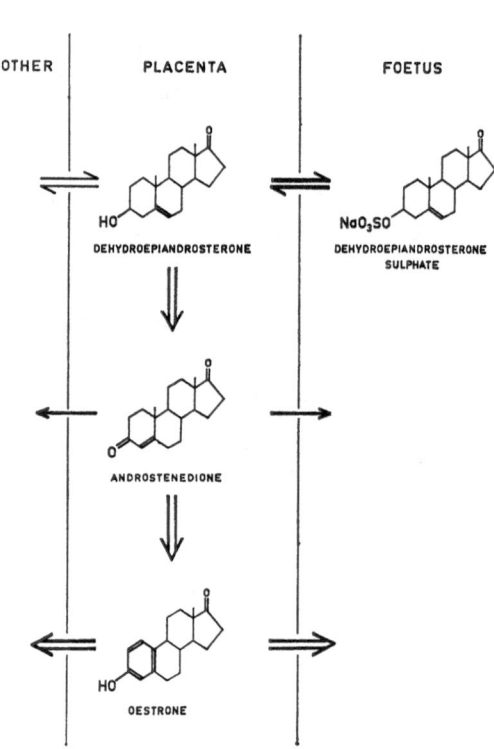

*Fig. 6.*   The formation of oestrone in the placenta from a neutral steroid precursor.

product of 17α-OH-pregnenolone (15). Thus there was no evidence
of significant 17α-hydroxylase or side-chain splitting activity in these
*in situ* studies of the placenta. Both of these enzymes are, however,
active in the foetal adrenal. On perfusion of DHA and DHAS into
mid-term foetuses, the labeled DHA was almost completely sulfury-
lated and no DHAS was found to have been hydrolyzed to DHA (16))
The foetal tissues thus have extensive sulfokinase activities with no
neutral steroid sulfatase activity. The reverse is true of the placenta
where no sulfokinase activity is found but neutral steroid sulfatase is
highly active.

In the above mentioned study (16), in which foetuses were perfused
with DHA and DHAS, there was significant 16α-hydroxylation of
both DHA and DHAS by foetal liver tissue. 16α-OH-DHAS was
found in the perfusate and its C-17 reduced form, Δ 5-androstenetriol

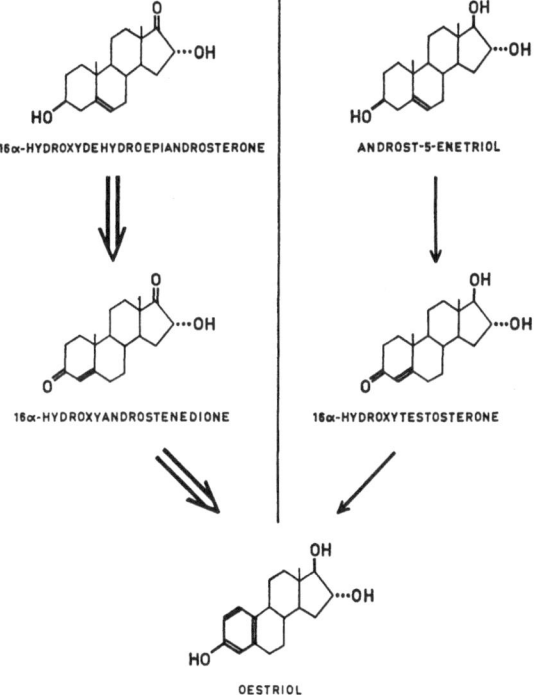

*Fig. 7.* The present concept of placental oestriol formation from 16α-hydroxylated
neutral steroid precursors.

sulfate (Δ 5-ATLS), was found in the liver. 16α-OH-DHA is converted by the placenta to oestriol, in good yield (17). Since 16α-OH-DHAS is present in large amounts in umbilical arterial plasma (14, 18) and since it has been estimated that at least 90 % of the oestriol excretion near term originates from neutral steroid precursors in the foetus (19), 16α-OH-DHAS can be considered the major foetal precursor of oestriol. Another neutral steroid pathway to oestriol involves Δ 5-ATLS, formed in the foetal liver by 16α-hydroxylation of DHA and DHAS (16) (fig. 7). Δ 5-ATLS was converted to oestriol in the placenta after its administration to intact foeto-placental units. Because the yield of oestriol was low and the amounts of Δ 5-ATLS in umbilical arterial plasma are low (14), this pathway was considered to be of minor importance. A third pathway to oestriol synthesis, though probably of less importance than the 16α-OH-DHAS pathway (20), involves 16α-hydroxylation of oestrone secreted to the foetus from the placenta (fig. 8). The 16α-hydroxylation of the oestrone takes place almost entirely in the foetal liver where 16α-OH-oestrone sulfate and its C-17 reduced derivative, oestriol sulfate, were isolated following foetal perfusion with labeled oestrone (21, 22). 16α-OH-oestrone sulfate is transported to the placenta where it is hydrolysed and reduced to oestriol.

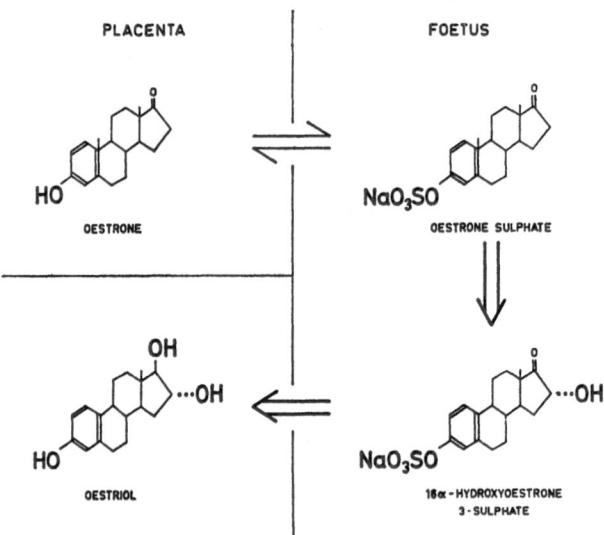

*Fig.* 8. The synthesis of oestriol from oestrone in the foeto-placental unit.

15α-hydroxylation is an important enzyme activity in the foetal liver. After foetal perfusion with oestrone sulfate (22) and administration of oestrone and oestradiol to foeto-placental units (21), 15α-OH-oestradiol-17β sulfate could be isolated from the foetal livers. In addition, a highly hydroxylated oestrogenic tetrol, isolated initially in large amounts from the urine after oestradiol-17β administration to young infants (23), has been isolated from late pregnancy and neonatal urine and recently has been identified as 15α-OH-oestriol (24). This same compound has been found after oestradiol-17β administration to pregnant women and has been shown to be synthesized almost completely by the foetus (25). 15α-hydroxylated steroid metabolites in pregnancy urine thus may serve as relatively specific chemical indicators of foetal steroid metabolizing activity.

The androgenic steroids, androstenedione and testosterone, are formed in the placenta as intermediates in the conversion of DHA and DHAS to oestrogens (11, 12). Small amounts are released to the foetal circulation where they are aromatized to a small extent in the foetal liver (26) and where they undergo various hydroxylation and reduction reactions (27). Whether the placenta is the sole source of circulating biologically active androgens in the foetus is not known because the role of the foetal testes *in situ* has not been evaluated.

The principal glucocorticoid, cortisol, and the salt retaining steroid, aldosterone, can not be synthesized *de novo* by the midterm foetus. On perfusion of mid-gestation foetuses with acetate, cholesterol and cholesterol sulfate, there was no evidence of significant conversion to pregnenolone or 17α-OH-pregnenolone (9). Neither pregnenolone (9), which can be transferred from the placenta, nor 17α-OH-pregnenolone (10) are converted by the foetus to the analogous Δ 4-3-keto steroids, progesterone and 17α-OH-progesterone respectively, indicating that the foetus lacks the 3β-HSD enzyme system. Thus, the progesterone required as a precursor for the foetal adrenal synthesis of cortisol and aldosterone has to be supplied by the placenta (fig. 5). The placenta, with a highly active 3β-HSD system, converts pregnenolone to progesterone in high yield (15) and the progesterone is released into the umbilical venous circulation. Pregnenolone sulfate carried to the placenta in umbilical arterial blood (28) and pregnenolone synthesized in the placenta from circulating cholesterol (7, 8) serve as the precursors *in vivo* to the progesterone of placental origin.

Progesterone is converted by the foetus to many products, including cortisol and corticosterone (29) (fig. 4). The mid-term foetus thus has active 11β, 17α and 21-hydroxylating enzyme systems. The adrenal localization of the 11β and 21-hydroxylase enzymes was shown by the absence of products bearing hydroxyl groups at C-11 and C-21 after progesterone was infused into adrenalectomized foetuses (30). Aldosterone was isolated from the adrenal glands after administration of corticosterone to a foetus (31), indicating the presence of an adrenal 18-hydroxylase system. Thus, the foetus at midpregnancy is capable of producing the physiologically active steroids, cortisol and aldosterone, from progesterone supplied by the placenta. Whether the production of cortisol by the foeto-placental unit is alone sufficient for the foetal requirements or whether there is a dependence on transplacental passage of maternal cortisol is not known.

Our present information concerning the distribution of foetoplacental steroidogenic enzymes is shown in Table 1. The foetus is unable to synthesize pregnenolone from cholesterol, lacks the sulfatase and the 3β-HSD system but has the other enzyme activities. Those enzymes lacking in the foetus are present in the placenta. Thus, the steroidogenic activities of the foetus and placenta complement each

Table 1. *Distribution of certain steroidogenic enzymes between the placenta and foetus based on in vivo studies at mid-gestation*

| Enzyme | Placenta | Foetus |
|---|---|---|
| Steroid sulfatase | yes | NO |
| Steroid sulfokinase | NO | yes |
| 3β-hydroxysteroid dehydrogenase system | yes | NO |
| Aromatising enzyme system | yes | yes |
| C-17-20 desmolase (side-chain splitting enzyme) | NO | yes |
| C-20-22 desmolase (cholesterol → pregnenolone) | yes | (very slight) |
| Steroid hydroxylating enzyme systems at: | | |
| C-2, C-7, C-11, C-15, C-16, C-17 | NO | yes |
| C-6 | yes | yes |
| Steroid UDPG-glucuronyl transferase | NO | yes |

other and the integrated foeto-placental unit is capable of synthesizing the biologically important hormonal steroids.

The physiological significance of the distribution of these enzyme activities is not fully understood at present. Certain of the foetal enzymes can be considered, from one viewpoint, as serving in part to protect the foetus from potentially harmful effects of the large amounts of steroids presented to it by the placenta. The active sulfokinases in the foetus, together with the lack of foetal sulfatases, lead to the sulfurylation of most of the circulating $\Delta$ 5-3$\beta$-hydroxy steroids and oestrogens, as well as some $\Delta$ 4-3-keto-steroids such as corticosterone (32). Conjugation is generally considered to inactivate physiologically active steroids, but there is no experimental confirmation of this hypothesis. The absence of the 3$\beta$-HSD system in the foetus prevents the conversion of non-sulfated $\Delta$ 5-3$\beta$-hydroxysteroids into their physiologically active $\Delta$ 4-3-keto-analogs and the active foetal hepatic 15$\alpha$-and 16$\alpha$-hydroxylation leads to marked lowering of the biological activity of the oestrogens. Progesterone is converted extensively in the foetus to 20$\alpha$-dihydroprogesterone (9), a compound with a lower progestational activity than progesterone. The enzyme activities localized in the placenta can be considered as promoting the transplacental passage of steroids to the mother. The active sulfatases in the placenta, with the lack of placental sulfokinase, lead to the rapid and extensive hydrolysis of sulfoconjugated steroids entering from the foetus. Since the transplacental passage of steroids is much faster when they are unconjugated (33), the hydrolysis of the sulfoconjugates allows the rapid egress of biologically active steroids which otherwise would accumulate in the foeto-placental unit.

The understanding of the essential role of the foetus in supplying the precursors for oestriol synthesis has led to the use of the maternal oestriol excretion as an indicator of foetal health. In cases with foetal death, the oestriol excretion falls to very low levels and a declining or constantly low excretion is interpreted to indicate that the foetus is in serious danger (34). Oestriol excretion has been used to help make the decision to terminate the pregnancy in cases of maternal diabetes (35) and postmaturity (36). Chronic abnormalities in the foetus can lead to marked decreases in maternal oestriol excretion, for instance, as was mentioned above, in anencephaly with adrenal hypoplasia (2), and in intrauterine growth retardation (37). Future investigation of the maternal excretion of 15α-hydroxylated oestrogens as an indicator of foetal health may prove useful since 15α-hydroxylase, in contrast to 16α-hydroxylase, appears to be almost completely a foetal enzyme activity (25).

There is evidence that a number of the steroidogenic enzyme activities which are characteristic of the foetus *in utero*, and which are very different from those in the adult, persist into the neonatal and early infancy period. By necessity, most of the *in vivo* evidence is less direct than that obtained in investigations of pre-viable foetuses. However, a few studies have been made of steroid metabolism in live-born anencephalic infants which are similar to studies possible in foetuses. Adrenal cortical capacity to synthesize pregnenolone from acetate or circulating cholesterol, and sufficient adrenal 3β-HSD system activity to allow cortisol and aldosterone synthesis are obvious prerequisites for viability. However, there is evidence from the blood and urinary steroid patterns of young infants that the 3β-HSD system activity is decreased compared with older children and adults. Δ 5-3β-hydroxysteroids are present in high quantities both in the circulating blood (28) and as sulfoconjugates in the urine (38, 39, 40, 41) in the first weeks of life. The Δ 5-3β-hydroxysteroids identified in the urine of normal young infants include DHA (42), 16α-OH-pregnenolone (43), 16α-OH-DHA (44) and its epimer 16-keto-androstenediol (45), 21-OH-pregnenolone (46), and Δ 5-androstenetriol (47). The roles of DHA, 16α-OH-DHA and Δ 5-androstenetriol as oestrogen precursors in the foeto-placental unit have been discussed in previous sections of this paper. 16-keto-androstenediol may serve as a neutral precursor to 16-keto-oestradiol-17β in the foeto-placental unit (48). 16α-OH-pregnenolone has been isolated from the foetal liver after administration of pregnenolone to a mid-gestation foetal-placental unit (9) but no precursor role has been defined. An *in utero* role for 21-OH-pregnenolone is also unknown at present. The most prominent of the neonatal urinary Δ 5-3β-hydroxysteroids, 16α-OH-pregnenolone and 16α-OH-DHA, continue to be excreted by full-term infants during the first 6 months of life (38) and are excreted in increasing amounts by premature infants during the first 5 weeks of life (49). (fig. 9 and 10). These large amounts of Δ 5-3β-hydroxysteroids could result from a subnormal activity of the adrenal 3β-HSD system, leading to the secretion of large amounts of pregnenolone sulfate and

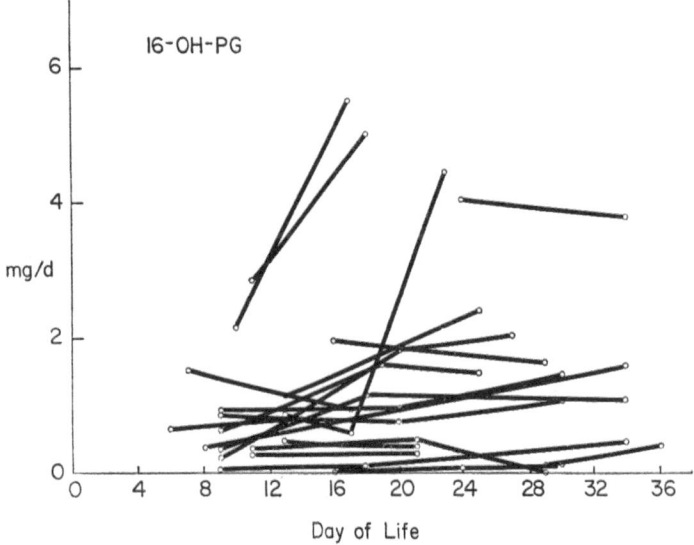

*Fig.* 9.   The daily urinary excretions of 16α-OH-pregnenolone (16-OH-PG) by 20 premature infants studied longitudinally. The lines connect the daily excretion values of individual infants. The figure is based on data reported in Ref. 49.

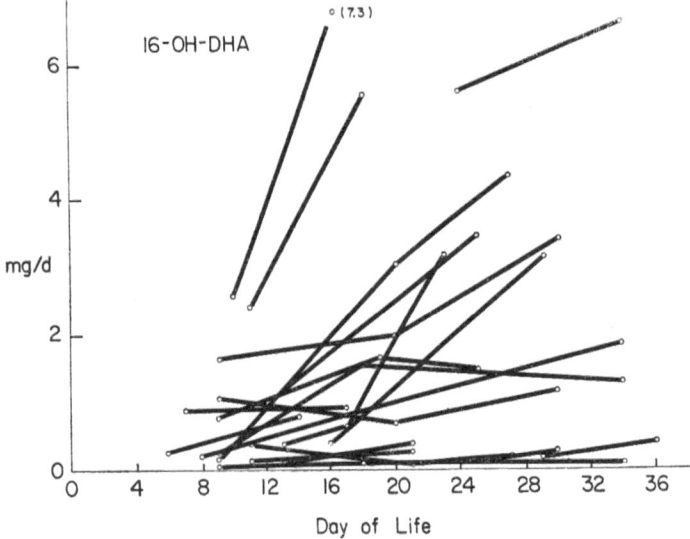

*Fig.* 10.   The daily urinary excretions of 16α-OH-dehydroepiandrosterone (16-OH-DHA) by 20 premature infants studied longitudinally. The lines connect the daily excretion values of individual infants. The figure is based on data reported in Ref. 49.

DHAS relative to the Δ 4-3-keto-steroids synthesized. In the presence of a continued inactivity of the peripheral (particularly hepatic) 3β-HSD system, the steroids would be excreted with no further metabolism except for 16α-hydroxylation. When a mixture of differently labeled DHA and androstenedione was perfused into a full-term anencephalic infant that lived a few hours, androstenedione and its C-17 reduced form, testosterone, were isolated from the liver and were found to be derived solely from the perfused androstenedione (50). Thus, there was no identification of hepatic 3β-HSD system activity in this infant. If the inactivity of the neutral steroid sulfatase enzyme persisted into early infancy, the action of the 3β-HSD system, if present, would be masked, since sulfo-conjugation at C-3 would prevent the action of the 3β-HSD system. Whether any one, or all, of these hypotheses is correct will require much further investigation.

The continued high activity of the 3β-hydroxysteroid sulfokinase enzyme into early post-natal life is indicated by the studies discussed above (38, 39, 40, 41, 49) which showed a prominent urinary excretion of sulfoconjugated Δ 5-3β-hydroxysteroids. That sulfoconjugation of oestrogens is more prominent in early life than in adulthood, has been shown in studies of the types of oestriol conjugates in urine from normal newborns (51) and in a study of the oestriol conjugates in the blood and urine of an anencephalic infant injected with labeled oestriol (52). Glucocorticoids and their metabolites also are excreted more as sulfoconjugates in the newborn than in adults (53). It is not known if the continued high sulfokinase activities for these several steroid groups is associated with a persistent inactivity of the respective sulfatases. The persisting high activity of 16α-hydroxylase is indicated by the 16α-hydroxylation of the most prominent neonatal urinary steroids, 16α-OH-pregnenolone and 16α-OH-DHA (38, 49). 15α- and 16α-hydroxylase activity for oestrogens continues at a high level in early infancy (23). Following intramuscular injection of labeled oestradiol-17β into 3 infants, ages 1 to 3 months, more than 15 % of the urinary radioactivity was present as oestriol and 16α-OH-oestrone and 16 % of the radioactivity was present as a highly polar compound recently identified (24) as 15α-OH-oestriol.

SUMMARY

The concept of the foeto-placental unit as an integrated endocrine organ has been defined recently by many *in vivo* studies at the 17th-20th week of gestation. A functioning foeto-placental unit is necessary for most of the increased oestrogen production of pregnancy and for the provision of glucocorticoids and aldosterone to the foetus. Neither the foetus nor the placenta alone have the necessary enzyme systems for the synthesis of these groups of steroids. However, when the foetus and placenta function as a unit, all of the enzyme systems are present for the synthesis of these steroids from circulating cholesterol. The placenta, but not the mid-gestation foetal adrenal, can synthesize physiologically significant amounts of pregnenolone from circulating cholesterol. Part of the pregnenolone is converted to progesterone in the placenta by the 3β-HSD system (absent in the foetus). The progesterone is transferred to the foetus where it is transformed by C-11, C-17, C-18 and C-21 hydroxylases (all absent in the placenta) to cortisol, corticosterone and aldosterone. Pregnenolone transferred from the placenta to the foetus undergoes 17α-hydroxylation, side-chain splitting and sulfurylation (absent in the placenta) and is converted to DHAS. The DHAS may undergo 16α-hydroxylation (absent in the placenta) in the foetal liver and be transported to the placenta as 16α-OH-DHAS. There it is subjected to a neutral steroid sulfatase (absent in the foetus) and is converted to oestriol by action of the 3β-HSD system and the aromatizing enzyme system. DHAS transported to the placenta from the foetus is converted in large part to oestrone and oestradiol-17β via the intermediates androstenedione and testosterone. A part of these androgenic steroid intermediates are released to the foetus.

By the age of viability, the foetal adrenal has developed the enzymatic capability to synthesize pregnenolone from endogenous precursors or circulating cholesterol and to convert at least a fraction of that synthesized to progesterone by means of an adrenal 3β-hydroxysteroid dehydrogenase enzyme system. However, certain features of the neonatal urinary steroid pattern suggest that there is a persistence into the newborn period of steroid metabolizing enzyme activities characteristic of the foetus. The newborn infant excretes large amounts of 16α-OH-pregnenolone sulfate, 16α-OH-DHAS and other

Δ 5-3β-OH steroids. The excretion of these steroids may result from a low activity of the adrenal 3β-hydroxysteroid dehydrogenase system relative to the amounts of pregnenolone synthesized, a lack of the extra-adrenal 3β-HSD system and/or a lack of neutral steroid sulfatase, and a persisting highly active hepatic 16α-hydroxylase. Sulfoconjugation of both neutral steroids and oestrogens is prominent and there is a continuing active 15α- and 16α-hydroxylation of oestrogens in early infancy.

ACKNOWLEDGEMENT

Theauthor wishes to thank Professor EGON DICZFALUSY for the opportunity to refer to a number of papers prior to their publication and for much assistance in the preparation of this paper.

NOTE 1 FROM PAGE 3

The following trivial names are used in this paper:
*pregnanediol*: 5β-pregnane-3α,20α-diol; *oestriol*: oestra-1,3,5(10)-triene-3,16α,17β-triol; *cholesterol*: cholest-5-en-3β-ol; *pregnenolone*: 3β-hydroxypregn-5-en-20-one; *dehydroepiandrosterone* (DHA): 3β-hydroxyandrost-5-en-17-one; *17α-OH-pregnenolone*: 3β,-17α-dihydroxypregn-5-en-20-one; *progesterone*: pregn-4-ene-3,20-dione; *androstenedione*: androst-4-ene-3,17-dione; *17α-OH-progesterone*: 17α-hydroxypregn-4-ene-3,20-dione; *cortisol*: 11β,17α,21-trihydroxypregn-4-ene-3,20-dione; *corticosterone*: 11β,21-dihydroxypregn-4-ene-3,20-dione; *aldosterone*: 11β,21-dihydroxypregn-4-ene-3,20-dion-18-ol; *oestrone*: 3-hydroxyoestra-1,3,5(10)-trien-17-one; *oestradiol-17β*: oestra-1,3,5(10)-triene-3,17β- diol; *16α-OH-DHA*: 3β,16α-dihydroxyandrost-5-en-17-one; *Δ5-androstenetriol*: 3β,16α,17β-trihydroxyandrost-5-ene; *16α-OH-oestrone*: 3,16α-dihydroxyoestra-1,3,5(10)-triene-17-one; *15α-OH-oestradiol-17β*: oestra-1,3,5(10)-triene-3,15α,17β-triol; *15α-OH-oestriol*: oestra-1,3,5(10)-triene-3,15α,16α,17β-tetrol; *testosterone*: 17β-hydroxyandrost-4-en-3-one; *20α-dihydroprogesterone*: 20α-hydroxypregn-4-en-3-one; *16-ketoandrostenediol*: 3β,17β-dihydroxyandrost-5-en-16-one; *21-OH-pregnenolone*: 3β,21-dihydroxypregn-5-en-20-one.

REFERENCES

1. CASSMER, O. (1959) *Acta endocrinol.* (Kbh) Suppl. 45.
2. FRANDSEN, V. A. and G. STAKEMANN (1961) *Acta endocrinol.* (Kbh) 38 : 383.
3. DICZFALUSY, E. (1964) *Fed. Proc.* 23 : 791.
4. DICZFALUSY, E., R. PION and J. SCHWERS (1965) *Arch. Anat. Microscop. et Morph. Expérim.* 54 : 67.
5. LEVITZ, M., S. EMERMAN and J. DANCIS (1962) *Excerpta Medica Internat. Cong. Series* 51 : 266.

6. VAN LEUSDEN, H. and C. A. VILLEE (1965) Steroids 6 : 31.
7. JAFFE, R. B., G. ERIKSSON and E. DICZFALUSY (1965) Excerpta Medica Internat. Cong. Series 99 : 182.
8. JAFFE, R. B. and E. P. PETERSON (1966) Steroids 8 : 695.
9. SOLOMON, S., C. E. BIRD, W. LING, M. IWAMIYA and P. C. M. YOUNG (1967) Recent Progress Hormone Res. 23 : 297.
10. PION, R., R. B. JAFFE, N. WIQVIST and E. DICZFALUSY (1967) Biochim. Biophys. Acta 137 : 584.
11. BOLTÉ, E., S. MANCUSO, G. ERIKSSON, N. WIQVIST and E. DICZFALUSY (1964) Acta endocrinol. (Kbh) 45 : 535.
12. LAMB, E., S. MANCUSO, S. DELL'ACQUA, N. WIQVIST and E. DICZFALUSY (1967) Acta endocrinol. (Kbh) 55 : 263.
13. MIGEON, C., A. R. KELLER and E. G. HOLMSTROM (1955) Bull. Johns Hopkins Hosp. 97 : 415.
14. COLÁS, A., W. L. HEINRICHS and H. J. TATUM (1964) Steroids 3 : 417.
15. PION, R., R. B. JAFFE, G. ERIKSSON, N. WIQVIST and E. DICZFALUSY (1965) Acta endocrinol. (Kbh) 48 : 234.
16. BOLTÉ, E., N. WIQVIST and E. DICZFALUSY (1966) Acta endocrinol. (Kbh) 52 : 583.
17. DELL'ACQUA, S., S. MANCUSO, J. RUSE, S. SOLOMON and E. DICZFALUSY (1967) Acta endocrinol. (Kbh) 55 : 401.
18. MAGENDANTZ, H. G. and K. J. RYAN (1964) J. Clin. Endocrinol. & Metab. 24 : 1155.
19. SIITERI, P. K. and P. C. MacDONALD (1966) J. Clin. Endocrinol. & Metab. 26 : 751.
20. KIRSCHNER, M. A., N. WIQVIST and E. DICZFALUSY (1966) Acta endocrinol. (Kbh) 53 : 584.
21. SCHWERS, J., G. ERIKSSON and E. DICZFALUSY (1965) Acta endocrinol. (Kbh) 49 : 65.
22. SCHWERS, J., M. GOVAERTS-VIDETSKY, N. WIQVIST and E. DICZFALUSY (1965) Acta endocrinol. (Kbh) 50 : 597.
23. HAGEN, A. A., M. BARR and E. DICZFALUSY (1965) Acta endocrinol. (Kbh) 49 : 207.
24. ZUCCONI, G., E. SIMONITSCH, B. P. LISBOA, L. ROTH, A. A. HAGEN and E. DICZFALUSY (1967) Acta endocrinol. (Kbh) (in press).
25. GURPIDE, E., J. SCHWERS, M. T. WELCH, R. L. VANDE WIELE and S. LIEBERMAN (1966) J. Clin. Endocrinol. & Metab. 26 : 1355.
26. MANCUSO, S., S. DELL'ACQUA, G. ERIKSSON, N. WIQVIST and E. DICZFALUSY (1965) Steroids 5 : 183.
27. BENAGIANO, G., F. A. KINCL, F. ZIELSKE, N. WIQVIST and E. DICZFALUSY (1967) Acta endocrinol. (Kbh) 56 : 203.
28. EBERLEIN, W. R. (1965) J. Clin. Endocrinol. & Metab. 25 : 1101.
29. BIRD, C. E., N. WIQVIST, E. DICZFALUSY and S. SOLOMON (1966) J. Clin. Endocrinol. & Metab. 26 : 1144.
30. WILSON, R., C. E. BIRD, N. WIQVIST, S. SOLOMON and E. DICZFALUSY (1966) J. Clin. Endocrinol & Metab. 26 : 1155.
31. PASQUALINI, J. R., N. WIQVIST and E. DICZFALUSY (1966) Biochim. Biophys. Acta 121 : 430.
32. BIRD, C. E., S. SOLOMON, N. WIQVIST and E. DICZFALUSY (1965) Biochim. Biophys. Acta 104 : 623.
33. LEVITZ, M. (1966) J. Clin. Endocrinol. & Metab. 26 : 773.
34. FRANDSEN, V. A. and G. STAKEMANN (1963) Acta endocrinol. (Kbh) 44 : 183.

20    J. W. REYNOLDS

35. GREENE, J. W., K. SMITH, G. C. KYLE, J. C. TOUCHSTONE and J. L. DUHRING (1965) *Am. J. Obstet. & Gynec.* (1965) 91 : 684.
36. LUNDWALL, F. and G. STAKEMANN (1966) *Acta Obst. et Gynec. Scand.* 45 : 301.
37. YOUSEM, H., J. SEITCHIK and D. SOLOMON (1966) *Obstet. & Gynecol.* 28 : 491.
38. REYNOLDS, J. W. (1965) *J. Clin. Endocrinol. & Metab.* 25 : 416.
39. MATSUMOTO, K., K. OKANO, T. UOZUMI and T. SEKI (1966) In: *Steroid Dynamics*, PINCUS, G., T. NAKAO and J. F. TAIT, eds., Academic Press, New York, p. 379.
40. GARDINER, W. L., C. J. W. BROOKS, E. C. HORNING and R. M. HILL (1966) *Biochim. Biophys. Acta* 130 : 278.
41. CATHRO, D. M., K. BIRCHALL, F. L. MITCHELL and C. C. FORSYTH (1965) *Arch. Dis. Childh.* 40 : 251.
42. CATHRO, D. M., K. BIRCHALL, F. L. MITCHELL and C. C. FORSYTH (1963) *J. Endocrin.* 27 : 53.
43. REYNOLDS, J. W. (1963) *Proc. Soc. Exper. Biol. Med.* 113 : 980.
44. BONGIOVANNI, A. M. (1962) *J. Clin. Invest.* 41 : 2086.
45. REYNOLDS, J. W. (1964) *Steroids* 3 : 77.
46. BIRCHALL, K. and F. L. MITCHELL (1965) *Steroids* 6 : 427.
47. REYNOLDS, J. W. (1966) *Steroids* 8 : 719.
48. REYNOLDS, J. W., N. WIQVIST and E. DICZFALUSY (1967) unpublished data.
49. REYNOLDS, J. W. (1966) *J. Clin. Endocrinol. & Metab.* 26 : 1251.
50. MANCUSO S., B. FRÖYSA and E. DICZFALUSY (1967) unpublished data.
51. TROEN, P., B. NILSSON, N. WIQVIST and E. DICZFALUSY (1961) *Acta endocrinol.* (Kbh) 38 : 361.
52. DICZFALUSY, E., M. BARR and J. LIND (1964) *Acta endocrinol.* (Kbh) 46 : 511.
53. DRAYER, N. M. and C. J. P. GIROUD (1965) *Steroids* 5 : 289.

# PROBLEMS IN THE PATHOLOGIC
# STUDY OF THE PLACENTA

P. GRUENWALD*

Pathologic examination of the placenta has been neglected for a long time, perhaps largely because the correlation of observed lesions with indications of functional impairment has been poor. One reason is incomplete knowledge of normal architecture, and another difficulty is the selection of those placentas which should be examined with some expectation of significant findings, among the overwhelming numbers of mostly normal ones (1). It has been relatively easy to find pathologic evidence of premature separation, infection, malformations associated with oligohydramnios, or peculiarities of twin pregnancy (2). However, the most important function of the placenta is concerned with the exchange between mother and fetus, and this is where the knowledge of normal and pathologic morphology is greatly deficient.

One of the obstacles to the meaningful interpretation of pathologic findings has been the variation even among nearby points of the same placenta. With newer knowledge of the lobular architecture and of the relation of structural differences to the placental lobule (3) (which is, in man, not identical with the cotyledon seen on the maternal surface) it should be possible to interpret these differences more satisfactorily (fig. 1, 2). The dense, outer part of the lobule may, for instance, show syncytial knots in a much higher proportion of villi than other areas, and the same portion may form the well-known spherical, hollow infarcts (fig. 3). The center of the lobules is selectively occupied by intervillous thrombi in some placentas whereas the

* Departments of Pathology, Sinai Hospital and The Johns Hopkins University, Baltimore, Maryland, U.S.A.

Work supported by research grant HD-00547-06 of the National Institute of Child Health and Human Development, U.S. Public Health Service.

interlobular tissue may contain fibrin deposits along villous stems. Maternal arteries and veins open into the intervillous space between lobules (3).

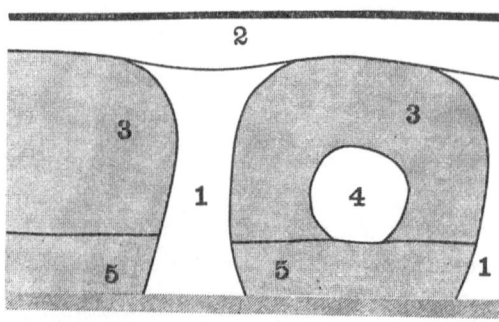

*Fig.* 1. Diagram of the regions of the human placenta which differ in the villous structure, as seen on a section at a right angle to the fetal (top) and maternal surface (bottom). 1, intervillous area; 2, subchorial area; 3 and 5, dense part of the lobule; 4, loose center of the lobule. From Gruenwald (3), courtesy *Bulletin of the Johns Hopkins Hospital.*

Pathologic-anatomic examination cannot be expected to correlate well with indications of an insufficient supply line as seen in the fetus, for several reasons. Firstly, many instances of fetal deprivation are due to maternal rather than placental insufficiency. Secondly, the fetus outgrows its supply line at some time during the third trimester and the metabolic support of the fetus becomes inadequate before term even in the average pregnancy as will be discussed in the following chapter. Thirdly, there is a considerable variation in placental size and a larger placenta will become insufficient later, or tolerate more pathologic change than a smaller one.

Any extensive, gross pathologic change is likely to result in fetal deprivation. Infarcts, hemangiomas, areas of premature separation, or thrombosis of large fetal vessels may do this when sufficiently large or numerous. Microscopically, multiple 'microinfarcts', or groups of avascular villi (fig. 4) may be seen; these may have similar effects. Many changes which frequently occur in the human placenta during the last month of the usual gestation time, have been considered as 'degeneration' or 'senescence'. Some of these, such as calcification in or near the decidua, or subchorionic fibrin plaques, are almost cer-

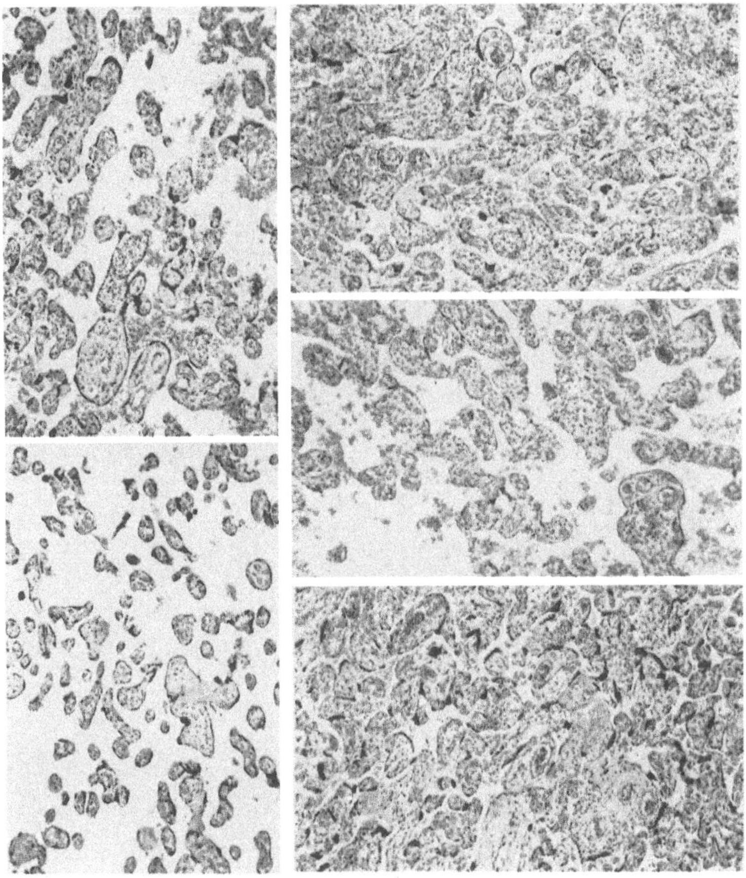

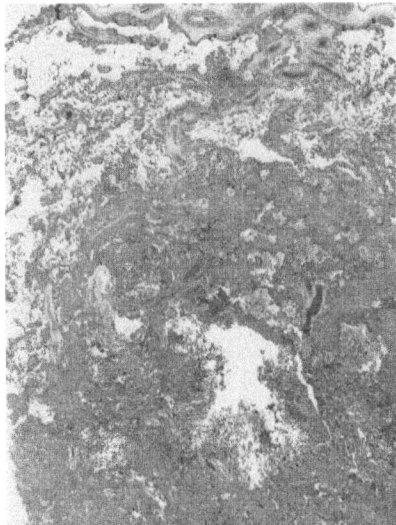

*Fig.* 2.   Placental structure as seen on one section of a mature placenta. *a—e* correspond to areas 1—5, respectively, in fig. 1. All were photographed at the same magnification.

*Fig.* 3.   Placental lobule with infarction of its dense portions, producing a spherical, hollow infarct. Chorion at the top. From GRUENWALD (3), courtesy *Bulletin of the Johns Hopkins Hospital*.

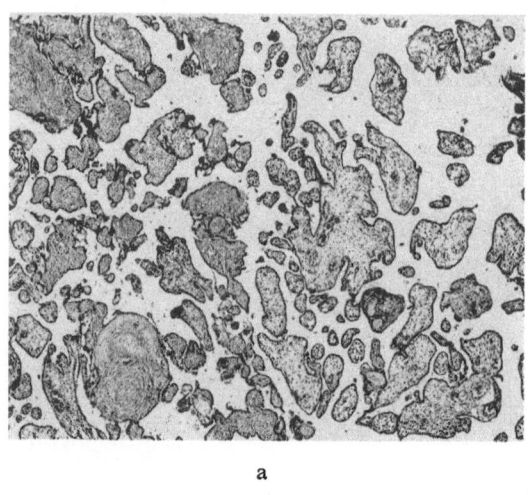

a

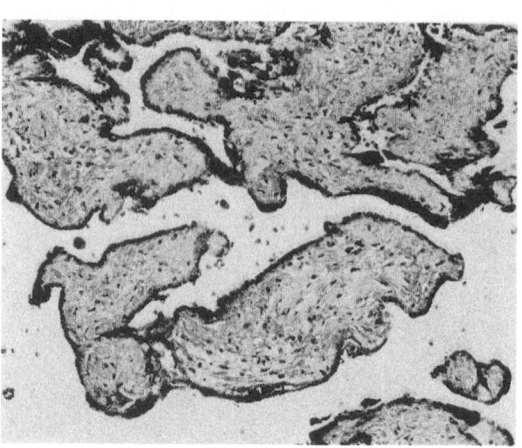

b

Fig. 4. a, group of avascular villi (left) compared with vascularized villi (right) from the placenta of a growth-retarded, mature fetus. b, avascular villi from the same placenta at higher magnification.

tainly of no functional significance unless present to an excessive extent. Others need further study.

The parameter by which to judge functional adequacy of the placenta, and to which to relate pathologic findings, is the growth and nutritional state of the fetus. Much has been learned in recent years about pathologic indications in the fetus of an impaired supply line. When such indications are present, the disturbance is not necessarily placental. It may well lie in the maternal organism or environment. A relative inadequacy (maternal or placental) may develop without pathologic changes in a previously adequate supply system when the fetus outgrows its capacity. This occurs particularly in prolonged pregnancy, and it has been common experience that in this situation there are no characteristic pathologic lesions.

At this time pathologic examination of the placenta can supply information on infection, premature separation, etc., and to a limited extent on impairment of the transfer function. Methods for satisfactory study of large numbers of placentas have not been agreed upon. Much work needs to be done before pathologic examination of the placenta will become a highly useful tool for evaluating the conditions under which a given fetus subsisted *in utero*. At the moment the principal value of placental studies lies in the acquisition of badly needed information for future use.

## REFERENCES

1. GRUENWALD, P. (1964) *Arch. Path.* 77: 41.
2. BENIRSCHKE, K. and S. G. DRISCOLL (1967) In: *Handbuch der speziellen pathologischen Anatomie und Histologie*, Springer Verlag, Berlin-Heidelberg-New York. 7/5: p. 97.
3. GRUENWALD, P. (1966) *Bull. Johns Hopkins Hosp.* 119: 172.

# DISCUSSION

DISCUSSION PAPER DR. REYNOLDS

*Prof. Kloosterman* (in the chair): I thank Dr. REYNOLDS for his beautiful introduction. We now all know why the name of KAROLINSKA is so often mentioned in connection with studies of human production. Also you made an important point by mentioning to us those functions the placenta can do and the foetus can not. In the third place you gave us a very interesting introduction to the problem of post-maturity. Thank you very much. Who likes to ask some questions to Dr. REYNOLDS?

*Dr. Sereni:* Since oestriol is synthetized mostly by the foetus, as you have clearly shown, some obstetricians believe that frequent determinations in the maternal blood of the concentration of this compound might be taken as a good index of the clinical conditions of the foetus. In other words, a fall in maternal oestriol concentration should indicate foetal distress. Could you make a short comment on this point?

*Dr. Reynolds:* Yes, the use of maternal oestriol blood levels as indicators of foetal viability or foetal health does make sense. I am not sure whether in practice it will prove to be more useful or as useful as the urinary oestriol estimation.

*Dr. Valaes:* Could you explain in terms of teleological function the purpose of the placental and foetal unit for the continuation of pregnancy. Is the level of oestriol produced by the unit essential for the continuation of pregnancy? Our friends the obstetricians often use the oestriol excretion as an index of imminent termination of pregnancy and try to correct a decreased excretion by giving exogenous oestriol.

*Dr. Reynolds:* You asked me several questions here. The first question, as I interpreted it is a fundamental one, and very difficult if not impossible to answer: what is really the physiological role of oestrogens during pregnancy? This is a question that I really cannot answer. I hope perhaps one of the gynaecologists could give their opinion of this. I do know that oestrogens are produced in great excess during pregnancy, and pregnancy can come to term with reduced amounts of oestrogen production compared with the normal. The anencephalic infant is brought to term and the infant grows to essentially the normal size and the normal weight, if the weight of the normal cranium is taken into account. In such an anencephalic case the oestrogen production is much lower than it normally is. Yet the pregnancy proceeds. Just exactly what level of oestrogen is needed as an absolute minimum for maintenance of pregnancy and how it acts to maintain pregnancy, I don't really know. I am not an obstetrician so I cannot answer the point about the administration of oestrogens during pregnancy to counterbalance a low production. This, to me, would not accomplish much to help a sick foetus. In term of other aspects of teleology I feel I tried to answer some of that in my talk, when I discussed the enzyme distribution in terms of a series of detoxification mechanisms to protect the foetus from the amounts of oestrogens and progesterone produced by the placenta. Certainly many of these enzymes protect the foetus and promote excretion of steroids through the placenta as rapidly as possible.

*Dr. Koldovsky:* I have a question concerning the enzyme distribution. You have mentioned in one table the absence of sulfatase in the foetus and of glucuronidase in the placenta. How have the enzymes been estimated and are they specific?

*Dr. Reynolds:* The sulfatases are specific, in the sense that when I talked about sulfatases here I was talking about the sulfatases which hydrolyse a group at the C-3 position of neutral steroids and oestrogens. There are different enzymes for neutral steroids and for oestrogens. There also are other enzymes for sulfation and hydrolysis of the sulfate when it is at C-17. But in general the greatest proportion is sulfated at the C-3 position.

Secondly there is evidence from both *in vivo* and *in vitro* experiments, that there is an absence of sulfatase in the foetus and a very active sulfatase in the placenta. There also is very definitely glucuronic acid conjugation of steroids in the mid-term foetus. We are all aware of very low glucuronyl transferase activity in the newborn for bilirubin as a substrate, and certainly I think the activity in the newborn even for certain steroids is less than it is later in life; but it is present, even in the mid-term foetus.

*Dr. Koldovsky:* But how about the glucuronidase, not the glucuronyl transferase, not the glucuronidation but the enzyme with splitting activity?

*Dr. Reynolds:* Apparently glucuronide conjugates presented to the placenta are not split and they are forced through the placenta to the mother as glucuronide conjugates. (LEVITZ, M. (1966) J. Clin. Endocrinol. and Metab. 26: 773). This is a very slow transfer and thus the glucuronide conjugated steroids are not transferred well out of the foetal placental unit, but it can happen. Sulfates are apparently all split before they are transferred from the placenta. In other words, they are hydrolyzed in the placenta and then transferred as free compounds.

*Dr. Koldovsky:* We have estimated sulfatase and glucuronidase activity in foetus and placenta and we have estimated the sulfatase using catechol sulfate as substrate. Activity is present in the foetus in different organs. The glucuronidase activity using the phenolphthaleine glucuronate as substrate is relatively high in the placenta. If you compare the activity to that in the foetal liver, the activity of the placenta is approximately 50 to 70 per cent.

*Dr. Reynolds:* I can not explain your finding of sulfatase activity in the placenta. Again I am not sure about the specificity of the enzyme, and I think there is a great deal of substrate specificity. It may not be correct to transfer conclusions from the experiment with the compound you used to studies involving steroid substrates.

*Dr. Koldovsky:* No, all we can say is that this substrate has been split, and this is why I asked about the specificity of the enzymes.

*Prof. Visser:* I would like to congratulate Dr. REYNOLDS for this most beautiful work. Interested in steroids myself I know how difficult this work is. I have some questions. What is the role of cortisol and aldosterone in the foetus? You have said there is a role, and progesterone is the necessary precursor for these steroids. Do we really know what the role is and have you measured blood levels of cortisol and aldosterone in these foetuses? This also can answer your question of transplacental passage of these steroids.

Now the teleology of this whole foetal placental unit, could it be protection against androgens? As 3-beta-dehydrogenase enzyme activity is lacking, the foetus can not produce androgens. Transplacental passage of androgens from the mother is one of the dangers for the foetus. Would you like to comment on this? The third question is, is there another steroid which provides a better indication of foetal distress than oestriol. For instance this 15-hydroxylated compound, it might give a much more accurate indication than oestriol for the obstetrician.

*Dr. Reynolds:* I cannot give you any experimental evidence that cortisol and aldosterone are essential for the functioning of the mid-term foetus. I think that this work has not been done in the human. I am basing this conclusion on the perhaps mistaken assumption that many physiological processes in the foetus are much similar to those in the post-natal animal, that these same hormones are essential at this time of gestation. We know the concentration of cortisol in the newborn infant, I do not know the concentration of cortisol in the blood of the mid-term foetus. Perhaps this has been looked at but I am not aware of a specific figure.

Certainly the placenta functions as a rapidly acting detoxifying organ for androgens passed over from the mother. The placenta rapidly aromatizes and converts into oestrogens the androgenic compounds that might pass from the mother, for instance, androstenedione and testosterone. The oestrogens are detoxified in the foetus by the sulfation that I mentioned, and are then rapidly transferred back to the placenta. The problems come up when you consider some of the synthetic androgens, the 19 norcompounds for instance. These compounds have been studied relatively little, but what has been done shows that they are not aromatized in the placenta to anywhere near the extent that the normal androgens are (DELL'ACQUA et al. (1965) Acta Endocrinol. (Kbh) Suppl. 100: 81). Therefore the foetus is not protected in the same way from some of the synthetic androgens which may be transferred from the mother, as it is protected against the effects of the normal physiological androgens which may be transferred from the mother.

*Prof. Visser:* So you suggest that you can treat a mother with testosterone and will see no harmful effect on the foetus and if you give synthetic androgens with different molecular structure, there may be effects on the foetus?

*Dr. Reynolds:* It is difficult to know how much testosterone you can give to the mother. I don't know at what point the aromatization potential of the placenta may be exceeded. I think that from what is known that the foetus is likely to be much more protected against testosterone given to the mother than one of the synthetic androgens given to the mother.

*Prof. Kloosterman:* Thank you very much, Dr. REYNOLDS, for your introduction and for the discussions you raised and stimulated. I am especially grateful for the answer to the second question this morning about the teleological function of oestrogens. As a clinician I can assure you that we look only at oestrogens as a waste product or an intermediate product. I am not aware of any clinical value of oestrogens; up to now no experiments and investigations are known which indicate that oestrogens are of any value for treatment during pregnancy. I thank you once again.

DISCUSSION PAPER DR. GRUENWALD

*Prof. Kloosterman* (in the chair): Thank you for your interesting speech. I heard from it that you are living in a very specialized country where you have somebody for everything. I think however, that sometimes obstetricians can be expected to look at placentas as well! The first speaker after your lecture I can give the word to is Dr. WIGGLESWORTH who has to show us something.

*Dr. Gruenwald:* May I just say that I have no objections to obstetricians looking at placentas but I don't think that the examination should be done in the delivery room.

*Dr. Wigglesworth:* Firstly I would like to congratulate Dr. GRUENWALD on his masterly analysis of the problems involved in placental pathology and his demonstration of the very important concept of lobular architecture of the placenta.

Secondly I would stress that I agree with the majority of the facts Dr. GRUENWALD has presented. Finally, however, I would like to present a few slides on some recent work of my own which, I believe, throws some additional light on the vascular organization of the human placenta.

I have found it possible to locate and inject spiral arteries on the maternal surface of the delivered placenta. Before showing the results I would point out that it is perhaps fitting that I should present my results here in Holland, for the first injection study of vessels was performed 226 years ago, in 1741 in the city of Leiden by WILLEM NOORTWYCK. NOORTWYCK used an in-situ specimen for his study as have all later workers. Thirteen years later in London, JOHN and WILLIAM HUNTER studied similar specimens and in 1794 WILLIAM HUNTER published 'An Anatomical Description of the Human Gravid Uterus and its Contents', in which he described how the 'curling arteries' could be seen on the maternal surface of any fresh placenta by gently squeezing the placental substance so as to fill them the intervillous space. It was reading this description that prompted me to go and verify the finding and then to try to inject the vessels so displayed.

A nylon intravenous cannula is inserted into a spiral artery and injected with a barium gelatine solution. Figure 1 shows part of a placenta with an injected spinal artery. Slices through the entry of this and similar arteries shows that injection medium passes into the centers of the foetal lobules and may often be seen filling the intralobulair space.

Figure 2 demonstrates an X-ray of one of a series of dissections from a single placenta. It shows the spiral artery on the maternal surface (S), the foetal placental artery (F) and a mass of opaque injection medium within the placental lobule. Histological sections confirm that the barium has entered through the spiral artery and collected in the centre of the lobule with dense masses of terminal villi separating it from subchorionic and interlobular spaces. The venous side of the intervillous space is rather easier to inject than the arterial, as the openings are bigger.

We have also injected spiral arteries with barium and veins with blue barium. If these two solutions are of greater viscosity than that of blood there is little tendency for them to mix so that one can define arterial, capillary and venous areas of the intervillous space.

Figure 3 demonstrates the concept of placental organisation that emerges from these studies. Maternal blood entering the intervillous space through the spiral arteries passes directly to the centre of the lobule, diffuses through the tightly packed masses of terminal villi and drains back to the basal veins through subchorionic, interlobular and marginal venous pathways. The only postulate one needs to make to explain how this structure develops, is that the foetal placental lobules grow preferentially round the incoming streams of arterial blood.

The crowded masses of terminal villi form an intervillous capillary space and purely by default the areas between the lobules where there is no active growth, present loose spaces which form natural pathways for venous drainage. This is obviously wholly advantageous for placental exchange and means that the human placenta is just as logical in its formation as any other and is far more adaptable than most.

As I see it, this is the only way in which a villous haemochorial placenta could be designed so as to function efficiently. And it is to my mind against this structure that one has to explain pathological changes.

*Dr. Gruenwald:* As BOYD I think once said, the fact that something sounds nice and reasonable of course does not quite prove that it is so. In the last microscopic section of an artery that Dr. WIGGLESWORTH showed, it was quite obvious that the artery enters not into the centre of the lobule but between. But the material somehow got into the centre, and this is the big problem. I don't think there is any doubt that the arteries come in between the lobules but somehow apparently the blood manages to get into the centre. This is very interesting, and I have no idea how this actually can be accomplished. So I think the fact that is quite safe to assume is that the arteries enter between the lobules, but this does not prove that the blood does not get into the lobules. It must of course, because by far the greater part of the terminal villi concerned with the exchange function are in the dense part of the lobule. So obviously the blood must get there somehow. The interesting thing is that it is not all simple that the blood is just injected into the centre directly.

*Dr. Papadatos:* We have been studying lately placentography with a 20 per cent solution studying the morphology of the placenta and X-ray pictures of the placenta. We were struck lately by the unusual vascular bed that we had in a case of chromosomal abnormality. I want to ask two questions. Does anybody know what is the placental morphology in chromosomal anomalies, is there any specific morphological variation? And my second question is, would you say that placental aging causes the same degenerative changes that we get for example in toxaemia, infarcts and calcifications?

*Dr. Gruenwald:* I don't think that is to answer either. It has of course been suggested that just about every change you find in the maturing placenta is increased in toxaemia, but every time there has been somebody else who fails to find this. I think we all need studies with more regard to the lobular architecture, for instance the problem of counting syncitial buds, you can find them on every other villus in the dense part of the lobule and none at all a couple of millimeters away. So we have to repeat some of these studies. I don't think there is at the moment anything definite about changes that are absolutely characteristic of toxaemia. I don't know whether we are safe in saying that the changes in toxaemia are exaggerations of normal aging, and don't know anything about the chromosomal abnormalities.

*Dr. Wigglesworth:* The placentas are much smaller in some of these abnormalities, aren't they?

*Dr. Papadatos:* The picture was very unusual, and absolutely different from the usual vascular bed that we get in normal placentas.

*Dr. Wigglesworth:* Which chromosomal abnormality was this one?

*Dr. Papadatos:* 18-trisomy.

*Dr. Wigglesworth:* That is the one that is quoted as always having a small placenta, and also the babies are more growth-retarded in that variant than in the others. All 18-trisomies that I have seen were very much more retarded in size than the 13—15 trisomies or mongols. I don't know if Dr. GRUENWALD will agree with that.

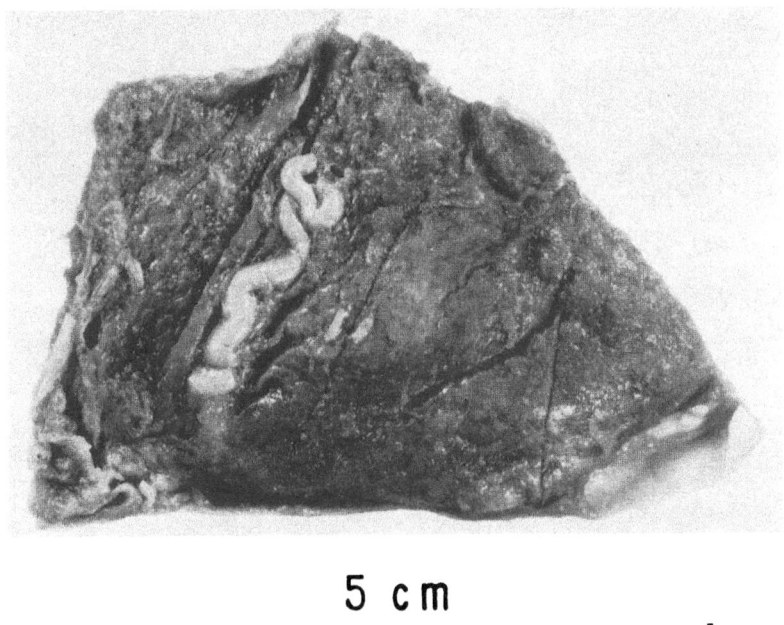

5 cm

*Fig.* 1.   Piece of fixed placenta showing injected spiral artery on maternal surface.

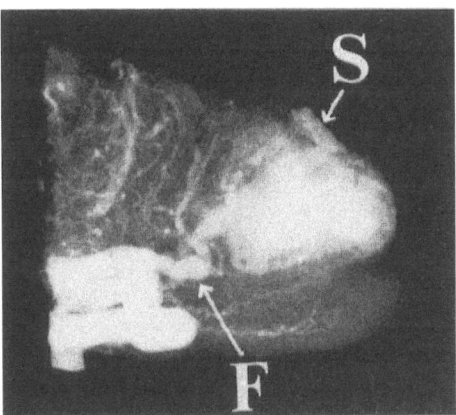

*Fig.* 2.   X-ray of dissected portion of placenta after injection of maternal and foetal arteries showing spiral artery S, foetal placental artery F and a mass of opaque injection medium within the placental lobule.

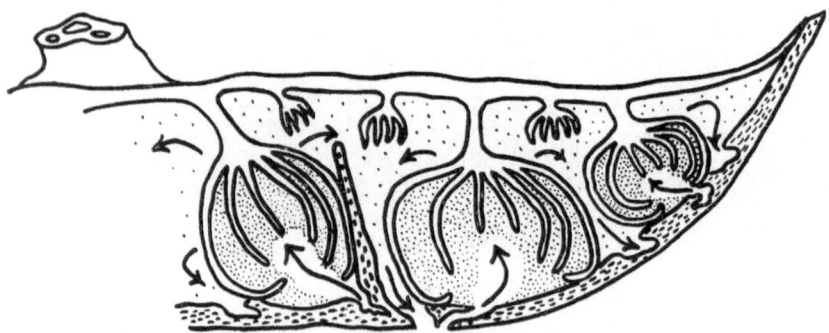

*Fig.* 3.   Diagram of maternal circulation through intervillous space. Density of stippling indicates density of villi.

*Dr. Gruenwald:* Yes, as far as I know this is true. Are you talking about the foetal or the maternal vascular bed?

*Dr. Papadatos:* I am talking about the foetal vascular bed.

*Dr. Wigglesworth:* I would say as far as degenerative changes of the placenta are concerned, one has a sort of paradoxical situation, in that in the normal placenta, if you get a normal maternal blood supply to the centre of the lobule, the villi will be at the most juvenile stage, as that is where they are actively growing, and those in the venous interlobular areas will tend to appear more degenerate. Whereas if you get occlusion of spiral arteries you will get a reversal of this pattern because immediately that area of the placenta has to be supplied by neighbouring vessels and you get more extensive degenerative changes in the dense central areas of the lobule. That is, if you don't get such severe reduction in collateral supply as to cause infarction. The whole picture is so complex because of this that untill you understand both the lobular architecture and the haemodynamic side of it you can't really begin looking at placental pathology. I feel that I can only now start to make sense of pathological changes in the placenta.

*Dr. Reynolds:* I would like to ask Dr. GRUENWALD a question. How frequently are completely normal but very small placentas associated with intra-uterine growth retardation compared with apparently the more common circumstance of microscopically abnormal placentas being associated with such retarded infants.

*Dr. Gruenwald:* That is not easy to answer because if we find a small placenta we have no right to assume that the foetus is small because the placenta is small. The placenta as far as its fixed tissue is concerned, it is an organ of the foetus and a small foetus can have a small placenta just as it has a smaller liver and smaller kidneys and smaller feet. This is the difficulty here. The association of birthweight with placenta weight is better than that of gestational age and placenta weight. But the question is what conclusions can be drawn from this. Now on the other hand, if for instance we look at perinatal mortality as a very crude indicator of embarassment of the foetus, we find that the mortality is higher if the weight of the placenta is below mean minus two standard deviations, either for particular week of gestation or for the particular birthweight group. But these changes must be quite severe, the placenta has to be terribly small, for just that alone to be a factor in foetal difficulties. On the other hand I would think that it certainly stands to reason that combined with other detrimental factors, the small placenta might give out sooner than a larger one. Another difficulty is that the ratio between foetus and placenta changes. If we look at the small foetus, the ratio may be adequate for the small foetus that is mature, but small for a small foetus of the same size that is immature, because the ratio changes during the third trimester from 1 : 5 tot 1 : 7. So it is very difficult to make anything out of this, just as it is with other pathological aspects of the placenta. We must study many more placentas. The difficulty of course is that we have no trouble finding plenty of placentas and plenty of normal children near term, but when we go into the smaller groups, such as the smaller babies, and we divide them up by birthweight for gestational age, adequacy of birthweight for gestational age or variations associated with pathologic changes of the mother, we can look at placentas in a large hospital for years and will not come up with very large groups. The abnormal cases are not all that numerous.

*Prof. Kloosterman:* Thank you very much. I should like to point to one thing. Dr. GRUNEWALD had raised a very important question when I heard him say, very distinctly, the placenta is just an organ of the foetus. Beforehand I heard a discussion going on between foetal parts of the placenta and maternal parts of the placenta. I never heard of an organ for two individuals combined. And I wonder whether we in the next days will raise the question again whether the placenta is just a normal organ of the foetus and the small placenta has something to do with the small foetus.

# ASSESSMENT OF FOETAL DEVELOPMENT

# GROWTH PATTERN OF THE NORMAL
# AND THE DEPRIVED FETUS

P. GRUENWALD*

This presentation is limited to the third trimester of human pregnancy. Much of the existing information on fetal growth is based on birth weights at various gestational ages. This is open to criticism because pregnancies terminating before term are not normal. Yet, as will be pointed out later, fetal growth retardation is unlikely to occur early in the third trimester and this reduces the largest source of error. Furthermore, no better information is available, and birth weight data will therefore be reviewed and interpreted. In addition, linear body measurements, and organ weights obtained at necropsy will be examined.

Growth curves constructed from birth weights are affected by a variety of factors (socio-economic state, maternal height, smoking, and other maternal characteristics), but these variants have usually not been regarded as pathologic. In fact, one is hard put to designate any one growth curve as universally normal in preference to all others. It is therefore technically expedient (though not scientifically sound) to contrast these *variations* which at term seldom differ from one another by more than 300 grams, with outright *pathologic* pregnancies in which much greater reductions of birth weight occur, often for unknown reasons.

All known data are consistent with the hypothesis that the fetal growth curve follows a straight course during the third trimester as long as the growth support available from the mother via the placenta is greater than, or equal to the needs of the fetus growing according

* Departments of Pathology, Sinai Hospital and The Johns Hopkins University, Baltimore, Maryland, U.S.A.
Work supported by research grant HD-00547-06 of the National Institute of Child Healt and Human Development, U. S. Public Health Service.

to its own growth potential. However, the requirements of the fetus
increase more rapidly than does growth support, and when the latter
falls below the needs for unrestricted growth, it becomes the limiting
factor in fetal growth, and the growth rate declines (1). According to
this supposition fetal size at term depends largely on the time at which
this departure from the straight growth curve occurs (fig. 1). Limitation of growth support has frequently and loosely been called
'placental insufficiency', but it is likely that more often the maternal
organism is the cause. McKEOWN and RECORD (2) showed long ago
with regard to multiple pregnancy, that growth support becomes
the limiting factor when the combined body weights come close to
3,000 grams (that is, 1,500 grams for each of twins, etc.) and their
own as well as the present author's data are in good accord with this.

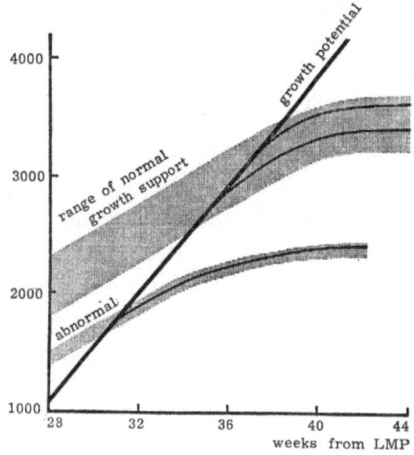

*Fig.* 1. Diagram showing the relationship of growth potential (heavy, diagonal
line) and growth support coming from the mother via the placenta (dotted areas)
of the fetus. Actual growth after limitation by growth support is shown by thin
lines.

In the foregoing it was assumed that the fetal growth potential is
about the same in all pregnancies, but there are certain exceptions to
this, apart from the sex difference in fetal body weight which is
unexplained as far as its mechanism is concerned. The incidence of
growth retardation among malformed fetuses is very high. Since the
same is found in experimentally produced as well as hereditary mal-

formations in animals, it may be surmised that a reduced growth potential is part and parcel of malformation. If this is true, then malformed fetuses will be small even in the presence of adequate growth support. For this reason malformed fetuses are excluded from further consideration.

Obviously, birth weight can be properly evaluated only in relation to gestational age, and pathologic growth retardation is usually recognized if birth weight is below an arbitrary limit such as the 10th percentile, or mean minus 2 standard deviations for the respective week of gestation. The former limit includes 3 to 4 times as many cases as the latter. The question then arises what standards should be used, and the answer depends largely on the problem to be studied. There are three practical possiblities: If one were to study pregnancy outcome in relation to prevailing conditions of living, or medical care, standards based on that particular population would be adequate. If socio-economic, racial, or other widely prevailing conditions were under study in different populations, then the highest known standards of any population (presently the Swedish) might be used as representing the values which would be approached, perhaps only after several generations, under favorable circumstances. Finally, an extrapolated growth curve, derived from the straight portion of the curve prevailing in most populations up to 36 or 38 weeks, is useful in studying the slowing of fetal growth late in pregnancy (3).

Several groups of growth curves may serve to illustrate what was characterized above as variations of fetal growth. Figure 2 compares Swedish, British, American and Japanese populations: the latter are shown for the immediate post-war period of deprivation and for 1963-64 when pre-war levels had been surpassed. The increase of birth weight in Japan during this time is entirely due to a changed fetal growth rate and not to increased gestation time: the mean length of gestation actually decreased slightly between 1945 and 1964 (4). Figures 3 and 4 show differences of fetal growth curves related to maternal height, and to smoking habits, both from the British Perinatal Mortality Survey of the National Birthday Trust in 1958. All these groups of curves are consistent with the hypothesis that departure from a common, straight-line growth curve occurs at different times in pregnancy, depending on a variety of factors which influence the growth support of the fetus. Unfortunately the numbers

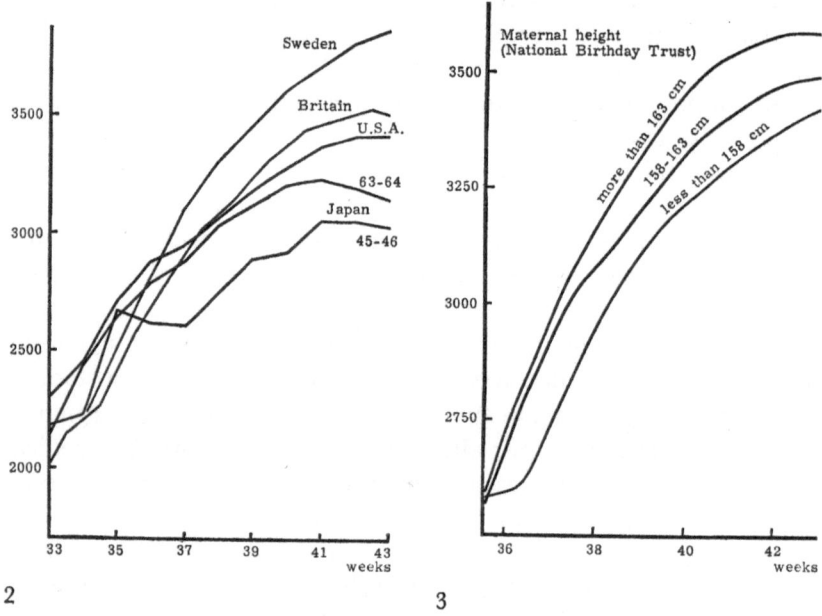

2

3

*Fig. 2.* Growth curves derived from birth weights of Swedish (Lindell, *Acta Obstet. et Gynec. Scand.* 34: 136, 1956), British (1958, courtesy National Birthday Trust), American (1) and Japanese (4) infants.

*Fig. 3.* Fetal growth curves from birth weights, for groups of mothers of different height. Courtesy National Birthday Trust.

of births early in the third trimester are insufficient to make this point with complete assurance.

Twin pregnancy is (depending on one's point of view) not truly pathologic, but the frequency and extent of fetal growth retardation exceeds that characterized above as variation. Figure 5, again taken from data of the National Birthday Trust, as well as this author's data from Baltimore, supports the above mentioned contention of McKeown and Record (2) that growth retardation sets in when the combined weight approaches 3000 grams. The same figure illustrates what is also true for singletons, namely, that growth retardation is on the average more severe in cases of perinatal death than in survivors or, expressed differently, that the mortality of growth-retarded fetuses

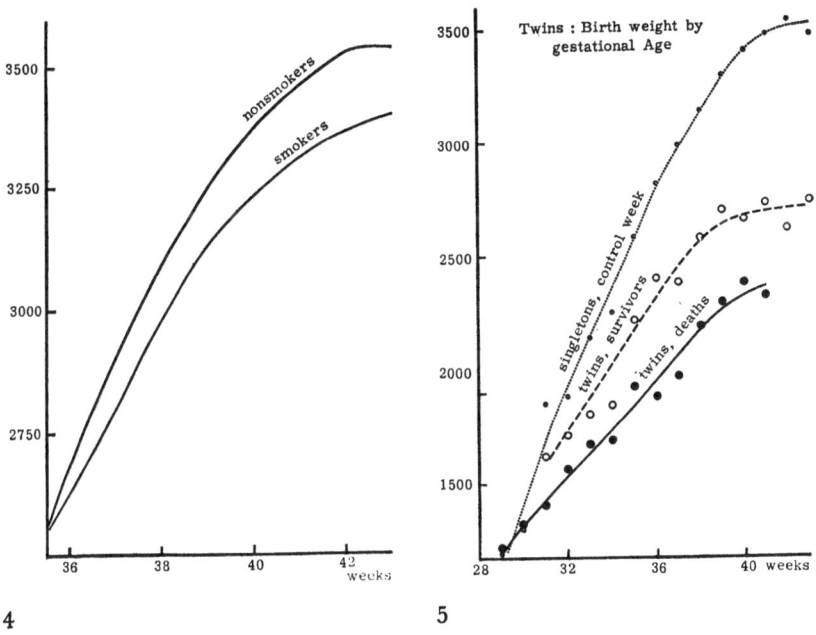

4

5

*Fig. 4.* Fetal growth curves from birth weights, for non-smoking and smoking mothers. Courtesy National Birthday Trust.

*Fig. 5.* Fetal growth curves from birth weights of twins (survivors and perinatal deaths) compared with singleton births. Courtesy National Birthday Trust.

is inordinately high. It would, of course, be meaningless to construct empirical growth curves of severely growth-retarded singleton fetuses *per se* since these are recognized by definition by an arbitrarily defined deficit of birth weight for their gestational age.

The proportion of growth-retarded fetuses among infants of low birth weight is, depending on the criteria used and the population studied, one-third to one-half of the total or even higher (5). Neonatal morbidity of pre-term infants is related mainly to difficulties in adaptation to extrauterine life (for instance, respiratory distress) and that of growth-retarded infants to fetal deprivation (for instance, hypoglycemia). Pathologic causes of death also show different trends, as illustrated by the predominance of pulmonary findings of hyaline membranes in pre-term, and pulmonary hemorrhage in growth retarded groups (fig. 6) There are indications that each of these two major causes of low birth weight carries the risk of different types of brain damage. This needs to be established in the future when the results of follow-up of significantly large series are interpreted with due regard to the relationship of birth weight and gestational age.

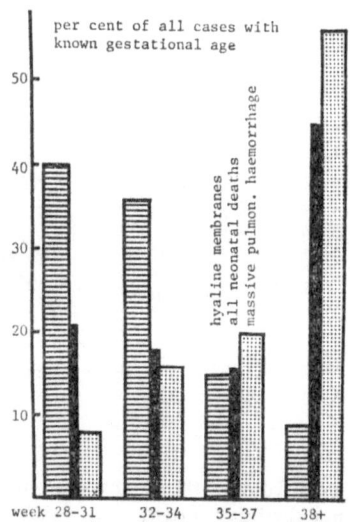

*Fig.* 6.   Gestational age distribution of autopsy finding of hyaline membranes and massive pulmonary hemorrhage. Courtesy National Birthday Trust.

Not all fetal deprivation is of sufficient severity and duration to result in a detectable deficit of birth weight. A classification of fetal distress (in a very wide and non-specific sense) as chronic, subacute and acute has therefore been suggested (6) on the basis that deprivation of a duration sufficient to produce obvious growth retardation must be chronic. Fetuses with malnutrition and wasting, but without obvious growth retardation are in the subacute category, and the well known perinatal distress without either growth retardation or wasting is classified as acute. Chronic fetal distress is recognized by a deficit of birth weight in relation to gestational age, usually in the order of either the 10th percentile or 2 standard deviations below the mean. Subacute fetal distress may be more conspicuous than the chronic form because of wasting, producing the 'long, thin' baby. Yet it has not been defined by objective criteria. The best known example is that occurring in prolonged pregnancy. Acute perinatal distress related to the birth process, does not concern us here.

The *growth pattern* in chronic fetal distress shows surprisingly little change of body proportions when growth retarded neonates are compared with normally grown pre-term infants of similar weight by means of the usual measurements. Both body length and head circumference of growth retarded infants are within 1 cm of those of pre-term ones in most weight groups (7). This may be statistically significant, but is of little use to the physician attempting to differentiate the two kinds of low birth weight. In subacute fetal distress, on the other hand, the infant is light for its length (or long for its weight). This difference between chronic and subacute distress is particularly apparent when one considers birth weight in relation to the third power of length (fig. 7). In normal development this ratio increases up to term as the fetus gains more weight than length; the ratio is

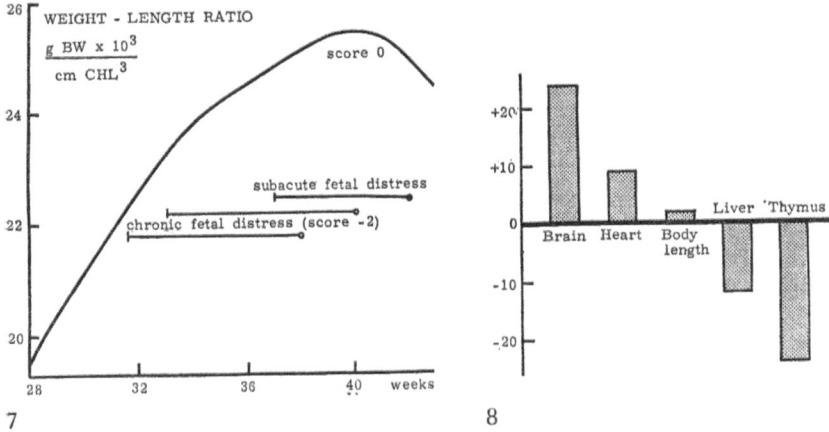

*Fig. 7.* Ratio of birth weight to the third power of crown-heel length for neonates with a birth weight within one standard deviation from the mean for their respective week of gestation (score 0). Courtesy National Birthday Trust. Data for groups of fetuses in chronic distress, and a representative case of subacute fetal distress are shown by circles. The horizontal lines connect these with the points on which they would fall if gestational age were commensurate with their actuel birth weight.

*Fig. 8.* Body length and organ weights of cases of chronic fetal distress (birth weight below mean minus 2 standard deviations for gestational age) expressed as per cent of values for normally grown infants of similar weight (within 1 standard deviation from the mean).

lower both in chronic and in subacute distress, but when such infants are placed in a position in the graph which they would occupy if their gestational age were appropriate for their birth weight, those in chronic fetal distress are much closer to the normal curve than are those in subacute distress (fig. 7). This possibility of characterizing subacute fetal distress has so far not been used for systematic classification.

When organ weights are studied at necropsy, marked abnormalities are found in chronic fetal distress and, to a lesser degree, in the subacute form. The trends are the same as those found in experimentally deprived animal fetuses: in comparison with normal-size infants of the same gestational age, the growth-retarded ones have smaller organs, but to varying degrees. This is particularly obvious when the latter infants are compared with normally grown infants of the same weight; the brain is considerably, and the heart somewhat larger (that is, less growth-retarded) whereas liver and thymus are markedly smaller (that is, more deficient in weight) (fig. 8). Similar trends are found, though to a slighter extent, in post-term infants that are normal in body weight by empirical, but not by extrapolated standards (3). The small thymus of neonates suffering chronic fetal distress shows the same severe involution that would occur in severe postnatal malnutrition. The brain of these undergrown infants is not only large in relation to body size, it also has well developed convolutions more in line with gestational age than with birth weight. Histologic maturation in various organs, such as kidneys or lungs, is also little or not affected by growth retardation. Existing standards are not sufficiently discriminating to permit us to determine whether maturation is entirely unaffected by chronic deprivation.

In the past, the immediate and late sequelae of pre-term birth were not distinguished from those of fetal deprivation because birth weight was used as the sole criterion. Much of this work will have to be repeated with a better appreciation of these factors. Cerebral damage is, of course, most important and it must be kept in mind that periods of poor oxygenation of the pre-term infant and hypoglycemia of the growth-retarded one may cause brain damage not present at birth, and therefore potentially preventable. The extent and frequency of permanent growth retardation following intrauterine deprivation also need to be investigated.

## REFERENCES

1. GRUENWALD, P. (1966) *Am. J. Obst. & Gynec.* 94: 1112.
2. McKEOWN, T. and R. G. RECORD (1952) *J. Endocrin.* 8: 386.
3. GRUENWALD, P. (1964) *Am. J. Obst. & Gynec.* 89: 503.
4. GRUENWALD, P., H. FUNAKAWA, S. MITANI, T. NISHIMURA and S. TAKEUCHI (1967) *Lancet* 1 : 1026.
5. GRUENWALD, P. (1964) *Pediatrics* 34: 157.
6. GRUENWALD, P. (1963) *Biol. Neonat.* 5: 215.
7. GRUENWALD, P. (1967) *Recent Adv. Reprod. Physiol.* 2 : 279.

# THE ASSESSMENT OF FOETAL AGE BY THE EXAMINATION OF THE CENTRAL NERVOUS SYSTEM

A. MINKOWSKI, S. SAINT-ANNE DARGASSIES, C. DREYFUS-BRISAC, J. CL. LARROCHE J. VIGNAUD AND C. AMIEL

In the human being, the assessment of foetal age can be done with a fair accuracy by the examination of the central nervous system (CNS). This has been proved to be a useful tool especially in over-grown infants (from diabetic mothers) or in undergrown infants (small for date infants). This has been confirmed by the anatomical aspect and the weight of the brain (9, 6).

There are four ways of assessing the foetal age from the study of the C.N.S.

1. Neurological examination
2. E.E.G.
3. X-Ray of the skull
4. Anatomical examination. This, of course, gives just a confirmation in cases terminated by death.

Those 4 ways are fully described in various papers, in a movie (11), and finally, in the book *Human Development* (17). We will only here summarize and discuss the data published elsewhere.

## I. NEUROLOGICAL EXAMINATION

S. SAINT-ANNE DARGASSIES (15) has used ANDRÉ THOMAS's (16) technique originally described for the full-term newborn applying it to the premature infant. The original material consisted of 25 premature born at 28 weeks, 28 premature born at 32 weeks, 33 premature born at 35 weeks, 28 premature born at 37 weeks.

In all cases there were harmonious correlations between weight, height and head circumference; the infants were *normal* (not twins) at the time of examination; their neurological age was always corresponding to the foetal age calculated from the first day of the last

---

\* Centre de Recherches Biologiques Neonatales, Hôpital Port-Royal, Paris.

Table 1. *Neurological assessment of foetal age* *

### I. PASSIVE TONE

| Week | 28 | 30 | 32 | 34 | 36 | 38 | 41 |
|---|---|---|---|---|---|---|---|
| | Complete hypotonia | Flexion of the thigh | | Flexion of the lower limb | Flexion of the four limbs | Hypertonic | |
| Poplital angle | 150° | | 110° | 100° | 90° | 80° | |
| Heel to ear | In contact | | | | | | |
| Return to flexion of forearm | No | | Weak | | Strong | | |

### II. ACTIVE TONE

| Week | 28 | 30 | 32 | 34 | 36 | 38 | 41 |
|---|---|---|---|---|---|---|---|
| Neck flexors | No | No | No | Starts | | Good | |
| Neck Extensors | | | Starts | ⟶ | | Good | |
| Trunk | No | No | No | Starts | Good | ⟶ | |
| Straightening of lower limbs | No | No | Fair | Excellent | | | |

### III. REFLEXES

| Week | 28 | 30 | 32 | 34 | 36 | 38 | 41 |
|---|---|---|---|---|---|---|---|
| Grasp | Finger only | | Strong | | Extends to the upper limbs | | |
| Rooting | Slow and incomplete | | Complete | Excellent | ⟶ | | |
| Sucking | No or Weak | | Synchronized with deglutition | | Perfect | ⟶ | |
| Moro | Weak | | Complete | | ⟶ | | |
| Walk | No | No | Starts | Good | ⟶ | | |
| Crossed extension | Random rattern | | Extension | | Adduction | ⟶ | |

*For discussion see text.

periods, with a few understandable exceptions: breech delivery, skin retraction or hip dislocation, fractures of the humerus or the clavicle.

The technique and the results have been so often described elsewhere that we think it is sufficient to give a summary (table 1):

As one can see, this is a result of a combined study of the so-called 'primary reflexes' and of the tone ('passive' when the observer stimulates motions, 'active' when the infant moves by himself). In our hands and others ones, (KONIGSBERGER, 8, a.o.) it has proved to be almost constantly reliable and it corresponds to whatever we know (very little indeed) on the neurological behaviour of the newborn; it almost constantly corresponds with the E.E.G. in a double blind test.

However, ROBINSON (13), in a rather interesting study advocated the isolated study of each reflex. He thinks that the appreciation of muscle tone is somewhat imprecise and practically difficult. He described a stydy of 219 neurological examinations based on the sole study of the reflexes on 62 infants born at known gestational ages between 25 and 42 weeks (37 of normal birth weight for the gestational age, 25 below 25 % of the mean birth weight for their gestational age). He indicated that some reflexes were almost constantly present, whatever the gestational age: palmar and plantar grasp, abduction phase of the Moro, withdrawal of the footsole, blink response to light.

He described 5 reflexes which have a clear cut time of appearance and are the same in 'small for date' babies: pupil reaction to light (appearing at 29—31 weeks), traction response (33—36 weeks); glabellar tap reflex (32—34 weeks), head straightening reflex (34—37 weeks), head turning to light (32—36 weeks).

However, after 18 years of study in which we examined 3000 infants, we think it would be very adventurous to base any assessment of the foetal age on one reflex. There is no doubt there would be variations on a larger scale than the one produced by ROBINSON (13).

On the other hand, the muscle tone is too much a part of the neurological behaviour of the newborn to be omitted; as a matter of fact, in trained hands, it has proved to be, by far the most reliable and accurate index of foetal age.

In all cases of dysmaturity (infants below the 10th percentile) the neurological assessment agrees with the real foetal age.

II. E.E.G. ASSESSMENT

## A. E.E.G. in normal premature and full term infants

This has been fully described in various papers by C. DREYFUS-BRISAC (1, 2) and co-workers from a total of 740 tracings from 344 infants:

1. 20 previable fetuses born between 20 and 26 weeks (24 tracings);
2. 60 infants born between 28 and 32 weeks, and followed up to the presumed term of 41 weeks (241 tracings);
3. 147 infants born between 32 and 37 weeks and followed up to the time of normal term (210 tracings);
4. 117 infants between 37 and 41 weeks (265 tracings).

As the results have been fully published elsewhere we think it is sufficient to give the following figures 1, 2 and 3.

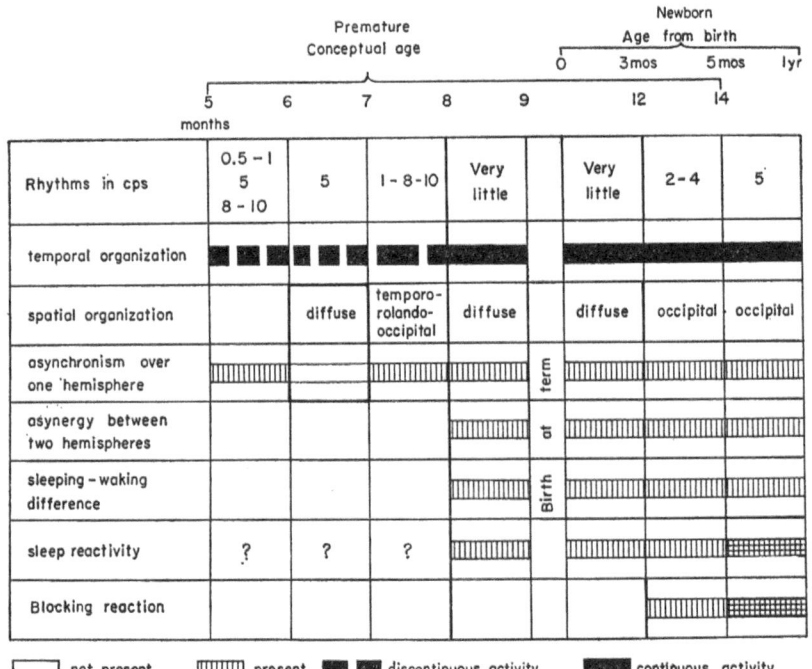

*Fig.* 1.

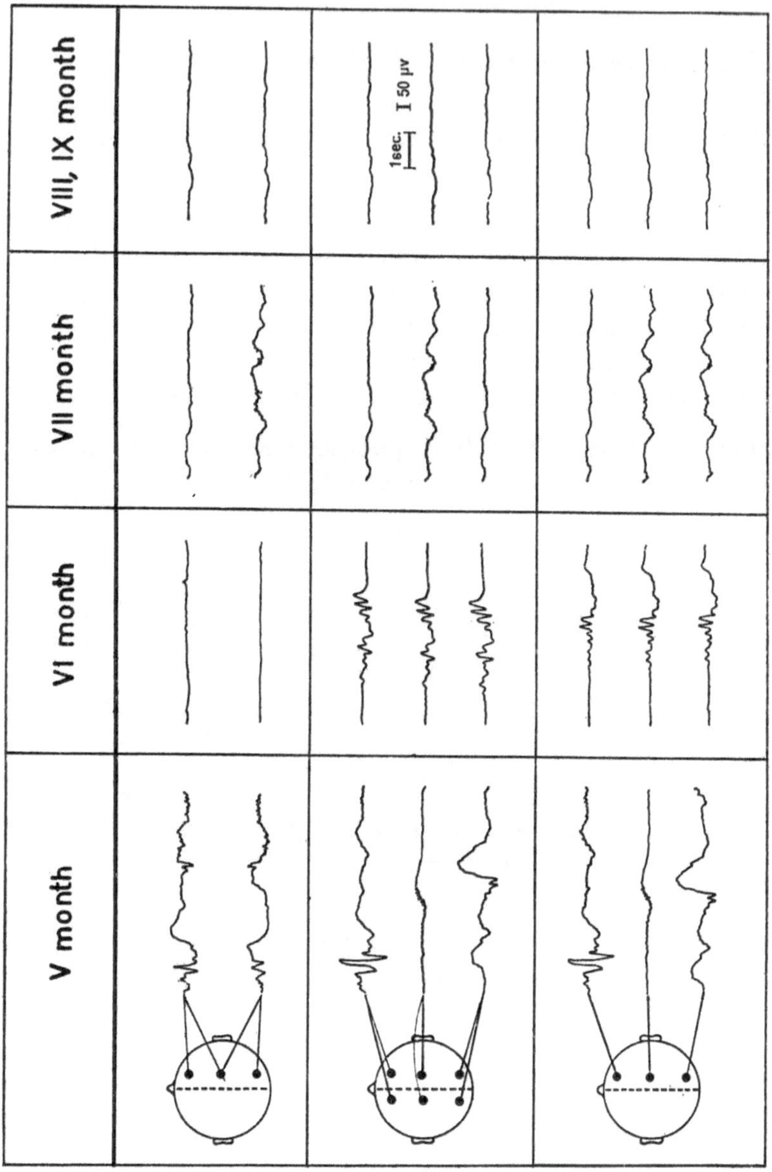

A. MINKOWSKI ET AL.

*Fig. 2.*

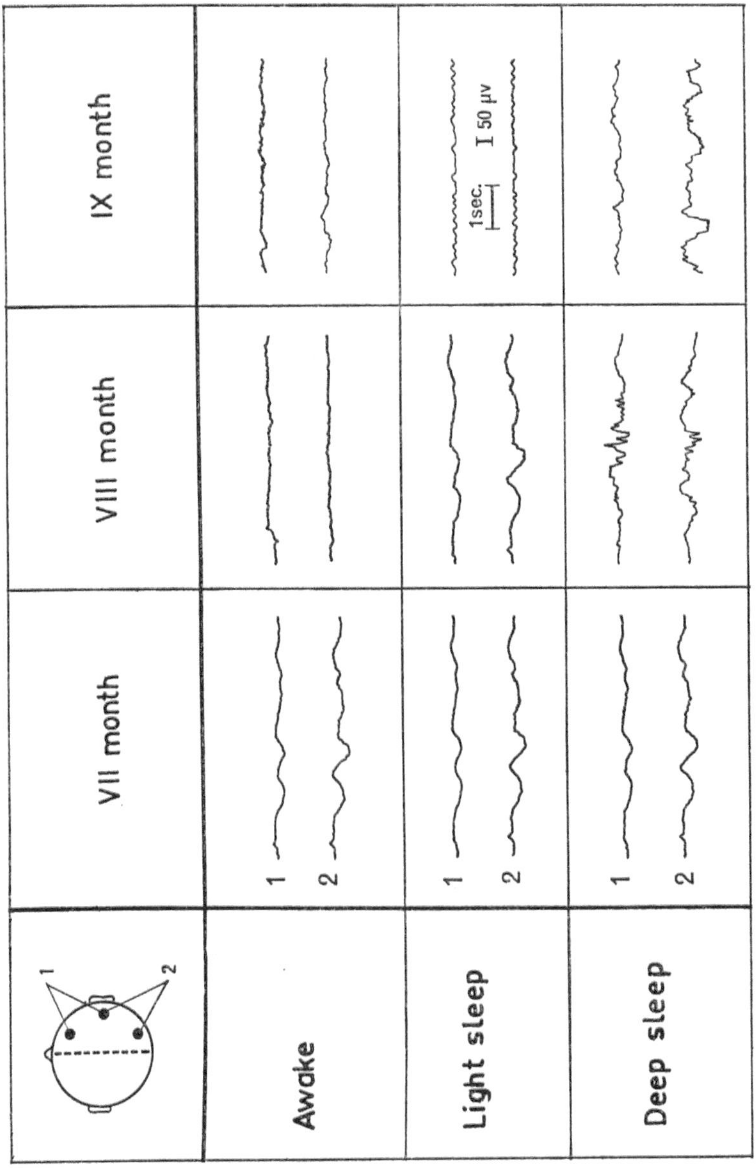

*Fig.* 3.

Relations between the gestational age and the development of the central nervous system have also been detected by recording visual and auditory evoked potentials in human prematures, the latency of the response being clearly correlated with the gestational age (3, 4, 5, 7, 18, 19).

### B. E.E.G. in dysmature infants

96 Small for date infants have been studied, 91 were born between 37 and 43 weeks, 5 were born before 37 weeks (mean 39,1 weeks). Birth weight ranged between 890 g and 2570 g (mean 1895,4 g), the body length was between 33 cm and 45 cm (mean 43,5 cm) and the occipito-frontal circumference was between 25 and 36 cm (mean 30,7 cm).

The results of the electroencephalographic study have been classified in 4 groups: correct, correct but not precise, incorrect and unclassifiable (table 2). 85 E.E.G.'s gave a correct appreciation of the gestational age with the criteria already described by DREYFUS-BRISAC (2a). Among them, twelve were not precise, mainly by simultaneous presence on the same record of two sleep patterns normally present at different gestational age. This makes it impossible to differentiate between infants of 37—39 weeks of gestational age, and those of 40 weeks or more. 7 E.E.G.'s were unclassified, being either incomplete, without waking or sleeping patterns, or too pathological. There were four errors of classification.

E.E.G. findings in a special series of 13 infants (below the 10th percentile) have been recorded on days 3, 7, 14, 21, during waking, drowsiness, sleep and arousal, in combination with metabolic studies. We missed the sleep tracing once (at day 3) and the waking tracing twelve times.

Main features on a total of 50 tracings were:

1. The electroencephalographic age in 12 infants corresponded to the gestational age. In only one case, there was a discrepancy at days 7 and 14, whereas the correspondence was satisfactory at days 3 and 21. That discrepancy occurred after a severe episode of hypoglycaemia, associated with transient convulsions and followed by a long disturbance of the waking tracing: it was in advance of the defined gestational age (32 weeks instead of 37) giving the picture

of heterochronism, described as a major pathological finding in the premature infant.

2. 7 Infants showed the following disturbances of the waking tracing:
   a. A true abnormally slow anterior dysrythmia has been seen at days 5 and 7 in one infant who developed hypernatraemia on day 2 (176 mEq/L), followed by hyponatraemia on day 7 (127 mEq/L).
   b. Bifrontal sharp transient waves (slow diphasic isolated spikes) have been noticed in 5 infants and specially in the ones who had blood glucose levels below 20 mg per 100 ml at days 3 and 7; these persisted at day 14 in the infant whose tracing showed a heterochronism after an episode of severe hypoglycaemia.
   c. The occipital activity was too slow in 2 infants at days 3 and 7. One of those infants had sharp waves, and the other one a low anterior dysrythmia.

3. Anomalies of sleep tracings, as a whole, were minimal with the exception of the presence of slow diphasic frontal spikes at a high voltage (more than 100 microvolts up to 300 microvolts), perhaps a constant characteristic of the E.E.G. in small for date infants: many of those spikes were observed in 4 children, a little less in 6 others. Only 3 children out of 13 have had no humps on their tracings.

The frequency of bifrontal bivolted spikes during sleep seems specific for 'small for date' infants; that anomaly has bot been encountered in 121 various neurological and obstetrical conditions, or in respiratory distress syndrome.

*Late follow-up of the E.E.G. tracings*
Five infants have been followed up to now: 2 at 5 months, at 1 year, at 18 months; 1 at 5 months, and at 1 year; 1 at 5 months and at 18 months; 1 at 5 months only.

Five tracings have been taken at 5 months and three respectively at 1 year and 18 months.

In alle these infants, the waking and sleep tracings have been normal. Some unusual features have been seen during drowsiness: in two infants, at 1 year and 18 months, there was a regular and ample hypersynchronic activity at 4 c/sec for some minutes, persisting in clinical sleep.

In two infants at 5 months of age, another particularity has been a rythmic hypersynchronism at 4 c/sec, unexpected at this age; in one case, this feature increased at 1 year and 18 months; in the other one, it has disappeared at 1 year.

### III. SKULL X RAY ASSESSMENT

Some fair information can be derived from this method as the development of the skull closely parallels the development of the brain. In fact the so called 'digital markings' represent the development of the convolutions; the sutures open; the skull volume increases.

The original material collected by VIGNAUD (17) consisted of 73 infants from 24 to 41 weeks of gestational age

1. *Sutures.* The sagittal, metopic, coronal and temporal sutures grow very equally whereas the lambdoïd suture decreases.
2. The *volume* of the skull can be grossly calculated from the Mackinnon's equation:

$$V = 1/2\, I \times L \times H + 1/2\, I \times L \times B \times 0,51$$

   I  = greatest diameter (either biparietal or bitemporal)
   H  = vertex through auditory canals
   L  = greatest anteroposterior diameter
   B  = bregma through occipital fossa.

   The curve of growth in intracranial volume from 24 to 41 weeks parallels the curve of the increase in weight of the brain.
3. *Digital markings* are absent up to 28 weeks, rare and hardly visible at 28—37 weeks and constantly present at 37—41 weeks.

   This is very important as most of the small for date infants are born after 37 weeks. The X-ray appearance of the skull contributes then to the estimation of the real age.

### IV. ANATOMICAL EXAMINATION

The aspect and the values of the weight of the brain during fetal development have been described by LARROCHE in various papers (see 9). Cortical cells have been counted for each period by RABINOWICZ (12).

Table 2. *Result of electroencephalographic studies in several groups of 'small for date' infants. See text.*

| Gestational age at birth | Electroencephalographic age | | | |
|---|---|---|---|---|
| | Correct | Correct but not precise | Incorrect | Unknown |
| 30-36 weeks 5 cases | 4 | | | 1 |
| 37-39 weeks 54 cases | 41 | 7 | 2 | 4 |
| 40-43 weeks 37 cases | 28 | 5 | 2 | 2 |
| Total 96 cases | 73 (76 %) 85 (89 %) | 12 (13 %) | 4 (4 %) | 7 (7 %) |

REFERENCES

1. DREYFUS-BRISAC, C., J. FLESCHER and E. PLASSART (1962) *Biol. Neonat.* 4: 154.
2. DREYFUS-BRISAC, C. (1964) In: *Neurological and electroencephalographic correlative studies in infancy*, KELLAWAY, P. and I. PETERSEN, eds., Grune & Stratton Inc., New York, p. 186.
2a. DREYFUS-BRISAC, C. (1962) *World Neurol.* 3: 5.
3. ELLINGSON, R. J. (1960) *Electroenceph. Clin. Neurophysiol.* 12: 663.
4. ELLINGSON, R. J. (1964) In: *Neurological and electroencephalographic correlative studies in infancy*, KELLAWAY, P. and I. PETERSEN, eds., Grune & Stratton Inc., New York, p. 78-115.
5. ENGEL, L. R. and B. V. BUTLER (1963) *J. Pediat.* 63: 386.
6. GRUENWALD, P. (1963) *Biol. Neonat.* 5: 215
7 HRBEK, A and P. MARES (1964) *Electroenceph. Clin. Neurophysiol.* 16: 575.
8. KONIGSBERGER, M. R. (1966) *Pediat. Clin. N. Amer.* 13: 823.
9. LARROCHE, J. CL. (1962) *Biol. Neonat.* 4: 126.
10. MINKOWSKI, A. (1962) *Biol. Neonat.* 4: 121.
11. MINKOWSKI, A., C. DREYFUS-BRISAC, J. CL. LARROCHE, S. SAINT-ANNE DARGASSIES and J. VIGNAUD (1964) *The development of the C.N.S. from the fetal period to term.* Service du Film de Recherche Scientifique Paris.

12. Rabinowicz, Th. (1967) In: *Techniques for the establishment of an atlas of the cerebral cortex of the premature.* Blackwell Scient. Publ., Oxford, p. 91.
13. Robinson, R. J. (1966) *Arch. Dis. Childh.* 41 : 437.
14. Saint-Anne Dargassies, S. (1955) *Etudes Neonat.* 4: 71.
15. Saint-Anne Dargassies, S. (1962) *Biol. Neonat.* 4: 174.
16. Thomas, A. and S. Saint-Anne Dargassies (1952) *Etudes neurologiques sur le nouveau-né et le jeune nourrisson,* Masson, Paris.
17. Vignaud, J. (1966) In: *Human development,* F. Faulkner, ed., Saunders, Philadelphia, Pa., p. 277—285.
18. Weitzman, E. D., N. Fishbeen and L. Gruzioni (1965) *Pediatrics* 35: 458.
19. Weitzman, E. D., K. Ungar, L. Duhamel and L. Graziani (1966) *Electroenceph. Clin. Neurophysiol.* 21: 405.

# DEVELOPMENTAL CHANGES IN
# FETAL HEMOGLOBIN

H. C. SCHWARTZ, T. J. GRIBBLE, F. WELLAND, W. NIJHOF
AND J. H. P. JONXIS

About 100 years ago, KÖRBER observed the resistance of cord blood to alkali denaturation when compared with blood from adults. Since that time we have gained considerable insight into the biochemistry of adult (Hb A) and fetal (Hb F) hemoglobin, as reviewed recently by JONXIS (1) and BAGLIONI (2).

Hemoglobin F, like hemoglobin A, is composed of two identical pairs of polypeptide chains to each of which a heme group is attached. One pair, the alpha chains, is identical with the alpha chains in hemoglobin A; however the second pair, designated as gamma chains, have an amino acid sequence which is different from the beta chains of hemoglobin A. Thus, hemoglobin F has two alpha chains and two gamma chains ($\alpha_2 \gamma_2$); hemoglobin A has two alpha chains and two beta chains ($\alpha_2 \beta_2$). These structural differences between hemoglobins A and F are reflected not only in their electrophoretic, chromatographic, and immunologic properties, but in such chemical characteristics of hemoglobin F as the resistence to alkali denaturation. These properties have permitted measurements of the quantitative changes in fetal hemoglobin at various periods in development. More than 90 percent of the hemoglobin in the human fetus is Hb F and at birth 80 per cent of the cord blood hemoglobin is Hb F. However erythrocytes released from the bone marrow in the first days of life already contain 50 per cent Hb A. Apparently, the 'switch-over' from gamma to beta chains begins before birth. As a result, the Hb F concentration decreases rapidly in the first six months of life and at one year of age only 1 to 5 per cent of the hemoglobin is Hb F (1).

* Department of Pediatrics, Stanford University School of Medicine, Palo Alto, California, U.S.A. and Department of Pediatrics, State University, Groningen, The Netherlands.

It is noteworthy that the advantageous shift to the left of the oxygen dissociation curve for fetal erythrocytes is probably due to differences in the environment of the fetal red blood cell, rather than in the hemoglobin. When solutions of hemoglobin F and hemoglobin A are dialyzed to the same hydrogen ion concentration and ionic strength, the dissociation curves are identical.

Many clinical observations have contributed to our knowledge of the developmental changes in hemoglobin. Among these have been the description of the alpha and beta thalassaemia syndromes, hemoglobin H with four beta chains and its associated abnormal fetal hemoglobin (Bart's) with four gamma chains, amino acid abnormalities in the alpha and gamma chains, the intrauterine deaths associated with homozygosity for alpha thalassaemia and the syndrome of persistence of high fetal hemoglobin. Recently an embryonic hemoglobin with two alpha chains and two epsilon chains has been described in small embryos and in babies with the 13—15 trisomy syndrome (3).

Although these clinical conditions, where hemoglobin F synthesis is altered, are well recognized, little is known about the mechanism for the control of fetal hemoglobin synthesis. Even in simple microbial systems where the mechanism for the genetic control of protein structure has been worked out, knowledge about the control of protein synthesis is incomplete. In such systems protein synthesis appears to be partially under genetic and partially under environmental control (4).

During the past year I (Dr. Schwartz) have had the pleasure of working with Dr. Nijhof and Professor Jonxis in trying to design an experimental model for studying some of the environmental factors which might influence hemoglobin synthesis. We have used newborn Friesian and Groningen calves. In order to obtain a large population of reticulocytes, stippled cells, and other immature erythrocytes, calves were phlebotomized to hemoglobin concentrations of about 3 grams per 100 ml over a three day period as shown in fig. 1. Shock was avoided by performing an exchange transfusion of the blood with plasma and Macrodex[R]. This was done with a Pharmaseal Exchange Transfusion Set[R] through an indwelling polyethylene catheter in the external jugular vein. Samples of blood could be removed easily through the catheter. Fetal and adult hemoglobin synthesis were

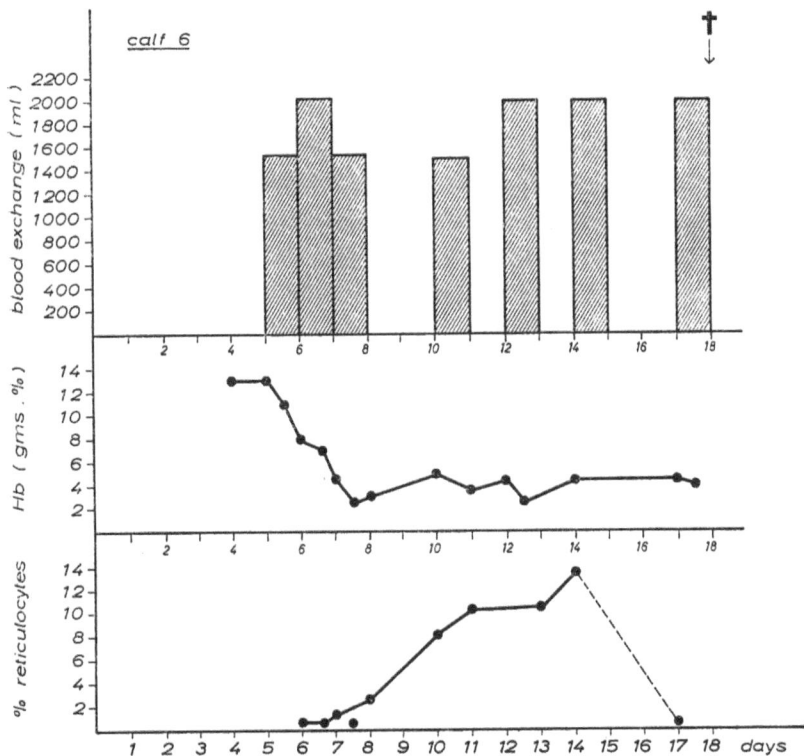

*Fig.* 1. Changes in the hemoglobin concentration and reticulocyte count after exchange transfusion of blood with plasma and Macrodex[R].

measured by incubating whole cells with radioactive leucine and then determining the specific activity of chromatographically separated hemoglobins A and F. The results of such an experiment are shown in fig. 2. This experimental model permits the investigation of certain environmental effects on hemoglobin synthesis. Studies on the effect of testosterone, cortisone, thyroxin and chorionic gonadotropins are in progress. These studies are prompted by the clinical observation of increased erythropoiesis after cortisone and testosterone therapy in certain anemic states and of changes in fetal hemoglobin concentration in aplastic anemia, during thyroxin induced metamorphosis and in association with high chorionic gonadotropin levels in molar pregnancies and choriocarcinomas.

The study of hemoglobin synthesis in this 'whole cell' system is

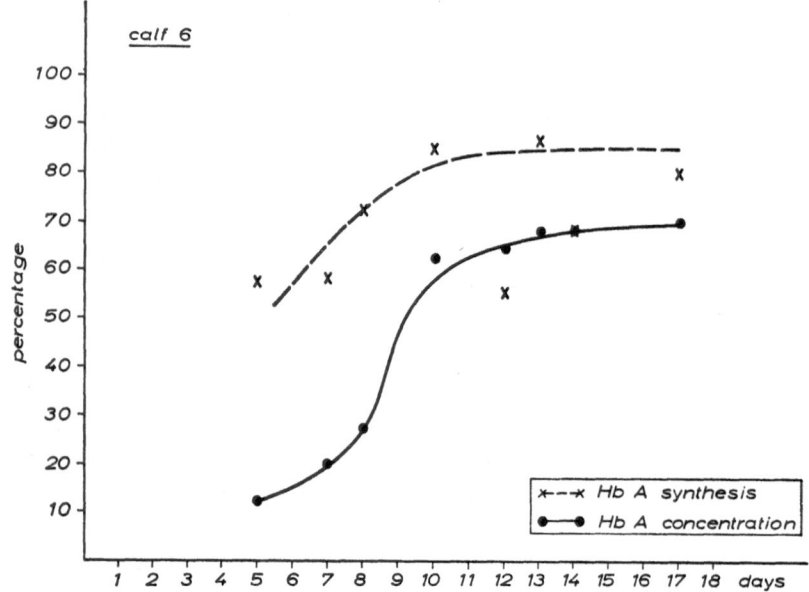

*Fig.* 2. Comparison of hemoglobin A synthesis, the rate of incorporation of radioactive leucine into Hb A, with changes in the concentration of Hb A.

however limited by such variables as the transport of substrate into the cell and the maintenance of energy systems within the cell. Some of these problems are circumvented when 'cell-free' systems are utilized. A few years ago, Dr. T. J. Gribble and I began studies with the 'cell-free' system described by SCHWEET, LAMFROM and ALLEN (5). This system consists of ribosomes, a protein fraction which contains the amino acid activating enzymes ('pH 5 enzymes') and the pH 5 supernatant solution prepared from hypotonically lysed rabbit reticulocytes. When these fractions are incubated with radioactive leucine, an amino acid mixture, and an energy generating system (ATP, GTP, creatine phosphate and creatine kinase), hemoglobin synthesis can be measured as the rate of incorporation of leucine $C^{14}$ into protein precipitated with trichloroacetic acid.

Although this system efficiently synthesizes hemoglobin, it is unsatisfactory for studying fetal hemoglobin synthesis for the rabbit makes only adult hemoglobin. Therefore we studied hemoglobin synthesis initially in nucleated avian erythrocytes and reticulocytes from babies who received an exchange transfusion for hemolytic disease of the newborn. These cells have some capacity to synthesize adult and a fetal form of hemoglobin. A comparison with the activity of rabbit whole cells, hemolysate, 12000 x gravity supernatant fraction and the 'cell-free system-complete' is shown in table 1. The synthesis of hemoglobin in whole cells was comparable in the three species, especially when one allowed for the differences in reticulocyte and

Table 1. *Comparison of hemoglobin synthesis by whole cells and various 'cellfree' fractions prepared from avian, human and rabbit immature erythrocytes*

| Cell fraction | Rabbit | Chicken | Human |
|---|---|---|---|
| | Total Counts per minute $\times$ $10^3$ | | |
| Whole cells | 19000 | 4500 | 1500 |
| Hemolysate | 3600 | 830 | 610 |
| Supernatant solution (12000 $\times$ gravity) | 4300 | 17 | 61 |
| Precipitate 12000 $\times$ gravity | 100 | 204 | 81 |
| Supernatant & precipitate (Recombined) | 3100 | 239 | 164 |
| Ribosomal system 37° (Complete) | 1400 | 19 | 5 |
| Ribosomal system 0° (Complete) | 14 | 2 | 1 |

normoblast counts. The phenylhydrazine induced hemolytic anemia of the rabbit was accompanied by almost 100 per cent reticulocytosis, the human reticulocyte counts were between six and ten per cent, and the avian erythrocyte is normally nucleated. The relative losses of activity after hemolysis were also comparable. The significant difference was in the activity of the supernatant solution after centrifugation at 12000 x gravity where both the avian and human systems had very little activity when compared with the rabbit. Since so great a loss was sustained in the preparative methods, the avian and human 'ribosomal' systems promised to be of limited value in studying hemoglobin F and A synthesis.

In the course of these studies, we were prompted to search for variations in substrate or cofactor concentrations which might affect hemoglobin synthesis. Since the heme groups lie in separate folds of the polypeptide chains, PERUTZ et al. had suggested that once the polypeptide chain is synthesized and provided with a heme group around which it can coil, it takes up its configuration spontaneously (6). Therefore we attempted to determine whether heme might be a factor limiting the synthesis of globin.

This effect of heme was studied in the rabbit 'cell-free' system. Since protoporphyrin is more soluble and has less tendency to dimerize, it was used as substrate instead of heme. Dr. F. Welland and I were able to show that the protoporphyrin and iron present in the incubation mixtures could be converted to heme, since the enzyme heme synthetase (ferrochelatase) is present in the 12000 x gravity supernatant solution. When the activity of heme synthetase was studied in various centrifugal fractions, it was found to have the same distribution as cytochrome oxidase, a known mitochondrial enzyme (fig. 3).

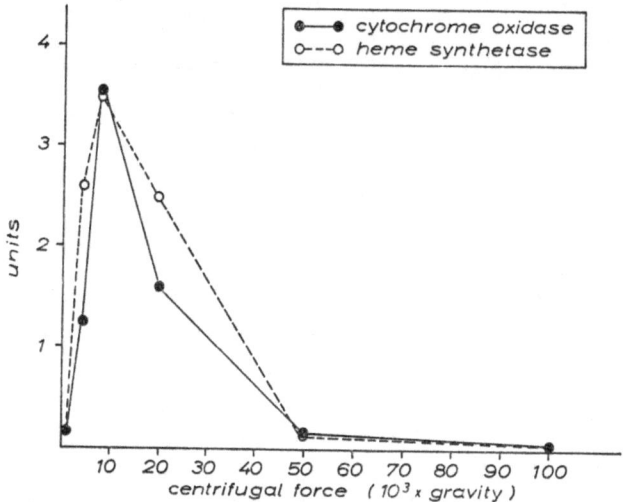

*Fig.* 3. Comparison of heme synthetase and cytochrome oxidase activity in various centrifugal fractions from a rabbit hemolysate.

Protoporphyrin and/or heme stimulated globin synthesis. This effect was most evident when it was studied at various final magnesium concentrations (fig. 4). When the concentration of magnesium was low at the end of the incubation i.e. at the trichloroacetic acid precipitation step in the assay, the protoporphyrin caused an increase in the radioactivity of the soluble protein, suggesting that the release

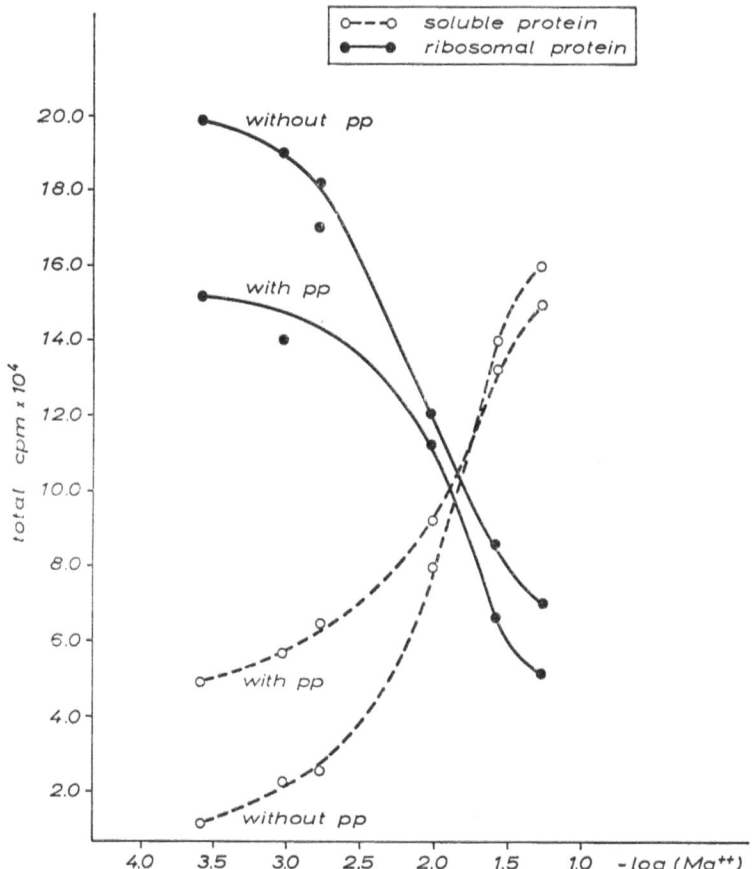

*Fig.* 4. The effect of added protoporphyrin on globin synthesis at various final magnesium concentrations in a rabbit 'ribosomal' system.

of protein from the ribosomes had been augmented. At high magnesium concentrations the ribosomes were probably stripped of partially synthesized polypeptide chains and the effect of protoporphyrin was obliterated. The increase in soluble protein was maximal at a protoporphyrin concentration of $3.2 \times 10^{-5}$ M (7). It was interesting that this concentration was similar to the protoporphyrin concentration, $5 \times 10^{-5}$ M, which was optimal for the enzymic synthesis of heme and the formation of hemoglobin from iron, protoporphyrin and globin (8).

In order to determine whether hemoglobin or a highly labeled non-hemoglobin protein was being formed, the soluble protein from an incubation mixture was chromatographed on Amberlite IRC-50 (9). Aliquots which contained protein were then assayed for radioactivity (fig. 5). When protoporphyrin was added, 67 per cent of the radio-activity was present in the major hemoglobin fraction. When the radio-activity was compared with the hemoglobin fraction of the control, there was a 36 per cent increase in the formation of soluble hemo-globin. The chromatographic fraction which contained non-hemo-globin proteins and minor hemoglobins had 33 per cent of the radio-activity. Whether this fraction contained a globin subunit or a highly labeled globin intermediate as well requires further elucidation.

These studies suggest that heme may play a regulatory role in the synthesis of hemoglobin by augmenting the release of polypeptide chains from the ribosomes. Several observations have been made recently on the possible role of heme in the regulation of hemoglobin synthesis and indicate several different mechanisms. In iron deficient rabbit reticulocytes, the stimulation of globin synthesis was accom-panied by an increase in the specific activity of both the ribosomal protein and the soluble protein (10). Furthermore, the size and pro-portion of polyribosomes was increased (11), apparently stabilizing them in a synthetically active form (12). Studies on the rate of poly-peptide chain synthesis in rabbit reticulocytes (13) and human bone marrow (14) indicated that the individual globin chains were synthe-sized at a relatively fast initial rate and after reaching a control point were formed at a second slower rate (15).

It was suggested that heme insertion might act as the control point (14) and that a coordinated control between heme and globin syn-thesis might exist (10). Such a control probably regulates the synthesis of the heme moiety and apoenzyme of tryptophane pyrrolase (16). In a 'cell-free' system of pigeon erythrocyte nuclei, the coordinated synthesis of heme and globin may in turn be regulated by the demand for oxygen. It was found that the inhibition of globin synthesis by oxygen could be overcome with heme (17).

There is very little knowledge about how the organization of sub-

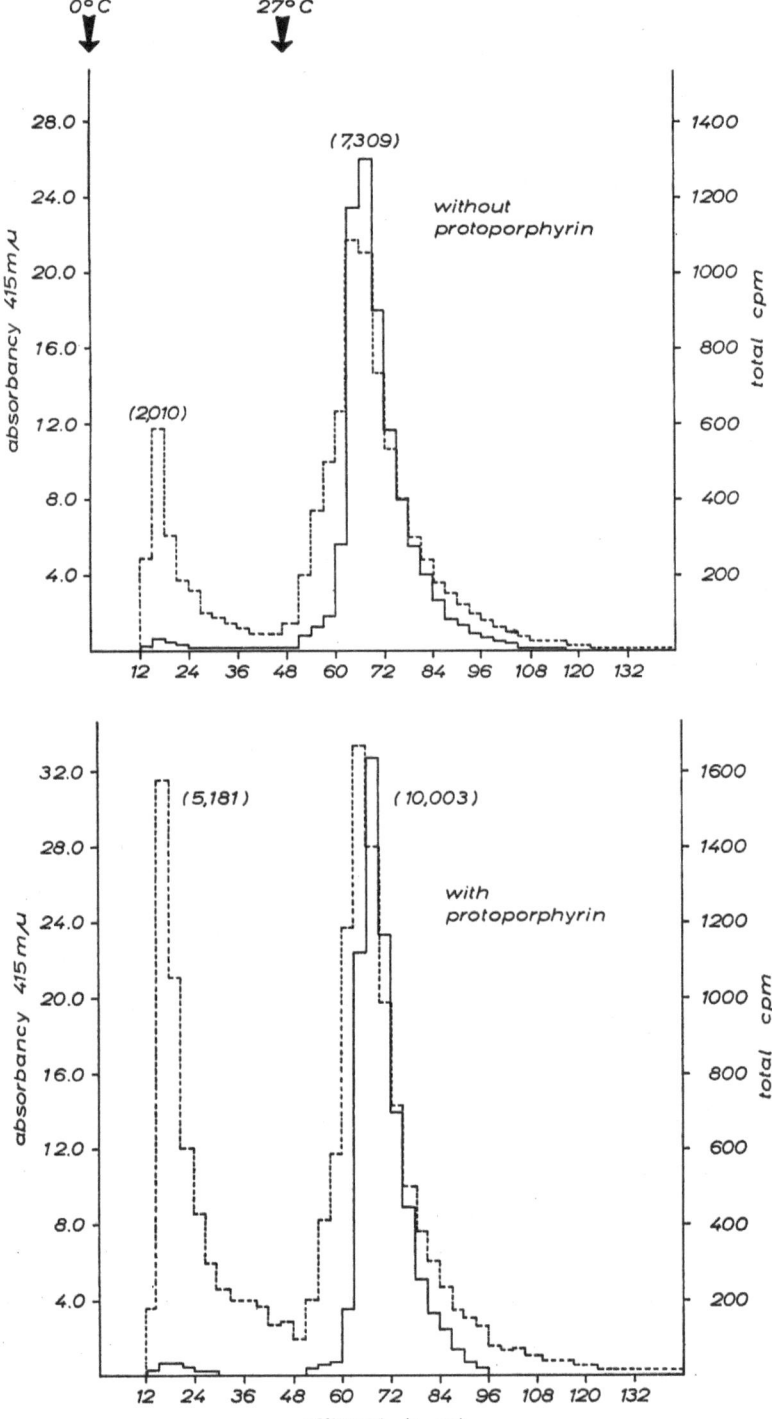

*Fig.* 5. Comparison of the radioactivity and hemoglobin concentration in the chromatographically separated soluble protein from a rabbit 'ribosomal' system.

cellular particles relates to the control of hemoglobin synthesis. Heme is synthesized from iron and protoporphyrin in the mitochondria and must be assembled with the newly synthesized polypeptide chains of the ribosomes. If the synthesis of heme and globin are under reciprocal control, then the localization of the heme synthetase (ferrochelatase) system in the mitochondria may be critical. The mitochondrial localization of delta-aminolevulinic acid synthetase, the rate limiting enzyme in heme synthesis may have similar significance.

It has been suggested that in Rhodopseudomonas spheroides two different enzyme pathways for the synthesis of the heme moiety of chlorophyll and that of the other hemoproteins may exist (18). It has been similarly proposed that separate pools and/or pathways may exist for the heme synthesized for alpha, beta and gamma chains, since in a splenectomized patient with beta-thalassaemia, the specific activities of heme and globin of hemoglobin F were consistently higher than those of hemoglobin A after the administration of glycine-2-$C^{14}$ (19).

It would appear that although hemoglobin synthesis may be regulated like other proteins at the gene level, the messenger RNA level and/or the polyribosome level, unlike most proteins, its heme moiety may also play a regulatory role. One might ask to what aspect of dysmaturity do these speculations on the control of hemoglobin refer? It is possible, that the well studied fetal protein, hemoglobin F, could serve in part as a model for developmental changes in other proteins; especially since the synthesis of type II hexokinase appears to be related to that of the gamma chain of hemoglobin F in dysmature and normal infants and adults with hereditary persistence of fetal hemoglobin (20, 21).

## REFERENCES

1. JONXIS, J. H. P. (1966) In: *Advances in Pediatrics*, Vol. XIV, Year Book Medical Publishers Inc., Chicago, Ill., p. 91.
2. BAGLIONI, C. (1966) *J. Cell. Physiol.* 67, sup. 1, 169.
3. HUENNS, E. R., F. HECHT, J. V. KEIL and A. G. MOTULSKY (1964) *Proc. Natl. Acad. Sci. U.S.* 51: 89.
4. WATSON, J. D. (1965) *Molecular Biology of the Gene*, Benjamin Inc., New York, N.Y., p. 390—414.
5. SCHWEET, R., H. LAMFROM and E. ALLEN (1958) *Proc. Natl. Acad. Sci. U.S.* 44: 1029.

6. PERUTZ, M. F., M. G. ROSSMANN, A. F. CULLIS, H. MUIRHEAD, G. WILL and A. C. T. NORTH (1960) *Nature* 185: 416.
7. GRIBBLE, T. J. and H. C. SCHWARTZ (1965) *Biochim. Biophys. Acta* 103: 333.
8. SCHWARTZ, H. C., R. GOUDSMIT, R. L. HILL, G. E. CARTWRIGHT and M. M. WINTROBE (1961) *J. Clin. Invest.* 40: 188.
9. ALLEN, D. W., W. A. SCHROEDER and J. BALOG (1958) *J. Amer. Chem. Soc.* 80: 1628.
10. LONDON, I. M., G. P. BRUNS and D. KARIBIAN (1964) *Medicin* 43: 789.
11. GRAYZEL, A. I., P. HÖRCHNER and I. M. LONDON (1966) *Proc. Natl. Acad. Sci. U.S.* 55: 650.
12. WAXMAN, H. S. and M. RABINOVITZ (1965) *Fed. Proc.* 24: 838.
13. NAUGHTON, M. A. and H. M. DINTZIS (1962) *Proc. Natl. Acad. Sci. U.S.* 48: 1822.
14. WINSLOW, R. M. and V. M. INGRAM (1965) *J. Biol. Chem.* 241: 1144.
15. ENGLANDER, S. W. and L. A. PAGE (1965) *Biochem. Biophys. Res. Commun.* 19: 565.
16. MARVER, H. S., D. P. TSCHUDY, M. G. PERLROTH and A. COLLINS (1966) *Science* 154: 501.
17. HAMMEL, C. L. and S. P. BESSMAN (1966) *Science* 152: 1080.
18. LASCELLES, J. (1966) *Biochem. J.* 100: 184.
19. KREIMER-BIRNBAUM, M. and R. B. BANNERMAN (1967) *Science* 155: 1116.
20. SJOSTEDT, S., G. ENGLESON and G. ROOTH (1958) *Arch. Dis. Child.* 33: 123.
21. HOLMES, E. W. Jr., J. I. MALONE, A. I. WINEGRAD and F. A. OSKI (1967) *Science* 156: 646.

# DEVELOPMENTAL CHANGES IN LIVER ENZYME ACTIVITIES WITH SPECIAL REFERENCE TO THE PERINATAL PERIOD OF LIFE

FABIO SERENI AND BENEDETTA LUPPIS*

INTRODUCTION

The rapid passage from intrauterine to extra-uterine life involves the performance by the liver of mammals of a series of new metabolic functions which are essential to accomplish the main goal to mantain homeostasis and to supply the peripheral tissues with optimal amounts of substances which are needed for life and growth.

In relationship to these new and very important duties the liver of all mammal fetuses till now studied undergo in the late part of gestation and in the first period of extra-uterine life very sharp histologic and metabolic modifications.

DAWKINS has written a rather comprehensive review on various aspects of fetus and newborn liver biochemistry (1). Our purpose is to recall some of the main topics of this chapter of developmental biochemistry discussing in more detail both those aspects which seem to us of primary importance and those problems to solve which, in recent years, we tried to give a contribution with our own experimental work.

Following these premises this paper will deal primarily with some aspects of liver nucleic acid and protein synthesis and metabolism during the perinatal period of life. Some of the most important recent acquisitions on carbohydrate and lipid metabolism will also be discussed.

* The Pediatric Department of the Milano University, Milano, Italy.
This work was supported by grants from the National Institute for Child Health and Human Development (HD 01895) and from the Association for the Aid of Crippled Children, New York, U.S.A.

PECULIARITIES OF NUCLEIC ACIDS AND PROTEIN SYNTHESIS
IN FETUS AND NEWBORN LIVER

The rate of nucleic acid and protein synthesis and catabolism by liver tissue undergo very sharp variations in fetus and newborn animals at certain critical periods of development. In the following paragraphs some of these variations will be discussed in some detail, specially emphasizing the importance of birth determining some very striking modifications of liver cell function.

*Synthesis and breakdown of nucleic acids in fetus and newborn liver*

From a very general point of view it can be stated that in the fetal liver, which rapidly increases in size during the second half of the gestation period, most of the more important enzyme activities which are involved in the synthesis of nucleotides and of nucleic acids are very active, whereas those which catalize nucleic acid breakdown are low.

More in detail aspartate transcarbamylase (2), deoxycytidylate deaminase (3) and thymidilate kinase (4) were all found very high in the liver of the fetus rat, whereas in the same tissue thymidine and uridine phosphorylase (5) and the overall rate of thymidine and uracil catabolism (6) were found to be very much reduced in early stages of development.

KRETCHMER and coworkers (7) recently investigated the efficiency of pyrimidine synthesis in rat fetal tissues, namely in liver and heart, evaluating the conversion of radioactive precursors in many intermediates till uridine-mono-phosphate (UMP). From their data the following main conclusions, as far as the liver is concerned, may be deduced:

– the synthesis of carbamyl-aspartate, starting from radio-active bicarbonate is very much reduced in fetal tissue. Since, as above mentioned, the activity of aspartate transcarbamylase is very high, a lack of activity of carbamyl-phosphate synthetase is therefore postulated;

– carbamylaspartate is efficiently converted to orotate, and orotate to UMP.

It seems therefore that the fetal liver has most of the enzyme activities which are needed for the 'de novo' synthesis of pyrimidine nucleotides, even if the in vitro conversion of orotic acid to UMP is almost completely dependent from an optimal exogenous supply of high energy bond phosphates (5-phosphoribosyl-pyrophosphate — PRPP).

Much more difficult appears to be an evaluation of the in vivo rate of liver RNA and DNA synthesis in the fetus and newborn animal. BRESNICK et al. (8) had the opportunity to investigate the fate of labeled orotate injected either in the pregnant rat or in the amniotic sac of 16—18 days old fetuses (the pregnancy lasts in rats 22 days). Their results may be interpreted as an index of a relatively low in vivo conversion of orotate to UMP by the fetal liver; the latter compound was however very well incorporated into RNA, suggesting at this period of intrauterine life a fairly high liver RNA synthesis activity.

In agreement with these results, interesting data were published few years ago by STEVENS (9) on nucleotide distribution in fetal rat liver. These data show a relatively small concentration of UMP, whereas no significant differences were found for other nucleotides.

Furthermore the rate of liver DNA synthesis, measured as the in vitro thymidine incorporation into deoxyribonucleic acid, was also found much higher in rat liver from fetuses than from adult animals (5)

It appears from many experimental data that shortly after birth liver nucleic acid synthesis and catabolism undergo sharp quantitative modifications. In recent years our group in Milano was actively engaged in investigating some aspects of liver RNA synthesis and metabolism during the perinatal periode of life (10, 11).

The rate of RNA synthesis was evaluated by two different techniques, i.e. measuring the incorporation of radioactivity from labeled precursors ($6^{-14}$ C-orotate, $2^{-14}$ C-uridine, $^{32}$P) into nuclear RNA and by determining the DNA dependent RNA polymerase activity of isolated nuclei. The rate of RNA breakdown was evaluated in nuclei and in the microsomal fraction determining both the ribonuclease activity and the autohydrolysis of endogenously labeled RNA.

Figures 1 and 2 show some of our data. They refer respectively the $6^{-14}$ C-orotate incorporation rate into the nuclear RNA of rat liver and the RNA polymerase activity of nuclei isolated from the liver of the same animal. Soon after birth a significant increase of both these parameters was found; the incorporation rate of pyrimidine precursors into nuclear RNA reaches a peak at about three days of

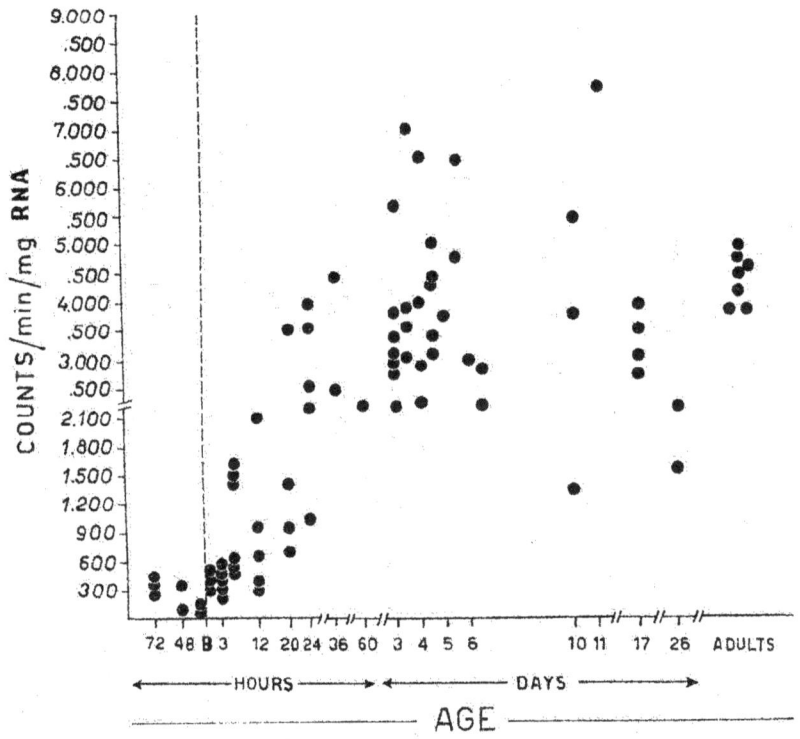

*Fig.* 1. Incorporation of radioactivity from 6⁻¹⁴ C-orotate into nuclear RNA of the liver of fetus, newborn and adult rat (From SERENI et al. 10).

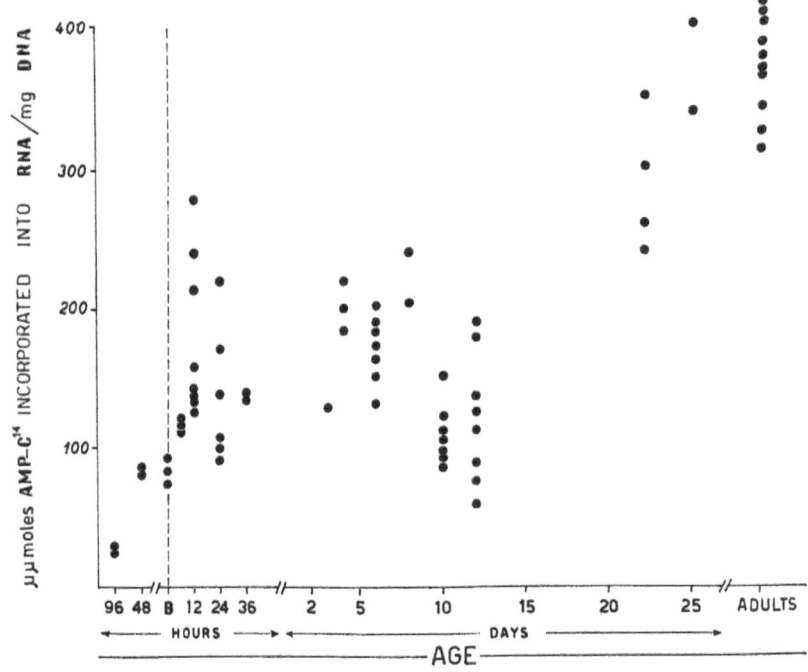

*Fig.* 2. RNA polymerase activity of isolated uuclei from liver of fetus, newborn and adult rats. (From SERENI et al. 10.

age, whereas liver RNA polymerase activity reaches the adult values only at 20—25 days of life. Conversely the rate of hydrolysis of endogenous and exogenous RNA is higher in newborn than in adult liver. However no significant variations seem to occur in this respect soon after birth.

Our observations on the role of birth activating liver RNA synthesis partially agree with two other series of data which OLIVER and BLUMER (12) and STEVENS and STOCKEN (5) recently published.

OLIVER and BLUMER (12) measured the rate of incorporation of radioactivity from 6-$^{14}$ C-orotate both in nuclear and cytoplasmic RNA and in DNA of liver cells at various periods of time after birth. A peak in the incorporation rate was obtained in every instance 1—2 days after birth; a second peak was found in livers of animals 10 days old.

From the data of STEVENS and STOCKEN (5) it clearly results that birth induces a very sharp increase of liver dehydroorotase activity, which is a key enzyme in pyrimidine synthesis, catalizing the conversion of carbamylaspartate to dehydroorotate.

*To summarize* from ours and other investigators data, it clearly results that the passage from the intrauterine to the extrauterine life is followed by a sharp activation of both liver RNA and DNA synthesis. The physiologic significance of the early activation of liver RNA synthesis is very likely to be, in our opinion, the primary event leading thereafter to a more active synthesis of many specific protein molecules. By this means the liver can accomplish the new metabolic functions related to the extrauterine life.

Two series of data must be remembered in this regard. The first one concerns the early postnatal activation of the synthesis of certain fractions of plasma proteins, as the vitamin K dependent factors, which are poorly synthetized by the fetal liver. This important chapter of biochemical development of the liver will be discussed in detail later on.

The second series of data, which very likely are closely related to the early postnatal activation of nucleic acid synthesis, are represented by the sharp increase in activity, soon after birth, of many enzyme systems of protein, carbohydrate or lipid metabolism, as well as some detoxication processes. It must be however stressed that only for some of these enzymes a dependency between postnatal increase in activity and protein synthesis activition was demonstrated by in vivo experiments.

The sharp postnatal increase of tyrosine-alpha-ketoglutarate transaminase activity may be in effect inhibited in the newborn rat both by injecting ethionine (13) and actinomycin (14). The same is true for tryptophan pyrrolase, when puromycin is injected (15). RAIHA and SUIHKONEN (16) recently demonstrated that also the postnatal increase of arginine synthetase was blocked up to 80 % in the newborn rat by puromycin injection. Finally DAWKINS has shown (17) that the increase of liver glucose-6-phosphatase activity after birth is prevented by in vivo injection of protein synthesis inhibitors.

*Recent investigations concerning the importance of hormonal factors determining the postnatal activation of RNA synthesis*

It is still unknown if humoral factors are responsible for the postnatal activation of liver enzyme and protein synthesis. The role of those hormones which are known to control adult liver RNA and protein synthesis deserve special attention. The hypothesis that adrenal cortex plays a certain role is supported by the following series of data:

– it is well known, from our (18, 19) and other investigators data (see for a complete literature review ref. 20), that glucocorticoids deeply influence liver RNA metabolism.

More in detail it has been proved that cortisone increases, both in vivo and in the isolated and perfused rat liver, the rate of RNA synthesis, by activating the DNA dependent RNA polymerase activity; moreover glucorticoids decrease the rate of hydrolysis of RNA by the microsomal fraction.

– it has been shown by us many years ago (21) that in the newborn rat adrenalectomy at birth prevents the postnatal increase of tyrosine transaminase activity. Since this developmental change very likely reflects variations in the rate of enzyme molecule synthesis (13), the obvious implication was that adrenalectomy at birth interferes with the normal protein synthesis activity of the liver.

After these first observations other authors attempted to inhibit the postnatal increase of enzyme activities by adrenalectomizing newborn animals at birth. RAIHA and SUIHKONEN (16) have shown a strong inhibition of the arginine synthetase developmental curve, whereas NEMETH (22) and DAWKINS (17) did not find the same for tryptophan pyrrolase and for glucose-6-phosphatase.

– finally the free corticosteroid plasma concentration is usually high in newborn animals at birth. HALTMEYER et al. (23) for example recently found in the rat an average free corticosterone plasma concentration of 17.4 μg % on the first day of life, being the average adult value 3.4 μg %.

We recently tried to evaluate the importance of adrenal cortex on postnatal regulation of liver RNA synthesis by two different approaches (11).

In the first series of experiments we adrenalectomized newborn rats at birth, and consequently followed the development of the rate of RNA synthesis, by measuring the rate of incorporation of 6-14 C-orotic acid into nuclear RNA: a partial, but consistent inhibition of RNA synthesis was found in adrenalectomized animals.

In the second series of experiments we tried to increase the low rate of RNA synthesis in newborn rats soon after birth by glucocorticoid injections. Neither the DNA dependent RNA polymerase activity or the 6-14 C-orotate incorporation into nuclear RNA were effected in the first few days of life.

*To conclude* it seems therefore that the adrenal cortex plays indeed a role in the postnatal activation of liver RNA and protein synthesis. It is however very likely that this is not the only or the most important humoral agent to be considered. Other limiting factors must be present to explain why exogenous corticosteroids cannot induce in the newborns an early activation of RNA synthesis.

At this purpose some very preliminary data which we obtained puite recently on hypothyroid newborn rats seem to indicate that also the thyroid gland plays a certain role on the normal development of at least some steps of nucleic acid synthesis (24).

Newborn rats were made hypothyroid by injecting [131] I to the mother at the end of the gestation and to the newborns soon after birth, following the technique described by HAMBURGH and FLEXNER (25). As it is possible to observe from the data reported in figure 3 hypofunction of thyroid gland in newborn animals results in a very significant lower incorporation of radioactivity from 6-14 C-orotate in liver nuclear RNA. However the DNA dependent RNA polymerase activity was not inhibited by hypothyroidism, suggesting therefore that the low orotic acid incorporation values may have been due to a defective synthesis of prymidine nucleotides from orotic acid.

*Liver plasma protein synthesis in the fetus and in the newborn. Qualitative and quantitative variations during development*

Deep differences can be demonstrated, in animals as well as in man, in the amount and in the characteristics of plasma proteins synthetized by the liver of the immature subjects when compared with the adult-ones. From a qualitative point of view two plasma protein fractions are well known to be present in the serum of fetus and newborn animals but not in adults. Fetuin was first described by PEDERSEN (26), about 20 years ago, in the serum of newborn calf and it was later found

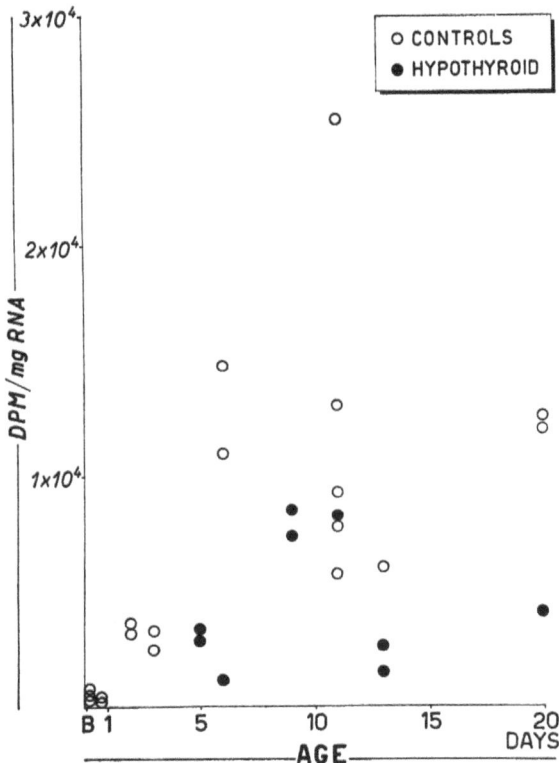

*Fig.* 3. ¹⁴C-Orotic acid incorporation into liver nuclei RNA of control and hypothyroid newborn rats.

also in the serum of other animals, as in the newborn goat and in the lamb, but not in man (27, 28). Fetuin is an acid glucoprotein, which migrates electrophoretically as an alpha globulin, and which contains glucosamine, mannose, galactose, galactosamine and sialic acid (29, 30). The presence of fetuin is largely responsible for the low albumin/ globulin ratio which is usually found in the serum of these animals in early periods of life. It gradually disappears after birth.

Postalbumin is the other specific foetal plasma protein up to now described. It was found in man (31), in the mouse (32) and in the rat (33): in man it disappears from serum after the fourth month of intrauterine life, whereas in the mouse and in the rat is it still present, although in minor concentrations, at birth. WISE and OLIVER (34) very recently demonstrated in the rat that the site of synthesis of postalbumin is the liver; furthermore KIRSCH et al. (35) have clearly shown that this plasma protein is both physicochemically and immunologically different from albumin. The sharp decrease of postalbumin in the rat serum after birth parallels the disappearance of hemopoietic tissue from the liver; the authors therefore put forward the hypothesis that this protein fraction may be synthetized by hemopoietic and not by liver parenchymous cells.

Although the synthesis of fetuin and of postalbumin is characteristic of immature liver tissue, no rapid switch-off of the synthesis of these molecules was shown at any critical period of life. In addition nothing is known of the mechanisms which regulate their rate of synthesis.

Few investigations were performed on the quantitative aspect of plasma protein synthesis by the liver of fetus and newborn animals. Some very significant data concern the rate of synthesis of albumin and of a certain number of protein clotting factors.

The rate of albumin production by rat liver slices is about equal in the fetus at term and in the adult; however it more or less doubles during the first five days of extrauterine life (36). This activation in liver albumin synthesis may very well account for the increase in concentration of serum albumin which is usually found after birth.

Much more is known of the rate of liver synthesis before and after birth of a series of specific proteins which play an important role in the clotting process. It is well established, since a long period of time, that the plasma concentration of many clotting factors is lower at birth than in later periods of life. This is true both for man (37) and for many other newborn animals (38). More specifically in man a deficiency in factors II, VII, IX and X was repeatedly demonstrated, while in newborn animals sofar studied, besides factors II, VII, IX and X, also factor V was found to be low in plasma.

The finding of a relatively low concentration of certain protein molecules in plasma does not necessarily mean that their rate of synthesis is also low. This is particularly true for protein clotting factors which biological half life is short. However in vitro experiments reported by GRODSKY et al. (39) indicate very clearly that at least for factor VII exists an impaired capacity of immature liver tissue to synthetize the protein molecule.

Still very open to discussion appears to be the problem of the intimate mechanism by which shortly after birth, in all newborn mammals till now studied, an increased rate of liver synthesis of deficient plasma clotting factors occurs. This phenomenon is apparently related at least in part with birth, since a significant, even less marked postnatal rise in plasma concentration of factors II and VII may be observed also in premature infants (37). It seems unlikely that a condition of vitamin K deficiency may account for low plasma concentration of clotting factors observed at birth in newborn animals, and, moreover, that vitamin K may be involved in the postnatal rise of these factors. As a matter of fact, also by administering large doses of vitamin K it is not possible to raise the low plasma concentration of factor II and factor VII in the very early periods of life to the adult value (40—43).

In contrast with previous reports (44) it seems now sufficiently proved that vitamin K acts at a level of protein synthesis which is subsequent to the formation of a specific messenger RNA but prior to the release of the complete protein from the liver. In fact both in vivo and in the perfused rat liver actinomycin D does not block the increase of clotting factors released by the liver, whereas a sharp inhibition is obtained with puromycin or cycloexymide (45—46).

Preliminary experiments performed by MASERA et al. (47) do in effect support the hypothesis that the increase in concentration of plasma clotting factors after birth is to be considered as an event which primarily depends on the more general phenomenon of postnatal activation of liver RNA and protein synthesis.

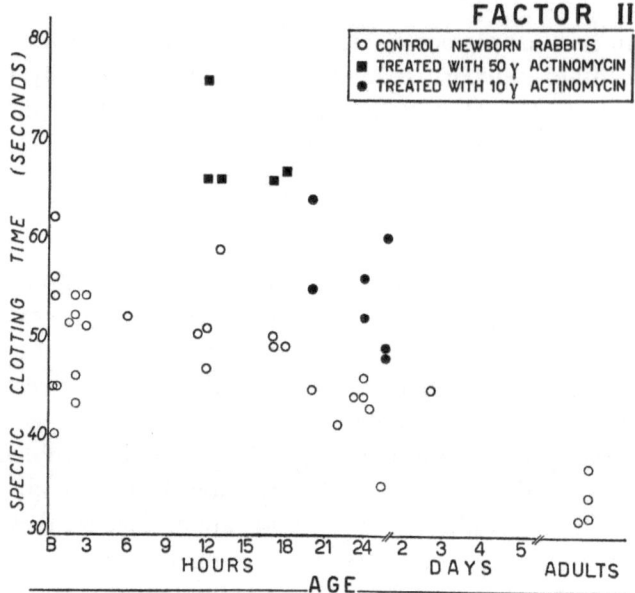

*Fig.* 4.  Influence of Actinomycin D injected at birth on the specific clotting time for factor II of plasma of newborn rabbits (from MASERA et al., 47).

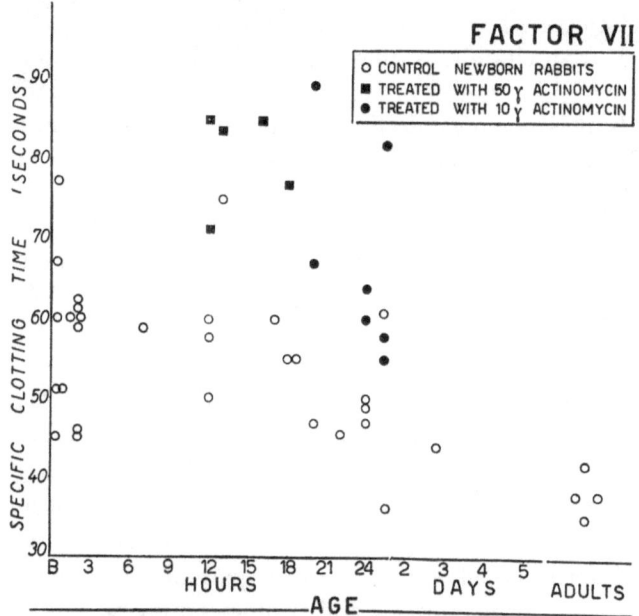

*Fig.* 5.  Influence of Actinomycin D injected ad birth on the specific clotting time for factor VII of plasma of newborn rabbits (from MASERA et al., 47).

Working on newborn rabbits we were able to establish the following points:

– The plasma concentration of both factor II and factor VI remains low during the first twelve hours of extrauterine life. A sharp increase in the concentration of these factors is usually observed starting from the twelfth hour of life; normal levels are usually reached in animals three-four days old.

– The postnatal physiologic increase in the plasma concentration of clotting factors is preceded by a very definite activation of nuclear RNA synthesis, which was evaluated by the rate of $6^{-14}$ C-orotate incorporation into RNA.

– Blocking liver RNA synthesis by in vivo administration of relatively low doses of Actinomycin D it is possible to prevent, totally or partly, the physiologic postnatal increase of both factor II and factor VII plasma concentration (figs. 4 and 5). The same strong inhibition was observed when puromycin was administered at birth.

*Additional aspects of liver protein metabolism which undergo sharp variations during the perinatal period of life*

Two series of investigations recently performed must be briefly mentioned, since both further confirm the deep influence of birth on many aspects of liver protein metabolism.

CHRISTENSEN and CLIFFORD (48) in the guinea pig studied the efficiency of amino acid transport mechanisms through cell membranes during the first 24 hours of extrauterine life. In order to evaluate this metabolic function quantitatively, they injected fetuses with cycloleucine (1-amino cyclopentane-carboxylic acid), which is a very poorly metabolized aminoacid analogue. The ratio between the intracellular and extra-cellular concentration of glycine was also measured. In both cases after 24 hours of life, the distribution ratio between liver cell water and plasma rose about two and half times. Nothing is known about the factors controlling these variations. It appears however very likely that these experiences must be considered as a further aspect of the more general phenomenon of the increase of liver protein synthesis in the immediate postnatal period of life.

The second series of data which must be mentioned at this point

## FETUSES CLOSE TO TERM

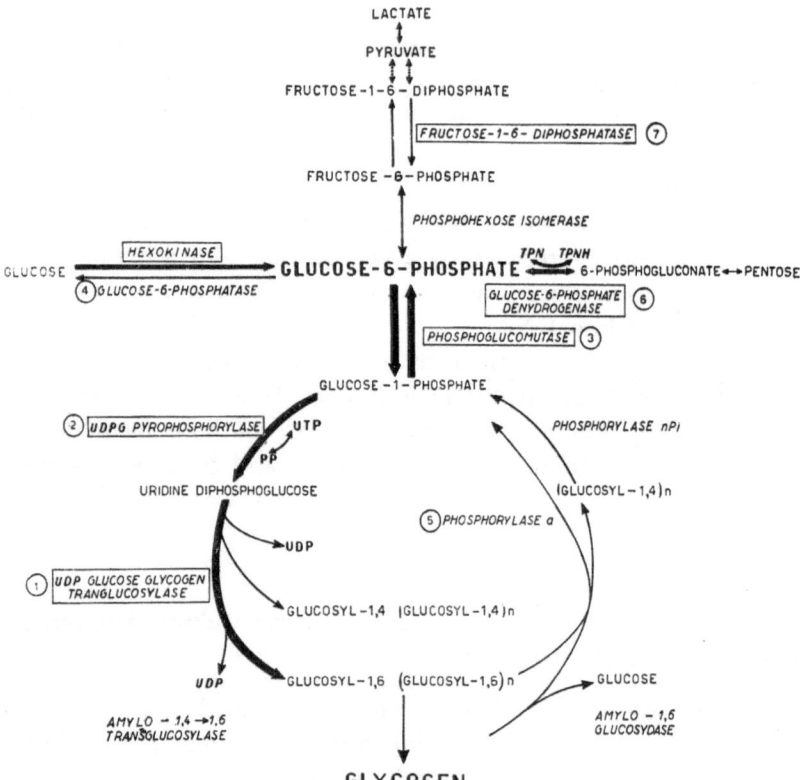

*Fig.* 6.   Scheme of glycogen metablism in the liver of fetuses close to term. Heavy lines indicate enzyme systems relatively more active at this stage of development.

concern the postnatal activation of the enzymes of urea biosynthesis. Two papers were recently published on this subject, by KRETCHMER, RAIHA et al. (7, 16) and by ILLNEROVA (49); both authors studied the activity of the various enzyme systems of the urea cycle, using different methods. The conclusions they reached were similar in some respect but differed in others. KRETCHMER, RAIHA et al. (7, 16), who reported data on rat fetuses and newborns till the seventh day of life, found that the in vitro rate of urea synthesis by liver slices increases very sharply in the first 24 hours after birth. The activity of arginine synthetase (i.e. the simultaneous evaluation of argininosuccinate synthetase and of argininosuccinase), an enzyme which controls the

## NEWBORNS AT BIRTH

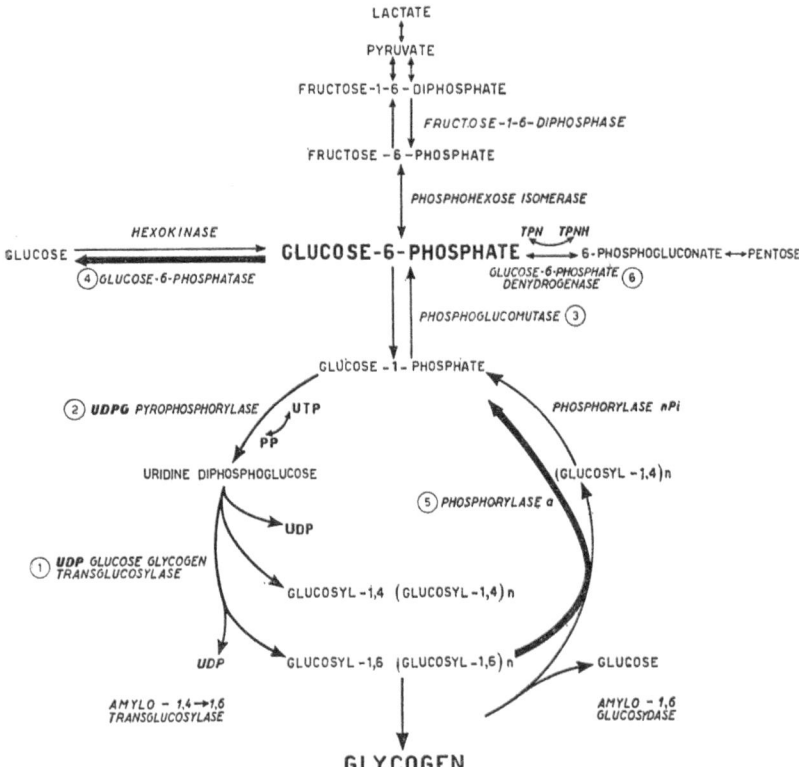

*Fig.* 7.   Scheme of glycogen metabolism in the liver of newborn mammals at birth. Heavy lines indicate enzyme systems relatively more active in this period of life.

rate of urea formation by the Krebs-Henseleit cycle, parallels very well the overall rate of in vitro urea production. ILLNEROVA (49) had the opportunity to study the postnatal period of life, from day 1 or 2 till after weaning. She observed a second period of sharp increase in liver urea formation, between day 14 and 19, i.e. just before newborns start to assume solid food. Finally it is interesting to remind that from the data of RAIHA and SUIHKONEN it results that not in all mammal species the liver urea formation capacity is very low before birth. As a matter of fact in human liver obtained from fetuses as young as 8 weeks old, the arginine synthetase activity was allready considerable; at birth it is about 40 % of the adult value, but it about doubles in the first four weeks of extrauterine life.

6

LIVER GLYCOGEN METABOLISM BEFORE AND AFTER BIRTH

It is well known for a long time that liver glycogen depots increase very sharply in fetuses during the late period of intrauterine life, whereas soon after birth a sharp decrease occurs, presumably to meet, at least in part, the metabolic requirements of the newborn prior the onset of an adequate food intake. Since this chapter of biochemical development was extensively discussed in many recent general reviews (1, 50, 51), we will not report in detail all the very important contributions which also recently were made on this subject. We will rather try to summarize some of the most important findings and to briefly mention some of the few questions still open to discussion.

The activity of most of the enzyme systems involved in glycogen metabolism varies very sharply during the late part of gestation and during the neonatal age (52, 58). It is roughly possible to state that those enzymes which play an important role on glycogen synthesis, as UDPG-glycogen transglucosylase, UDPG-pyrophosphorylase and phosphoglucomutase, are allways found very active in the liver of fetuses close to term; on the contrary the enzyme systems which have a great importance in glycogen breakdown and glucose release in the blood, as phosphorylase and glucose-6-phosphatase, become active only at term or soon after birth, These variations of enzyme activities involved in glycogen metabolism at different stages of maturity are schematically shown in figures 6 and 7.

Although these series of studies have undoubtely contributed to a better understanding of the mechanisms which determine the accumulation and the diminution of liver glycogen depots before and after birth, nevertheless many problems have still to be solved. Among them, first of all, the lack of quantitative relationship which by some respect exists between variations in tissue glycogen content and enzyme activities. This was stressed by NEMETH et al. (59) and by KORNFELD and BROWN (54); both worked on liver of fetus guinea pig, and both demonstrated that liver glycogen accumulation does not occur at a certain stage of fetal life when many important enzymes of glycogen synthesis are already active. DAWKINS, on the other hand, has pointed out (1) that the lack of activity of glucose-6-phosphatase cannot be considered, as NEMETH thought (58), as the major cause of liver glycogen accumulation in fetal life, since this enzyme activity is fairly high in some mammal species long before birth (as for example in man and in macacus rhesus).

Still not completely solved is also the problem of the precursors from which liver glycogen is preferentially formed during fetal life. The in vitro incorporation of radioactivity from labeled pyruvate in liver slices is very low through all the fetal life period, to increase very sharply soon after birth (60). This finding points against the existence during fetal life of an efficient gluconeogenesis from three-carbon compounds, and, conversely, indicates that glucose is probably the major source of fetal glycogen.

BALLARD and OLIVER (52) had in effect found in the fetus liver glycogen higher incorporation values from glucose than from pyruvate. Furthermore the fructose-1, 6-diphosphatase activity is low in the fetus andin creases only after birth (60, 61). This enzyme is essential in the conversion of pyruvate to glucose-6-phosphate.

The liver glucokinase activity is rather low in fetus and newborn rats till the age of 18 days, when it sharply increases (62). The conversion of glucose in glucose-6-phosphate is in the fetus and newborn liver probably almost completely due to an hexokinase which has a low Km for glucose (63, 64). The activity of hexokinase was found by BURCH et al. (57) rather high in the liver of fetus rats five days before term.

Finally a series of investigations by JOST, JACQUOT and KRETCHMER (56, 65) have very well demonstrated the fundamental role which the adrenal cortex and pituitary gland play on the process of fetal glycogen accumulation by the liver. The suppression of any maternal or endogenous supply of these hormones to the fetus inhibits both the formation of liver glycogen depots and the normal development of a series of enzyme activities which play a fundamental role in glycogen synthesis and metabolism.

PECULIARITIES OF LIVER LIPID METABOLISM DURING THE PERINATAL PERIOD OF LIFE

The very striking variations of lipid metabolism which occur in the mammalian liver during the perinatal period of life are much less studied than those concerning carbohydrate metabolism, but they are nevertheless equally important.

During the first period of intrauterine life, the liver of the fetus contains very scarce amounts of lipids. As gestation approaches to term FREEDMAN and NEMETH (66) have shown that total lipids, particularly triglycerides, do accumulate in significant amounts. This storage of lipids decreases very suddenly in the immediate postnatal period of life, stays low during all the suckling period, to rise again only after weaning.

These variations in liver fat content can be correlated very well with the metabolic requirements of fetus and newborn animals. Throughout intrauterine life the placenta maintains a rather constant blood glucose concentration in the fetus, and supplies therefore very well any energy need. The prepartum accumulation of triglycerides and the postpartum drop seem to have roughly the same nutritional meaning as the analogous variations in liver glycogen concentration. Both appear to contribute very efficiently to meet energy requirements of the newborn in the immediate postnatal period of life, when the very young animal does not yet take adequate amounts of food. Lipid storages increase again significantly after weaning.

A series of in vitro studies on lipogenesis and lipid catabolism on livers from fetus and newborn animals seem to substantiate this finalistic interpretation of changes in liver fat concentration before and after birth.

POPJACK (67) and VILLEE and HAGEMAN (68) allready showed many years ago a high rate of lipid synthesis, starting from acetate and from pyruvate, by the fetus liver close to term. These findings were essentially confirmed by BALLARD and HANSON (69) who very recently published a careful series of studies on changes in the rate of lipogenesis in the rat liver during development. Starting from glucose or acetate, the synthesis of both fatty acids and non saponifiable lipids was high in liver fetus close to term and dropped to negligible values shortly after birth. Throughout the suckling period the lipid synthesis remains low, increasing again only after weaning. When the non saponifiable lipids were analyzed, it was found that they change very much in composition during development; fetus liver contained much higher amounts of cholesterol, whereas adult rat liver contained much more phospholipids.

The same authors also investigated the activity of four enzyme systems which are considered to play a key role in liver lipogenesis.

While NAD-malate dehydrogenase and isocitrate dehydrogenase developmental changes did not bear any relationship to the rate of lipidogenesis found in liver, changes in ATP-citrate lyase closely followed the age dependent changes in liver lipogenesis. Finally the liver NADP-malate dehydrogenase activity was found to be negligible in the fetus at term, when lipogenesis is very active.

The authors interpretation of these data is that the generation of NADPH by the coupling of NAD and NADP-malate dehydrogenase is not appreciably present in fetal liver, as it is accepted to be in adult liver and adipose tissues.

The very noteworthy accumulation of tryglycerides (and cholesterol) in the liver of the fetus in the late part of gestation appears to be a phenomenon synchronous with the fat deposition in adipose tissue during the same period of time.

Not very much is yet known on free fatty acid metabolism by liver tissue before and after birth. The most significant series of investigations are probably those performed by DRAHOTA et al. (70) on the rat. These authors studied the aceto-acetate production by liver slices from newborn and adult rats, with or without the addition of either palmitate or acetate to the medium. The production of ketone bodies both from endogenous or exogenous lipids was found to be rather low at birth, increasing very sharply immediately afterwards. A parallel increase in aceto-acetate blood concentration was reported. Liver ketogenesis decreased to rather low values after weaning, if rats were fed with a normal diet. High fat diets on the contrary were effective mantaining high rates of liver fatty acid catabolism.

When these data on fatty acid catabolism are considered together with those previously reported on liver lipogenesis, a still incomplete, but we think reasonable. scheme on liver lipid metabolism during the perinatal period of life may be deducted. This scheme is reported in table 1.

Table 1. *Lipid metabolism by the liver at various stages of development*

| Maturity stage | Tissue lipid storage | Rate of lipogenesis (from glucose, aceta- te, pyruvate) | FFA oxidation |
|---|---|---|---|
| Early fetal life | Low | Low | Low |
| Late fetal life | Increases, especially triglycerides | High | Low |
| Shortly after birth | Drops | Decreases | High |
| Suckling period | Low | Low | Still high |
| After weaning | Increases again | Increases again | Low at a normal diet |

## SOME OTHER RELEVANT CHANGES OF LIVER ENZYME ACTIVITIES DURING THE PERINATAL PERIOD OF LIFE

Beside those discussed in the previous chapters, many other liver enzyme activities undergo sharp variations during the perinatal period of life. A complete list of them is far beyond the limits of this paper. We would like however briefly to mention the two following important aspects:

– The rate of in vitro respiration of liver slices falls, at least in the rat, very significantly in the last period of gestation, to rise again in the first 24 hours of extrauterine life (71). The activity of many oxidative enzymes were studied in the liver of most of the laboratory animals during the perinatal period of life. A general trend of postnatal rise was usually observed, even if marked differences between animal species were noted (1).

– With the noteworthy exception of sulphation, which is high in the fetus liver (72), all the other known liver conjugation activities, on exogenous or endogenous substrates, are low in the fetus at term and rise significantly soon after birth. This was found in all mammal species, and regards either conjugations with glycine or glucuronic acid, or acetylation (73, 74). The activity of many microsomal oxidative enzymes, which are responsible for the rate of inactivation of many drugs, also rises soon after birth (75). The practical implications of these findings in the field of developmental pharmacology is obviously very great, but their discussion is out of the purposes of this paper.

## CONCLUSIONS

We have purposely limited the topics discussed in this paper to a relatively small number, choosing those problems which seemed to us of major importance, more recently investigated and, may be, also less well known by pediatricians.

From an overall evaluation of the data at our disposal, the general consideration may be deduced that we have already reached a fairly good knowledge of the degree of activity of most of the main metabolic pathways, in relationship to the age or to the stage of maturity of the fetus and the newborn. This is especially true for the more commonly studied laboratory animals. Much less known are on the contrary the humoral or cellular factors which eventually play a role in determining the developmental variations in activity of the enzyme systems.

Most of the investigations that we have discussed were conducted on experimental animals; it appears obvious that the single obser- vations and their results cannot be transferred to humans in any case and without adequate controls, specially because the very diffe- rent maturity stage that any mammal reaches at birth. In addition in some newborn animals (for example in the rat) the presence of large amounts of hemopoietic tissue, in liver tissue at birth and its rapid disappearance in the first few days of extrauterine life, hampers the exact interpretation of the data in terms of liver parenchymous cell function.

Notwithstanding these limitations, we think that it is reasonable to state that some very fundamental biologic events influence the liver metabolism in the same direction in different animals. This was found for example as far as the influence of birth in regard of some aspects of glycogen and lipid metabolism, and of nucleic acid and protein synthesis is concerned.

In conclusion we think that the chapter of biochemical development we have discussed seems to be a very fruitful one in contributing to a better understanding of the physiology of growth and of the biochemical aspects of the neonatal age. It this is true, as we believe, its importance for the progress of modern pediatrics does not need to be furthermore stressed.

## REFERENCES

1. DAWKINS, M. J. R. (1966) *Brit. Med. Bull.* 22: 27.
2. NORDMANN, Y., R. HURWITZ and N. N. KRETCHMER (1964) *Nature* 201: 616.
3. MALEY, G. F. and F. MALEY (1959) *J. Biol. Chem.* 234: 2975.
4. HIATT, H. H. and T. B. BOJARSKY (1960) *Biochem. Biophys. Res. Comm.* 2: 35.
5. STEVENS, L. and L. A. STOCKEN (1963) *Biochem. J.* 87: 12.
6. STEVENS, L. and L. A. STOCKEN (1960) *Biochem. Biophys. Res. Comm.* 3: 155.
7. KRETCHMER, N., R. HURWITZ and N. RAIHA (1966) In: *Development of metabolism as related to nutrition*, HAHN, P. and O. KOLDOVSKY eds., S. Karger, Basel, p. 187.
8. BRESNICK, E., K. LANCLOS and E. GONZALES (1965) *Biochem. Biophys. Acta* 108: 586.
9. STEVENS, L. (1962) *Comp. Biochem. Physiol.* 6: 129.
10. SERENI, F., L. PICENI SERENI, V. TOMASI and O. BARNABEI (1967) *Arch. Biochem. Biophys.* 121 : 251.
11. SERENI, F. and O. BARNABEI (1967) In: *Advances in enzyme regulation*, G. WEBER ed., Pergamon Press, 5 : 165.
12. OLIVER, I. T. and W. F. C. BLUMER (1964) *Biochem. J.* 91: 549.
13. KENNEY, F. T. (1963) In: *Advances in enzyme regulation*, G. WEBER ed., Pergamon Press, 1: 137.
14. GREENGARD, O. (1963) In: *Advances in enzyme regulation*, G. WEBER ed., Pergamon Press, 1: 16.
15. NEMETH, A. M. (1963) In: *Advances in enzyme regulation*, G. WEBER ed., Pergamon Press, 1: 57.
16. RAIHA, N. C. R. and J. SUIHKONEN (1966) In: *Proceedings 36th Ann. Meet. Soc. Ped. Res.*, Atlantic City, 1966.
17. DAWKINS, M. J. R. (1963) *Ann. New York Acad. Sci.* 111: 203.
18. BARNABEI, O. and F. SERENI (1964) *Biochim. Biophys. Acta* 91: 239.
19. BARNABEI, O., B. ROMANO, G. DI BITONTO, V. TOMASI and F. SERENI (1966) *Arch. Biochem. Biophys.* 113: 478.
20. TATA, J. R. (1966) In: *Progress in Nucleic Acid Research and Molecular Biology*, DAVIDSON J. N. and W. E. COHN eds., Academic Press, 5: 191.
21. SERENI, F., F. T. KENNEY and N. KRETCHMER (1959) *J. Biol. Chem.* 234: 609.
22. NEMETH, A. M. (1963) *Ann. New York Acad. Sci.* 111: 199.
23. HALTMEYER, G. C., V. H. DENENBERG, J. THATCHER and M. X. ZARROW (1966) *Nature* 211: 1371.
24. PICENI SERENI, L., N. PRINCIPI and F. SERENI. Unpublished data.
25. HAMBURGH, M. and L. B. FLEXNER (1957) *J. Neurochem.* 1: 279.
26. PEDERSEN, K. O. (1944) *Nature* 154: 575.
27. BARBORIAK, J. J., G. DE BELLA, L. SETNIKAR and W. A. KREHL (1958) *Amer. J. Physiol.* 193: 89.
28. CHARLWOOD, P. A. and A. THOMSON (1948) *Nature* 161: 59.
29. DEUTSCH, H. F. (1954) *J. Biol. Chem.* 208: 669.

30. MOORE, D. H., R. M. DU PAN and C. L. BUXTON (1949) *Am. J. Obst. Gynec.* 57: 312.
31. ANDREOLI, M. and J. ROBBINS (1962) *J. Clin. Invest.* 41: 1070.
32. PANTELOURIS, E. M. and P. A. HALE (1962) *Nature* 195: 79.
33. WISE, R. W., F. J. BALLARDAND and E. EZEKIEL (1963) *Comp. Biochem. Physiol.* 9: 23.
34. WISE, R. W. and I. T. OLIVER (1966) *Biochem. J.* 100: 330.
35. KIRSCH, J. A. W., R. W. WISE and I. T. OLIVER (1967) *Biochem. J.* 102: 763.
36. WISE, R. W. and I. T. OLIVER (1967) *Biochem. J.* 102: 760.
37. OSKI, F. A. and J. L. NAIMAN (1966) *Hematologic Problems in the Newborn*, W. B. Saunders Co., Philadelphia, Pa.
38. HATHAWAY, W. E., H. S. HATHAWAY and L. P. BELHASEN (1964) *J. Lab. & Clin. Med.* 63: 784.
39. GRODSKY, G. M., M. KROPATKIN and J. G. POOL (1960) *Amer. J. Physiol.* 199: 139.
40. FRESH, J. W., J. H. FERGUSON, C. STAMEY, F. M. MORGAN and J. H. LEWIS (1957) *Pediatrics* 19:241.
41. ABALLI, A. J., V. L. BANUS, S. DE LEMERENS and S. ROZENGVAIG (1957) *A.M.A. J. Dis. Child.* 94: 589.
42. DYGGVE, H. (1958) *Acta Paed. Scand.* 47: 251.
43. ABALLI, A. J., V. L. BANUS, S. DE LEMERENS and S. ROZENGVAIG (1959) *A.M.A. J. Dis. Child.* 97: 524.
44. OLSON, R. E. (1964) *Science* 145: 926.
45. JOHNSON, B. C., R. B. HILL, G. S. RAHOTA and R. ALDEN (1965) *Fed. Proc.* 24: 453.
46. SUTTIE, W. (1967) *Arch. Biochem. Biophys.* 118: 166.
47. MASERA, A., L. PERLETTI, L. PICENI SERENI and F. SERENI. Unpublished data.
48. CHRISTENSEN, H. N. and J. B. CLIFFORD (1963) *J. Biol. Chem.* 238: 1743.
49. ILLNEROVA, H. (1966) In: *Development of metabolism as related to nutrition*, HAHN, P. and O. KOLDOVSKY eds., S. Karger, Basel, p. 197.
50. SERENI, F. and N. PRINCIPI (1965) *Ped. Clin. North. America* 12: 515.
51. KRETCHMER, N. and R. GREENBERG (1966) *Advances in Pediatries* 14: 201.
52. BALLARD, F. J. and I. T. OLIVER (1963) *Biochim. Biophys. Acta* 71: 578.
53. DAWKINS, M. J. R. (1961) *Nature* 191: 72.
54. KORNFELD, R. and D. H. BROWN (1964) *J. Biol. Chem.* 238: 1604.
55. JACQUOT, R. L., N. KRETCHMER, K. K. TSUBOI, I. C. TAYLOR and H. McNAMARA (1961) *A.M.A. J. Dis. Child.* 102: 476.
56. JACQUOT, R. L. and N. KRETCHMER (1964) *J. Biol. Chem.* 239: 1301.
57. BURCH, H. B., O. H. LOWRY, A. M. KUHLMAN, J. SKERJANCE, E. J. DIAMANT, R. S. LOWRY and P. VON DIPPE (1963) *J. Biol. Chem.* 238: 2268.
58. NEMETH, A. M. (1954) *J. Biol. Chem.* 208: 773.
59. NEMETH, A. M., W. INSULL Jr. and L. B. FLEXNER (1954) *J. Biol. Chem.* 208: 765.
60. LEA, M. A. and D. G. WALKER (1967) *Developm. Biol.* 15: 51.
61. BALLARD, F. J. and I. T. OLIVER (1962) *Nature* 195: 498.
62. WALKER, D. G. and G. HOLLAND (1965) *Biochem. J.* 97: 845.
63. WALKER, D. G. (1963) *Biochem. Biophys. Acta* 77: 209.
64. BALLARD, F. J. and I. T. OLIVER (1964) *Biochem. J.* 90: 261.
65. JOST, A. and R. JAQUOT (1958) *Compt. Rend. Acad. Sci.* 247: 2459.
66. FRIEDMAN, A. D. and A. M. NEMETH (1961) *J. Biol. Chem.* 236: 3083.
67. POPJAK, G. (1954) *Cold Spring Harbour Symp. Quant. Biol.* 19: 200.
68. VILLEE, C. A. and D. D. HAGERMAN (1958) *Amer. J. Physiol.* 194: 457.

69. BALLARD, F. J. and R. W. HANSON (1967) *Biochem. J.* 102: 952.
70. DRAHOTA, Z., P. HAHN and F. HANOVA In: *Development of metabolism as related to nutrition*, HAHN, P. and O. KOLDOVSKY eds., S. Karger, Basel. p. 124.
71. VAN ROSSUM, G. D. V. (1963) *Biochem. Biophys. Acta* 74: 15.
72. DICZFALUSY, E. (1964) *Fed. proc.* 23: 791.
73. YAFFE, S. (1966) *Ann. Rev. Med.* 17: 213.
74. DONE, A. K. (1966) *Ann. Rev. Pharm.* 6: 189.
75. FOUTS, J. R. (1965) In: *Embryopathic Activity of Drugs.* ROBSON, J. M., F. SULLIVAN and R. L. SMITH eds., J. & A. Churchill, London, p. 43.

# DEVELOPMENT OF ENZYMES AND ABSORPTION PROCESSES IN THE SMALL INTESTINE OF HUMAN FETUS

O. KOLDOVSKÝ, A. HERINGOVÁ, V. JIRSOVÁ, J. KRAML, H. PELICHOVÁ AND J. UHER*

In this communication I would like to summarize results from our laboratory dealing with the development of various functions of the fetal human intestine. We have relatively good access to this material, since abortions are performed for different medical and social reasons according to laws valid in our country (1). Most of our material comes from fetuses between 8 and 14 weeks of pregnancy, some fetuses are older up to 20 weeks. We have studied two main problems first how and when functions of the small intestine change in the period studied.

The other group of questions was mainly evoked by other studies performed in experimental animals. We have shown in experimental animals (2) that many functions develop differently in the jejunum and ileum. Hence we have examined the human jejunum and ileum separately to see whether this striking developmental pattern existing in experimental animals could also be found during fetal life in man.

First I would like to demonstrate developmental changes of two hydrolytic enzymes — alkaline phosphatase and nonspecific esterase. You can see (fig. 1) that nonspecific esterase activity does not change but is always higher in the ileum than in the jejunum during the period studied. On the other hand alkaline phosphatase activity undergoes substantial and different changes in the jejunum and ileum. In according with the results of FOMINA (3) and DAHLQVIST and LINDBERG (4) we find a steady increase in the jejunum. Values in the ileum are the same as in the jejunum in the youngest fetuses, later a rapid increase is found. Maximal activity was observed in 14 week old fetuses, after this age ileal activity again falls (fig. 2).

* Laboratory of developmental nutrition, Inst. Physiology, Czechoslovak Ac. Sci.; Institute of Mother and Child Care; I. Inst. Medical Chemistry, Charles University and Clin. Obstetr. Gynecol, Inst. Postgraduate Schooling of Physicians. Prague.

The other group of enzymes that I would like to describe are proteolytic and peptidase activities  The next figure (fig. 3) summarizes
our results. Proteolytic activity (substrate nitrocasein, pH of estimation 7.8) increases in the jejunum very slightly without significant

## NON SPECIFIC ESTERASE

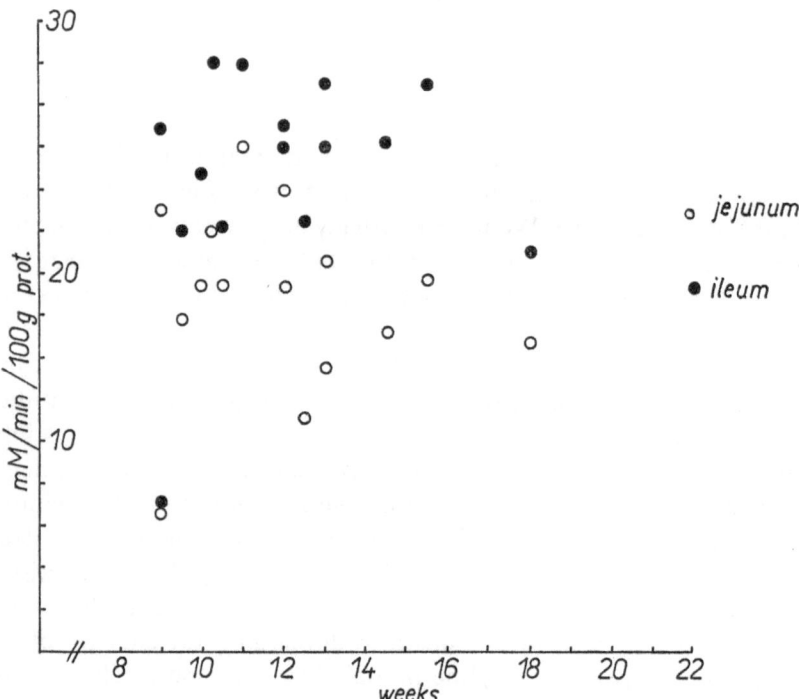

*Fig.* 1.    Nonspecific esterase in the proximal (o) and distal (•) third of the small
intestine of human fetuses. Ordinate: mMoles liberated β-naphtol per 100 g of protein
per min. Abscissa: age in postconceptional weeks. Symbols denote individual
values (PELICHOVÁ et al. 1966, ref. 11).

differences. In the ileum there is a large statistically significant increase
with age. In 9—10 and 11—12 week old fetuses there is no difference
in the activities of both parts, in the oldest fetuses significantly higher
values in the ileum than in the jejunum are found. Changes of aminopeptidase activity (substrate leucyl-β-naphtyl-amid) resemble changes
of proteolytic activity.

Tripeptidase activity (glycylglycylglycine at pH 7.8 served as
substrate) is the same in both intestinal parts and changes very little

during the period studied. Only the differences between activity in the ileum of 9—10 week old fetuses and 11—12 old fetuses is statistically significant.

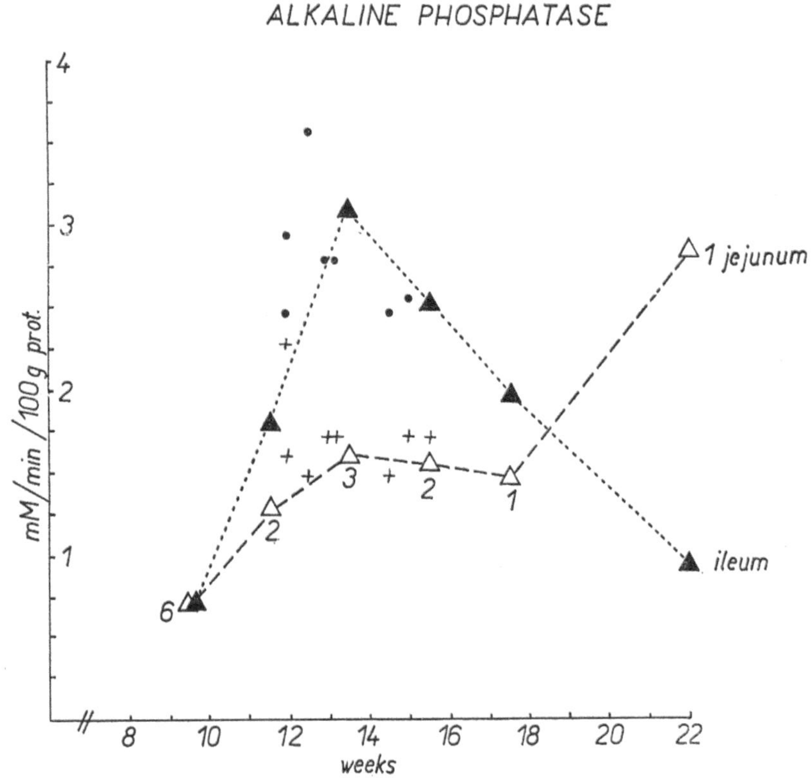

*Fig. 2.* Alkaline phosphatase activity in the supernatants of homogenates from the proximal and distal thirds of the small intestine of human fetuses. Abscissa: age in weeks after conception. Ordinate: mMoles of liberated β-napthol per min per 100 g of protein. The crosses denote individual values in the proximal third of the small intestine, the points denote individual values in the ileum, except the age group between 8,5 and 10,5 weeks where only the mean value is given. Triangles (white = proximal, black = distal third) denote the mean values of fetuses grouped according to age by two weeks. The figure at the proximal third mean value gives the number of individual determinations. The mean values are connected by lines (PELICHOVÁ et al. 1966, ref. 11).

Without attempting to comment these results at the moment I would like now to present another group of our results concerning with the development of mechanisms dealing with carbohydrates in the small intestine. First I would like — to stress again the different developmental pattern of different parts of the intestinal tract — to present a figure (fig. 4) showing changes of invertase activity in the jejunum and ileum and also in the large intestine. In agreement with findings of other laboratories (3, 5, 6) invertase activity increases in the jejunum substantially during the period studied. Up to the 12th week values in the ileum are the same in the jejunum, later activity

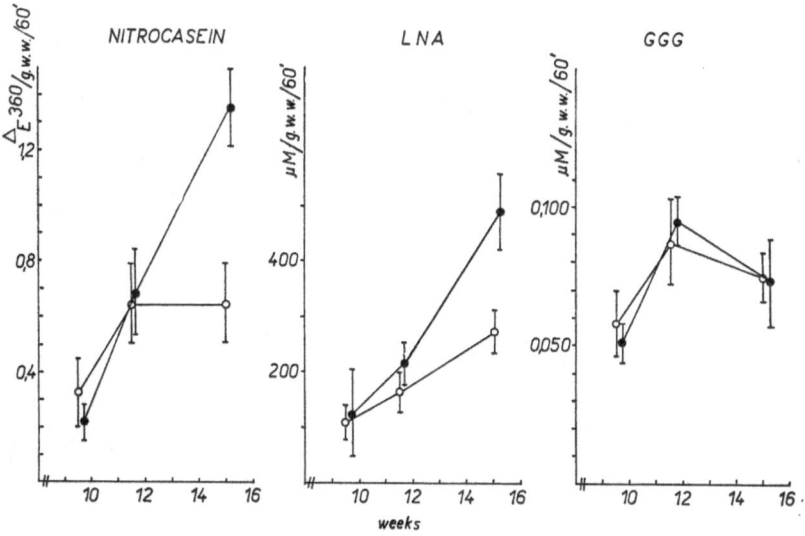

*Fig.* 3. Fetal development of proteolytic (left), aminopeptidase (middle) and tripeptidase (right) activities. Proximal half = o, distal half = ●. Ordinates:

left: $\Delta E \dfrac{360}{5\,\text{ml}}$ / g w.w. /60 min

middle: $\mu M/g$ w.w./ 60 min

right: $\mu M/$ g w.w./ 60 min

Each mean value represents 5 determinations on at least 5 cases (HERINGOVÁ et al. 1966, ref. 12).

no more increases and this leads to the appearance of the proximo-distal difference typical for adults and also for newborns, as you can see in the figure; values for the jejunum and ileum are given from material obtained surgically. Interesting is the developmental change of invertase activity in the large intestine. In agreement with findings of DAHLQVIST and LINDBERG (4) we have detected activity of invertase in the large intestine of human fetuses from 10 to 16 weeks of pregnancy. The values were the same as in the jejunum and ileum of 8 week old fetuses. This activity was found in newborn children (biopsy specimen) to be extremely low.

A developmental pattern similar to that of invertase in the jejunum and ileum is found for the absorption capacity for glucose of both

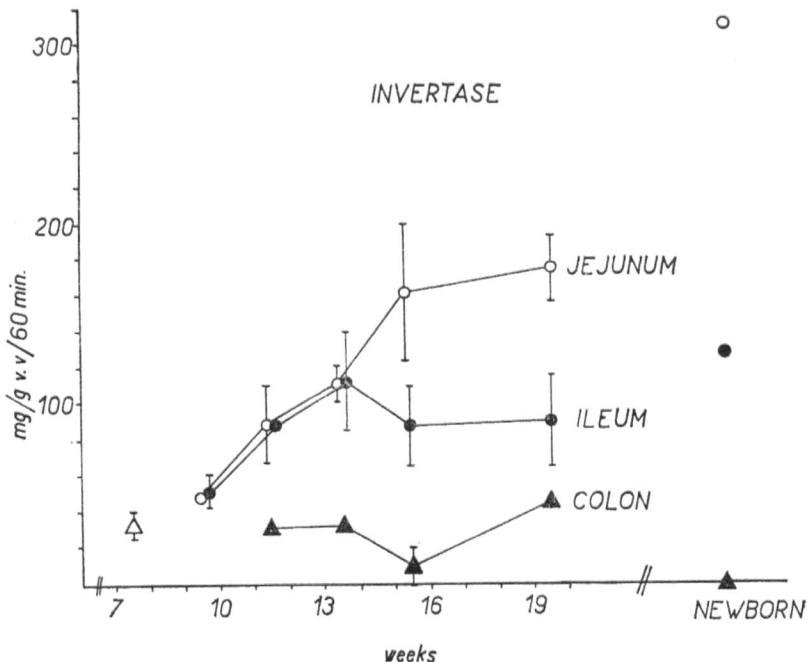

*Fig.* 4. Invertase activity of the jejunum (o), ileum (•) and colon (▲) of human fetuses of different ages. Activity is given as mg reducing substances liberated from 5.5 % sucrose solution at pH 6.25 per 60 min/g w.w. Small vertical lines denote 2 S.E. White triangle: small intestine not separated into jejunum and ileum. Data for newborns were obtained on fresh specimens from exencephalic monsters (HERINGOVÁ, JIRSOVÁ, JODL, KOLDOVSKÝ, UHER, to be published).

parts of the small intestine, using the method of everted sacs as introduced by WILSON and WISEMAN (7). In the next figure (fig. 5) you see the development of the capacity to transport glucose against a concentration gradient. In the jejunum active transport increases, in the ileum the values in the youngest fetuses are the same as in the jejunum but do not increase further. In adult animals the active transport of hexoses is accompanied by the increase of mucosal-serosal potential difference (8). We have found the same developmental pattern for this phenomenon as for glucose transport (fig. 5). Both methods thus show that the jejunum gains between the 3rd and 4th month of pregnancy a substantial capacity to absorb glucose. In adults active transport usually needs aerobic conditions; in human fetuses — as in newborn rabbits, as shown by WILSON and LIN (9) — active transport of glucose and also the glucose transfer potential difference (8) exist also in

GLUCOSE TRANSPORT

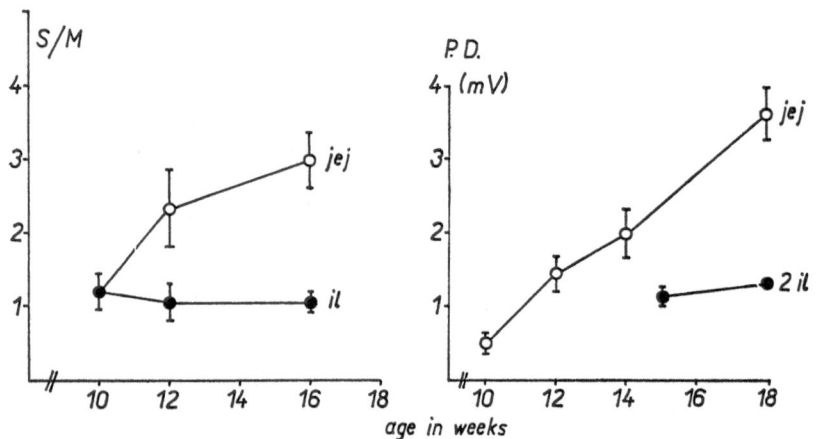

*Fig.* 5. Glucose transport in jejunum and ileum of human fetuses. Abscissa: age in postconceptional weeks. Left: S/M ratio = ratio of glucose concentration in serosal fluid to that in mucosal fluid. Right: the potential difference of glucose transfer across everted jejuna and ilea. Open circles = jejunum, black circles = ileum. Small vertical lines denote 2 S.E. (Data taken from ref. 13 and 14).

*anaerobic* conditions (fig. 6). Active transport in the jejunum using both criteria is practically the same in a nitrogen atmosphere as in an oxygen atmosphere.

The results described thus show that during the 3rd, 4th and 5th month of pregnancy different functions of the small intestine change. It is quite obvious that the jejunum differs in many respects from the ileum, this means that the formerly described special position of the ileum is not limited to experimental animals, but exists also in the human fetus.

These results are descriptive in character, but from some of them — especially the glucose transport — we can speculate also about their functional significance. I would like just to offer the following points for speculation: What is the significance of this absorption capacity? Is this absorption of glucose the goal or a means for other processes or — stated simplified — 'a training' for future function? Could we relate the increase of absorption capacity with the decrease of concentration of glucose in the amniotic fluid during pregnancy

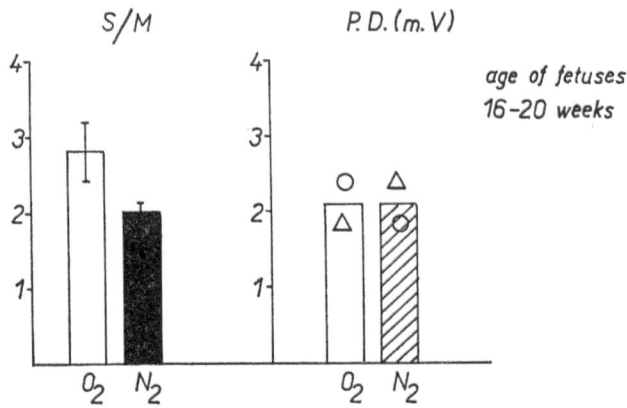

EFECT OF NITROGEN
ON GLUCOSE TRANSPORT
IN JEJUNUM

*Fig.* 6.    Effect of nitrogen on glucose transport and potential difference of glucose transfer across jejunum.
    Black column: nitrogen atmosphere, white columns: oxygen atmosphere. Left: S/M ratio. Right: potential difference in mV. Age of fetuses: 16—20 weeks. Circles resp. triangles denote individual values from corresponding fetuses. Small vertical lines = 2 S.E. (Data taken from ref. 13 and 14).

(10 and ČAPKOVÁ and JIRÁSEK — unpublished)? And from another approach: what does the presence of transport activity — usually functioning only in aerobic conditions — in anaerobic conditions mean? Do we have to think that this characteristic belongs only to the absorption process of the small intestine or could we ask whether a similar possibility exists also elsewhere — e.g. that the human fetus while going in anoxia could keep also some other functions which usually need oxygen in adults?

    The present state of our knowledge does not permit me to say anything more. The questions of factors responsible for developmental

7

changes remains open. In experimental animals we can and have studied the influence of hormonal regulation and also the effect of diet composition (for review see ref. 2). In the human fetus this is very difficult, but we have to try to find such circumstances where this also will be possible.

## SUMMARY

The paper summarizes results from the Prague laboratory dealing with the development of various functtions of the fetal human intestine.

Developmental changes of alkaline phosphatase, non specific esterase, proteolytic, aminopeptidase, tripeptidase and invertase activities are described for the jejunum and ileum separately.

Development of active glucose transport mechanism is also reported.

The results described show that during the 3rd to 5th month of pregnancy different functions of the small intestine change.

## REFERENCES

1. ČERNOCH, A. (1965) Gynaecologia 160: 293.
2. KOLDOVSKÝ, O., A. HERINGOVÁ, J. HOŠKOVÁ, V. JIRSOVÁ, R. NOACK, M. FRIEDRICH, G. SCHENK (1966) Biol. Neonat. 9: 33.
3. FOMINA, L. S. (1960) Vopr. med. Chim. 6: 176.
4. DAHLQVIST, A. and T. LINDBERG (1966) Biol. Neonat. 9: 24.
5. TACHIBANA, T. (1929) Jap. J. Obstet. Gynec. 12: 40.
6. AURICCHIO, S., A. RUBINO and G. MÜRSET (1965) Pediatrics 35: 944.
7. WILSON, T. H. and G. WISEMAN (1959) J. Physiol. 123: 116.
8. SCHACHTER, D. and J. S. BRITTEN (1961) Fed. Proc. 20: 137.
9. WILSON, T. H. and E. C. C. LIN (1960) Amer. J. Physiol. 189: 1030.
10. SCHREINER, W. E., A. BÜHLMANN and A. GUBLER (1963) Z. Geburtsh. 161: 149.
11. PELICHOVÁ, H., O. KOLDOVSKÝ, J. UHER, J. KRAML, A. HERINGOVÁ, V. JIRSOVÁ (1966) Biol. Neonat. 10: 281.
12. HERINGOVÁ, V., O. KOLDOVSKÝ, V. JIRSOVÁ, M. FRIEDRICH, R. NOACK, and G. SCHENK (1966) Gastroenterology 51: 1023.
13. JIRSOVÁ, V., O. KOLDOVSKÝ, A. HERINGOVÁ, J. HOŠKOVÁ, V. JIRSOVÁ and J. UHER (1966) Biol. Neonat. 9: 44.
14. LEVIN, R., O. KOLDOVSKÝ, V. JIRSOVÁ and J. HOŠKOVÁ (1967) Gut (in press).

# DISCUSSION

DISCUSSION PAPER DR. GRUENWALD

*Prof. Kloosterman* (in the chair): Thank you very much for this paper because of its substance and the way you brought it. I think that everybody present here will promise you not to use birthweight any more as a parameter for gestational age and that we all will know after this that dysmaturity and praematurity are two different things. I should like to defend the term dysmaturity a moment. These infants are mature, allright, but they came to maturity after starvation, therefore you could defend the word dysmaturity; moreover it is such a beautiful counterpart of praematurity.

*Dr. Papadatos:* On one of your slides you showed the growth-retardation of the liver. Is that due to decreased cellular mass or is it due to decreased glycogen content?

*Dr. Gruenwald:* Probably both. This has been studied by NAEYE. He studied the deficit in cell number versus cell size and this differs in various groups. I don't think this has completely been settled yet. There is certainly in some of them a decrease of cell size. There is definitely a difference in glycogen content, but I doubt that this can account for the entire deficit. I wonder about this myself and nobody has been able to give me the answer. May I say one more word that I forgot to mention before. Malformed infants are frequently growth-retarded. And in these cases, and this includes various types of dwarfs, such as Russel's or De Lange's, the growth potential of the foetus apparently is reduced. This is not a question of 'supplyline'. So in all studies of what you like to call dysmaturity, I think malformed infants in the widest sense should be excluded. I think the consistent thing then to say if we want to talk about something similar to dysmaturity, the term would really be dystrophy. But this term has been so mishandled in the past that I would not want to suggest it, but this would really indicate what happened. But as long as we all know what we mean it does not really matter what words are used.

*Prof. Minkowski:* Two questions. When you mentioned the twins, did you see any difference in the curves of the monozygous twins and the dizygous twins? I think there is a difference between the two curves.

*Dr. Gruenwald:* You could not tell this in the British perinatal mortality survey. In my own material I find that discordance at birth is greater in the monochorionic, but monochorionic development is a malformation and it affects perhaps one of the twins different from the other. The dissimilar monochorionic twins are a very peculiar group. We don't have tests to find out how many of the dichorionic likesex twins were monozygotic. This is rather difficult to establish.

*Prof. Minkowski:* Second question. You did not show the size or the volume of the adrenals. And as we are going to see later this is one of the organs which is functionally involved in the small-for-date infant.

*Dr. Gruenwald:* There is no significant difference. This was very disappointing to everybody. We would have expected that in chronic stress the adrenals might be large, the thymus small and all this, but it just does not come out this way. The differences are minimal and inconsistent between the groups.

*Dr. Nicolopoulos:* The thymus in one of your slides was markedly decreased in the dysmature infant. Do you have any observation about the lymphnodes and the rest of the lymphatic system, or any other studies, electrophoretic or immunological, of these infants.

*Dr. Gruenwald:* Lymphnodes, no; immune studies, no. It is likely that the colonisation of lymphocytes from the thymus to other lymphoid tissue in the human foetus probably occurs quite early. This is, as far as I know, not so in the rat and in the mouse. I wish somebody would make experiments and see if their thymus can involute and if they might show some immunologic abnormalities. Of course the thymus may produce a hormone as has been suggested, and this might even have an effect in the human.

*Dr. Wigglesworth:* I would like to ask what birthweight would come out when you extrapolate your charts.

*Dr. Gruenwald:* They get quite high. The empirical curve is about 1 standard deviation below the extrapolated at 42 weeks if we also extrapolate the standard deviation. By 44 completed weeks the extrapolated mean is 4575 grams, and only an occasional foetus grows that well. It is, of course, quite possible that different workers calculate somewhat different figures.

*Dr. Wigglesworth:* What is it at term?

*Dr. Gruenwald:* At term it is slightly higher than empirical, 3675 g. The difference at term is small, but it grows bigger each week.

*Dr. Wigglesworth:* Have you made any studies about the pattern of variation around your mean in the post-mature infants?

*Dr. Gruenwald:* The birthweight, yes. The spread of birthweight is somewhat wider in the post-term than in the full-term infant which you would expect because some foetuses still grow, some have begun to lose weight, others have just slowed down and this can be demonstrated.

*Dr. Loeb:* We have seen that the curves for the newborn infant are very different, for instance depending on the economical situation and probably on the racial situation also. I think in your groups you have children from different origins and you always put them on the same curve, let us say on the same standard curve, to determine if they are two standard deviations below the mean curve or not. We have a very great difficulty in our country because, as you probably know, we have got recently many Spanish workers and so we have a lot of Spanish children, and I am not sure that our standard curves for Belgian children are valuable for the Spanish children. We also have a lot of children now from North-Africa and I want to know what to do with all those children.

*Dr. Gruenwald:* This is a very appropriate question. You have to choose your standards depending on your purpose. If you want to see how one particular group makes out obstetrically and as newborns under existing and at the moment unalterable circumstances, then you should have standards based on that particular population. If, on the other hand, you are interested in differences associated with socio-economic status, racial properties and so on, affecting large groups, then you should use high standards. These might be Swedish, or the extrapolated growth curve. The latter two may differ from the local ones above 36 to 38 weeks, and from each other above 42 weeks.

I would say that if you are interested just in the performance of your clinicians, you should develop your own growth-curves for all your people or for each of these groups separately. Of course this a great difficulty we have in the United States, we have our Puerto Rican people and we have a lot of groups that differ both in their etnic background and in their socio-economic status. Unfortunately there is a lot of association of the two. Socio-economic status will not immediately affect foetal growth to the full extent. It will take two or three generations, because a mother who herself is stunted in growth and did not realize her growth potential, is also quantitatively not a good reproducer. One can feed her as well and give her as good medical care as possible, but she still can have small babies as you saw in my graphs on maternal height. These differences in maternal height are most likely socio-economic. Her children now will be larger when they grow up, and will have larger children again, and so on. The standards you use and I think you have to have the courage of your conviction, should be the standards that are appropriate to the question that you are asking.

*Prof. R. Schwartz:* I like to ask Dr. GRUENWALD again a question that I asked him the other morning, and that is whether he should not comment on another extrapolation and that is what you might call the supermature infant. It is interesting that when one looks at obstetrical patients with reference to their carbohydrate tolerance, one is amazed to find a significant number of previously undetected, I would call them gestational, diabetics whom we know have infants that are somewhat large in bodyweight. I wonder since he is refining his standards if he should not consider that he has perhaps a somewhat skewed population. Certainly his mixed population in Baltimore is very similar to the population that we deal with in Cleveland. He must have a significant number of undetected gestational diabetics.

*Dr. Gruenwald:* I think this was discussed in another session in Sweden, at which you were not present. I discussed at that time my way of correcting birthweights and eliminating secondary, higher peak of birtweight. I suspect that these were all babies that were for some reason or another four weeks older than was stated. It was pointed out to me that this might be a group of undetected gestational diabetics. However, the fact that these secondary peaks disappear about the middle of the third trimester is against that interpretation.

*Prof. Kloosterman:* Dr. GRUENWALD, I like to thank you once again for your most interesting paper and the discussion must have proved to you how many questions you have raised and how much interest you provoked. Thank you once again.

## DISCUSSION PAPER DR. H. SCHWARTZ

*Prof. Minkowski* (in the chair): I am very honoured to be the chairman of the afternoon. I think we have to thank Dr. HERBERT SCHWARTZ for his interesting paper. I remember, that at some meeting Dr. GRUENWALD referred to the tendency of some people presenting exact data without any comments. I think it is nice to see that Dr. SCHWARTZ has been thinking of so many hypotheses while discussing his own findings. I wonder if Prof. JONXIS, who is an expert in the field of haemoglobins, will start the discussion.

*Prof. Jonxis:* I don't suppose I have much to add. What was shown in the last picture is a bit quite true. The strange thing is that we now know about four normal haemoglobins of which three succeed each other, the early foetal haemoglobin, foetal haemoglobin, adult haemoglobin. Then there is still haemoglobin Bartt's, which we may or may not call abnormal. We don't know much about their physiological significance. Oxygen dissociation curves of the erythrocytes containing these forms of haemoglobin, may be a little bit different, but that difference is so small that it is unlikely to be of any significance. Of the young foetal form we know next to nothing. The interesting thing is that we see in nature an alpha chain combining with three other chains, one after another appear and disappear during development, but of the factors behind, what makes them appear and disappear, no one knows anything. We don't know what this internal clock is what makes them move. We only know some strange odds and ends of some hereditairy abnormalities as the persistent foetal haemoglobin peculiarity and some haemoglobinopathies in which early haemoglobin forms still occur. There are diseases as leucaemia in which they reoccur. One might suppose that the same persistance and reoccurrence of foetal forms can be seen with other isoproteins and enzymes.

*Dr. Gruenwald:* I would like to know to what extent the various environmental factors which were used in producing anaemia change the internal clock. Or else, do they just simply increase haemoglobin formation, according to whatever the clock says.

*Dr. H. Schwartz:* We do not know the answer to these questions; however, there are many interesting systems where such questions are being studied. In the tadpole, there is a change at metamorphosis from tadpole to frog haemoglobin. This change can be induced by thyroxin. In avian embryos, the initiation of haemoglobin synthesis appears to be associated with the induction of the enzymes required for heme synthesis, particularly the rate controlling enzyme, $\delta$-aminolevulinic acid synthetase. These observations can be contrasted with the studies on the differentiation of normoblasts to stem cells. In studies of splenic colonization after injection of bone marrow into irradiated mice, the formation of the erythroid colonies is erythropoietin dependent. In neither these nor similar systems, has the relationship of haemoglobin gene action, erythrocyte differentiation, and hormonal effects been elucidated.

*Prof. Minkowski:* May I ask you shortly one question? Could you tell us why you picked up the influence of magnesium in your study? I am interested in that because in our laboratory we have shown that the magnesium content of the foetal red cells is significantly higher than the one of the mother. Do you have any comment on that?

*Dr. H. Schwartz:* The effect of magnesium is well recognized in 'cell free' systems. What we studied was the effect of the magnesium concentration at the end of the incubation on the formation of soluble protein. The concentration of magnesium was so critical that this may indeed indicate the importance of the intracellular environment.

## DISCUSSION PAPER DR. SERENI

*Prof. Minkowski* (in the chair): Thank you Dr. SERENI. I think that this represents an enormous amount of work, for which Dr. SERENI has to be congratulated. As everybody of you knows the field of developmental biochemistry is in progress now. As I see that three experts in the field are sitting side by side, namely Dr. KOLDOVSKY, Dr. RÄIHÄ and Dr. EGGERMONT, I wonder if they want to start the discussion.

*Dr. Räihä:* I want to ask one more or less specific question and another one more general. If I take the specific question first: there are some studies by NEMETH on tryptophane-pyrrolase (J. Biol. Chem. 234, 2921, 1959), in which he delivered rat foetuses before normal term and then by giving progesterone, I think, he delivered them post-maturely and studied the increase in the activity of tryptophane-pyrrolase. He found that the process of birth as such was effective. In other words there was an increase in activity in the praematurely born rats after birth and if he prolonged the gestation, activity did not increase, until birth happened. I wonder if you have done such studies on RNA synthesis.

*Dr. Sereni:* We have no data of this kind, but we are planning to perform in the next future some experiments to establish more conclusively the role of birth 'per se' on the postnatal activation of liver RNA synthesis.

*Dr. Räihä:* Second question. Your studies raise very interesting speculations about possible clinical aspects of this increase in enzyme activity. We know of many diseases in the human, where we have enzyme defects, kinetic defects and also low activities of certain enzymes, which are important in the development of the human baby. According to the new theories of molecular biology, these could be either due to a defect in the genetic code or according to what you present, it could also be due to a defect in the regulation of the protein synthesis which is initiated at birth. Now if the latter is working, then it might be possible to influence this process, to do something therapeutically when we have a decreased activity of any enzymes. For instance by trying to induce activity by giving steroids. Do you know of any studies where this has been done in human subjects with defects in enzyme activities?

*Dr. Sereni:* This is a very important question, but unfortunately I don't think that our knowledge on this field is at the moment sufficient to allow a clear cut reply. As all of you certainly know, the only series of inborn errors of metabolism which can be medically treated are the so called vitamin $B_6$ dependent syndromes; in this case however the most likely pathogenesis is a defect in the cofactor-apoenzyme relation. A good example of inborn error of metabolism, where a defective regulation of enzyme synthesis may be hypothesized, is acute intermittent porphyria, but in this case we are too far from the subject of this discussion to go into more details.

*Dr. Koldovsky:* I would not like to speak on the liver enzymes, but make a comment on the adrenal regulation. I would like to use as an example an experiment that has been done in our laboratory. It is known that after day 15, there is an increase in invertase, as you have mentioned, in the small intestine and this increase occurs until day 25–30. On the other hand the beta-galactosidase lactase, the lactose splitting enzyme, is going down in this period. There is a change in the diet, the lactose disappears from the diet, the sucrose appears in the diet, so it is very nicely correlated. If you do adrenalectomy you prevent the increase of the invertase, if you do adrenalectomy and you give cortisone or corticosterone, you have normal development. This correlates very well with the liverstudies. We have been interested to know whether the decrease of the beta-glactosidase could be prevented by adrenalectomy, and indeed when we made the adrenalectomy in rats before weaning, we prevented the decrease of the beta-galactosidase. If we do adrenalectomy and give cortisone, we get a normal decrease. We also have done the adrenalectomy and have given aldosterone and both the invertase increases and the beta-galactosidase decreases. So where is the specific effect of the glucocorticoid if you get the same answer using aldosterone. Ten times less

aldosterone expressed per milligram is needed when you use aldosterone compared with corticosterone. I have not seen any other
papers on the effect of aldosterone on enzymes in development and
on the prevention of the effect of adrenalectomy. It might be that
the regulation or the normalization of the salt and water balance is
involved.

*Dr. Sereni:* Thank you, Dr. KOLDOVSKY. In relation to your remarks,
I think I must point out that in our experiments we did not use
corticosterone (which is, in the rat, the physiologic glucocorticoid)
but hydrocortisone.

*Dr. Koldovsky:* I would like to add that we have used both hydro-
cotisone and corticosterone and they both are needed in ten times
higher doses than aldosterone.

*Dr. Reynolds:* I have one comment to make on the point being discussed
here. It is a problem that has bothered me on reading papers in which
studies have been made on adrenalectomized animals. I think the
difficulty is that an adrenalectomized animal is basically a sick
animal. When you remove the cortisol and salt-retaining steroids, and
you have a sick animal, how much of the change you see is due to
the systemic illness of this animal and how much is really due to
the loss of a specific hormone. The fact that aldosterone is very
effective is interesting because it may well be that maintenance of
the salt- and water balance alone in this way prevents the generalized
illness to an extent that the hydrocortisone loss is not manifested.

*Dr. Sereni:* The only prove we have that the changes we observe after
adrenalectomy may be related to the lack of adrenal steroids is an
indirect one, i.e. giving hydrocortisone (or other steroids) the values
should return to normal. This was the case, for example, as far as
our experiments on liver tyrosine-transaminase are concerned. I must
also add that we usually inject to an adrenalectomized newborn
animal a supplement of sodium chloride solution.

*Dr. Reynolds:* Is their food-intake as normal as that of a non-operated
animal when they are on sodium chloride replacement?

*Dr. Sereni:* We had a high mortality rate in the animals operated
few hours after birth, but those who survive are usually in good

conditions. In some recent experiments we were able to keep alive newborn rats more than 24 hours after adrenalectomy; in alle cases the stomach was found full of milk.

*Dr. Eggermont:* I would like to ask Dr. SERENI if he has some data on the RNA polymerase in the newborn, as for instance the human foetus comes to birth with a very active glucose-6-phosphatase and also other enzymes.

*Dr. Sereni:* I have no data on liver RNA polymerase activity in new-born infants, neither I know any study published by other authors. It is obvious that big differences may exist between animals of different species and different degree of maturity at birth. Nevertheless I think that we have enough data to assume that in most of the mammals the passage from intra to extrauterine life brings along an activation of many aspects of liver protein synthesis.

*Prof. François:* I want to make two comments about the difference which exists in the maturation of different enzymes in the liver. For instance it is possible to have low levels of enzymes which have an action on catabolism of phenylalanine and tyrosine. In some new-borns you have a high level of phenylalanine and tyrosine for several weeks. The second question is, do you have an idea of the action of barbiturates on glucuronyltransferase.

*Dr. Sereni:* I am not quite sure that I understood your question quite correctly. If I understand it well you are asking now if I can draw a parallel between liver biochemistry of different species around birth. But I think this is too difficult to discuss in a few words. There are sharp differences as I told you. There is a beautiful paper by DAWKINS, the late DAWKINS, on glucose-6-phosphatase-activity in various animal species before and after birth (Brit. Med. Bull. 22, 1, 27). It can be very clearly seen that the degree of activity compared with the adult is very different. But for this specific enzyme, in every species there is a very sharp postnatal increase. The urea synthesis enzymes are very different because Dr. RÄIHÄ has shown in the human that the urea synthesizing capacity is already high before birth, whereas in animals this does only come up after birth.

It is now well proved that many drugs and chemicals can increase the activity of microsomal enzyme systems, probably enhancing the rate of synthesis of the enzyme protein molecule. An activation of liver glucuronyltransferase activity was demonstrated in experimental animals after barbiturates as well as other drug administration, both in adult and in foetus or newborn animals. We have recently published in Pediatrics (40: 446, 1967) a short note on this subject, but I would like to stress the potential danger to interfere with drug administration on the physiological development of the liver.

*Prof. Minkowski:* I think I just like to confirm what Dr. SERENI says on barbiturates in the newborn but I will go back to that subject after Prof. DE BRUIJNE's paper.

*Prof. Visser:* Just a little comment on this question of barbiturates. CRIGLER in Boston just published or is going to publish a case of Crigler-Najjar syndrome, who was treated very successfully with barbiturates. Now the point I would like to clear is the question which was brought up by Dr. KOLDOVSKY of aldosterone versus cortisone. What animal did you use in your experiment?

*Dr. Koldovsky:* Rats.

*Prof. Visser:* Well, this is I think not a problem to me. The difference between glucocorticoids and mineralocorticoids is a very relative one. Even in the human corticosterone and aldosterone have glucocorticoid acyivity, and in the rat corticosterone is the normal glucocorticoid. These animals have almost no cortisone. I am not worried about your problem.

*Dr. Koldovsky:* If you look at a glucocorticoid effect, for instance the effect of glucocorticoids as measured on the amount of liver glycogen, then corticosterone is hundred times more potent than aldosterone. In the regulation of mineral metabolism the opposite is true, and in the regulation of enzymes we are getting the ratio of aldosterone being ten times more active than corticosterone. This is the puzzle.

*Prof. Visser:* I understand this, but these molecules are chemically so very close in regard of their effect on enzyme maturation. I would not be too much worried, I think this is not a principal point.

*Dr. Räihä:* Would you give me permission to show two slides in regard to Dr. EGGERMONT's question. He asked about the possible

110 DISCUSSION SESSION II

differences in the increase of RNA polymerase between rats and human. These slides are not on RNA polymerase they are on the rate limiting enzyme in urea synthesis, the arginine synthetase system. I would like to show these pictures to you, because there is a striking difference between the development in the rat as compared with the human. Figure 1 shows the development in the rat. There is a very

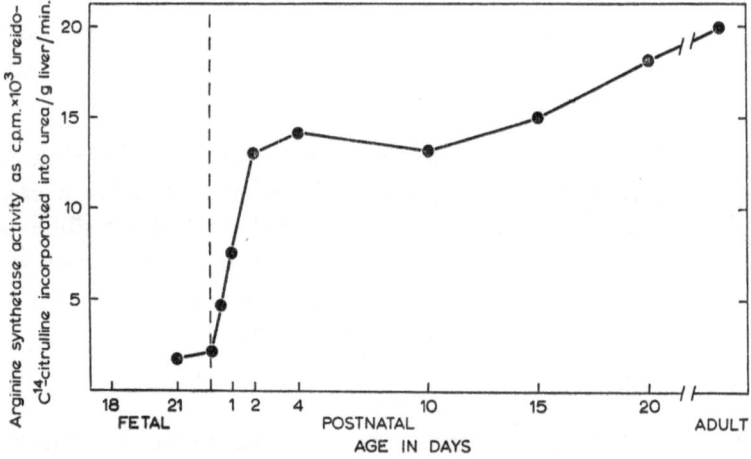

*Fig.* 1. Development of arginine synthetase activity in rat liver.

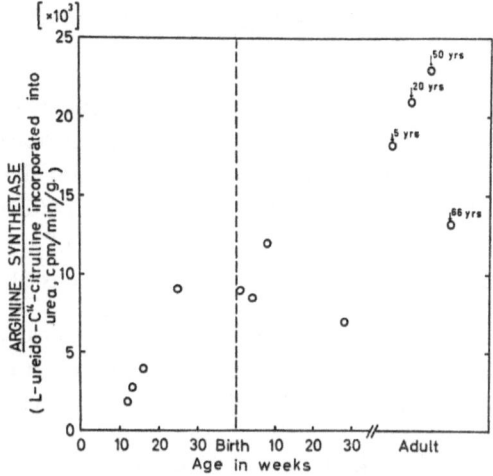

*Fig.* 2. Development of arginine synthetase activity in human liver.

rapid increase from birth, and adult activity is reached within one to two days after birth. Figure 2 shows the increase in the human during development. There is very little increase around birth and there is a distinct increase later after birth, but the post-parturation increase that we find in many enzymes of the rat we don't see in the human. So I think this gives some problems to us when we relate animal experiments to the human.

*Dr. Koldovsky:* One question to my neighbour, how did you get the values of the one to two years old children?

*Dr. Räihä:* The values right after birth were from two babies; one was 11 hours old, one 7 hours old. They were operated because they had liver rupture at birth and the surgeons were very kind to give me a piece of liver that I froze directly in the operating room. The other children that are older were subjected to abdominal surgery for various reasons. The foetal values are from cases of legal abortion.

*Prof. R. Schwartz:* I am not a developmental biochemist, but from the point of view of a physiologist, I wonder if Dr. SERENI would care to comment on another aspect of his slide which related to carbohydrate and lipid metabolism, particularly carbohydrate metabolism. What happens to gluconeogenesis? The implication of your slide is that only glycogen metabolism, increase and break-down of glycogen, increase of glucose-6-phosphatase activity etc. are important in maintenance of blood sugar. It seems to me that perhaps we should direct out attention more to what is happening with gluconeogenesis and the enzymes that are concerned with synthesis of glucose in the postnatal period.

*Dr. Sereni:* Liver gluconeogenesis is definitively low during foetal life, as it is shown by the low rate of incorporation of radioactivity from labelled 3-carbon compounds into glycogen. On the contrary, in the same stage of development, the hexokinase activity is rather high. The glycogen storage in the foetal liver during the final period of gestation is very likely derived, at least for the greatest part, from the glucose of maternal origin.

*Prof. Minkowski:* I thank you Dr. SERENI. Now I think this closes the discussion It is now the tea-time and so we can solve our own water and metabolism problems.

DISCUSSION PAPER DR. KOLDOVSKY

*Prof. R. Schwartz* (in the chair): Are there any questions for Dr. KOLDOVSKY?

*Dr. Eggermont:* The maturation of the gastro-intestinal tract can also be studied in another way. The meconium can be considered as a natural biopsy of the intestine. We proved that the enzymes alkaline phosphatase and maltase of meconium and intestinal mucosa have some properties in common. We did this mainly by studying their sedimentation behaviour in a density gradient. The sedimentation pattern of alkaline phosphatase from meconium is identical with the one observed from the small intestine. When measuring enzymes in the mecomium we have found a different trend for the glucosidases

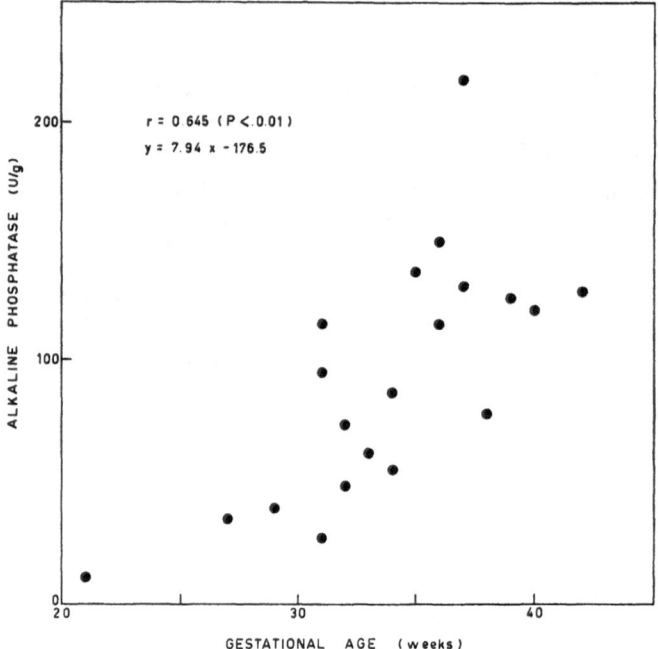

*Fig.* 3. The relation between alkaline phosphatase activity and gestational age of human foetuses. From EGGERMONT, E.: Enzymic activities in meconium from human foetuses and newborns. Biol. Neonat. 10: 266-280 (1966) with the permission of S. Karger, Basel/New York.

and alkaline phosphatase. Near term the glucosidases disappear from the meconium, while the alkaline phosphatase increases during the latter part of gestation. The values for maltase in newborn babies are lower than in praemature babies. The opposite is true for alkaline phosphatase. There is even a significant correlation between alkaline phosphatase in the meconium and the gestational age. It could be another biochemical parameter to obtain some information on the gestational age of the baby (fig. 3).

To explain this discrepancy I think it is due to the proteolytic activity of meconium. Maltase of meconium, and also the other glucosidases, are sensitive to the proteolytic enzymes of the pancreas, namely chymotrypsin and trypsin. When meconium was incubated with trypsin or chymotrypsin, maltase disappeared from the meconium while alkaline phosphatase was unaffected.

However there are some difficulties. When we were measuring these proteolytic enzymes in pancreatic tissue, we only found some traces of these enzymes. I think the proteolytic activity of meconium is very complex and may be due to other peptidase activity from the intestinal tract. So we should be very cautious with the diagnosis of cystic fibrosis based on unspecified determinations of proteases in the meconium. I think most of the proteolytic activity of meconium does not come from the pancreatic enzymes, but from the enzymes of the intestinal mucosa.

*Dr. Koldovsky:* I would like to make a comment. There is another difficulty with the determination of enzyme activity in the meconium. The enzymatic content is not only destroyed by other enzymes present in the meconium but perhaps there are also involved some other factors. You know that in newborn rats and also in human foetuses the so-called meconium particles in the mucosal cells have been described. There are perhaps lysozymes. These particles are characterized by high acid hydrolytic activity and also by acid proteolytic activity. As you have mentioned that meconium could be used as a natural biopsy specimen I want to add 'as a very speculative biopsy specimen'.

*Dr. Sereni:* I was impressed by the difference in development between the jejunum and the ileum of proteolytic enzymes and invertases.

8

Could you tell us something about histological appearance and changes during the same age of gestation?

*Dr. Koldovsky:* These histological changes develop differently. At the beginning between the 8th and 10th week of pregnancy from the classical histological studies and also from the histochemical determination of the usual enzymes the development seems the same. But later on there are differences in development, also morphological, that means presence of villi and microvilli. In this respect I would like just to mention the findings of a man whose name was Hilton published in 1910 or 1912. He has described villi in the large intestine of the human foetuses that are later on disappearing. We have studied similar things but with more modern methods in rats. We found that the histological and histochemical findings of the large intestine of the suckling rat or a newborn rat are very similar to those of the small intestine. We found that in microvilli area is present alkaline phosphatase activity; this disappears 7 or 8 days after birth.

In the human foetus the difference between jejunum and ileum appears during intra-uterine life. In the guinea-pig, where we have studied the same, the jejunal-ileal differences also appear before birth and are disappearing after birth.

*Dr. Räihä:* Dr. KOLDOVSKY raised the question that there might be other energy requiring processes in tissues other than the glucose transport in the intestine he was mentioning, which were not inhibited by total anoxia. I would like to report a small experiment we did in our laboratory. I am very happy to report this study following Dr. KOLDOVSKY's paper because he was the one who suggested we should do this.

Urea biosynthesis in the liver comprises a series of reactions that requires ATP in two places. We studied the capacity of the liver to synthesize urea when incubated in oxygen and when incubated in nitrogen. We compared adult to foetal or newborn liver slices from rats. In all cases the inhibition of urea synthesis during anoxia was over 90 per cent.

*Dr. Koldovsky:* I have no experimental data on human foetuses. But I know that experiments concerning active transport of potassium in the kidney are done under anaerobic conditions in newborn animals.

Some people have been able to show that this active transport of potassium against a concentration gradient exists under anaerobic conditions in kidney slices from newborn rats, newborn pigs and newborn puppies. Having your results and comparing these with the results from the literature, it is possible to speculate that the functions which could perhaps exist in anaerobic conditions could be related to some active transport processes.

*Dr. Widdowson:* Can you tell us something about the development of the fat splitting enzymes in the human foetus?

*Dr. Koldovsky:* We did not yet perform experiments in this field. We know however that there is present a non-specific esterase activity but we don't know the interpretation. We intend to study some lipolytic activities. I would just like to remember an old publication of TACHIBANA (Jap. J. Obstet. Gynec. 12, 40, 1929). This author studied lipase activity. The method was of course very old-fashioned, but he found an increase of lipase activity between the 3rd and 5th month of gestation. There exists also a paper by FOMINA from Moscow (Vopr. Med. Clin. 6, 176, 1960) who was studying the splitting of tributyrine. This is not a lipase but an esterase activity. This esterase activity was increasing during pregnancy. I admit the lipase activity would be more interesting for a nutritionist.

*Dr. Polman:* I should like to ask you a question about the invertase study. Did you study the activity of other $\alpha$-glucosidases? As you know the group of AURICCHIO presented a paper that at birth there are five different kinds of maltase activity well developed. Only maltase activity 1 is not developed at the time of birth. We have a few biopsies of infants 1 or 2 days old. We could not confirm the findings of AURICCHIO.

*Dr. Koldovsky:* We did not study anything else than invertase. But I think the situation is more complicated. In our laboratory we have found that the glucose-oxydase method for measuring the disaccharidase activity has some limitation if you are working with intestinal tissue. In the intestinal tissue there is present an inhibitor which gives lower values of glucose reading than actually is present. So for this reason we did not proceed with the glucose-oxydase method. We have used instead the old-fashioned method of Somogyi-

Nelson because this method is not inhibited. We have studied this inhibiting factor in rats and in human tissue. We have found that the inhibiting substance is very active in the jejunum of the suckling rat but practically not present in the ileum. In the human intestine of different ages this inhibitor was also present in different amounts.

*Dr. Eggermont:* In relation to maltase 1 and 2 we could show that these maltases are γ-amylases. That is a specific function: you can measure the reaction by the release of glucose from glycogen.

I think you measured the activity of maltase 1 and 2 by heat inactivation. I think we have to be cautious with this method. We could prove that after heat inactivation even at 45 degrees the residual enzymes do sediment very differently. You change all α-glucosidase enzymes with the exception of trehalase.

On the development of maltase 1 and 2 after birth I think there is a big difference between individuals. Some children have high γ-amylase activity very early in the first weeks of life. Others have still low activities at the age of one year. There must be some individual pattern.

# EXPERIMENTAL ASPECTS OF DYSMATURITY

# DYSMATURITY IN THE EXPERIMENTAL ANIMAL

J. S. WIGGLESWORTH*

Dysmaturity as it occurs naturally in animals in the form of runts has been recognised by farmers and stockbreeders for centuries. Runts have been considered a nuisance and as something to be discarded and there has been remarkably little study of them. Investigations of the mechanisms of growth control in experiments using the rabbit (1) and guinea-pig (2), and on the effects of cross-breeding horses of extreme size difference (3) were not concerned with causation of runts but with basic mechanisms of control of normal intrauterine growth.

There is in fact no sharp distinction between normal maternal constraint of intra-uterine growth and pathological foetal growth retardation but the purpose of this paper is to discuss pathological situations in animals which may throw some light on both physiological and pathological aspects of foetal growth in man.

*Spontaneous dysmaturity in rodents*

A study of runts in the mouse, McLAREN and MICHIE (4) revealed several interesting findings. The mouse has a double uterus with blood supply to each horn in the form of an arcade, the upper limb arising from the ovarian artery and the lower from the uterine artery. Runts were found to occur at specific sites in the uterine horn. Frequent sites are the ovarian end of the horn and the centre of the horn. In both the ovarian position and the centre of the uterine horn the maternal blood supply to the placenta was liable to be poorer than elsewhere, the ovarian position often sharing its supply with the ovary

* Nuffield Neonatal Research Unit, Institute of Child Health, Hammersmith Hospital, London W. 12

and the central one being at the junction of the vascular territories of ovarian and uterine arteries. Runts occurring in sites other than these were usually associated with placental fusion.

This work implied that runts in these animals occurred as a result of impairment in maternal blood supply to the placenta. An important point stressed by McLAREN and MICHIE was that runts in the mouse at least do not represent one end of a normal distribution. The distribution of birth weights in mouse litters is always skewed due to the occurrence of runts which are not compensated for by an equal incidence of large -for- dates foetal mice.

Observations of our own (BUTLER and WIGGLESWORTH unpublished) on the rat indicate that two distinct patterns of dysmaturity are seen. The one is the occurrence of sporadic runts in similar fashion to those already discussed in the mouse. The second pattern is one of uniform retardation in growth of all foetuses of a litter. The first situation is probably due to local factors such as variations in placental blood supply, the second is more likely to be related to some general factor.

We investigated the relationship between histological evidence of maternal disease and average foetal weight at term in two colonies of rats, one in Chicago U.S.A., and the other in London, England. The only disease found in the Chicago rats was chronic pulmonary infection and the incidence of this bore no relation to birth weight. In the London rat colony a proportion of the animals had evidence of disease in the liver in the form of patchy necrosis of parenchymal cells and small granulomas. The lesions were associated with enlargement of the spleen and were probably due to chronic low grade Salmonella infection although convincing bacteriological evidence of this could not be obtained.

One animal of a series of 96 appeared ill, had a dead stunted litter and widespread liver necrosis and was excluded from further consideration. Table 1 shows the mean average foetal weight at term of litters from rats with normal livers as compared to those of rats with histological evidence of liver damage, the histological study being carried out 'blind'. The mean foetal weights of the liver damage group are significantly lower than the normals. It must be stressed that all the animals with liver damage included here appeared quite healthy and would have been considered normal in the absence of careful pathological study. Only one animal in the normal group had a litter of dys-

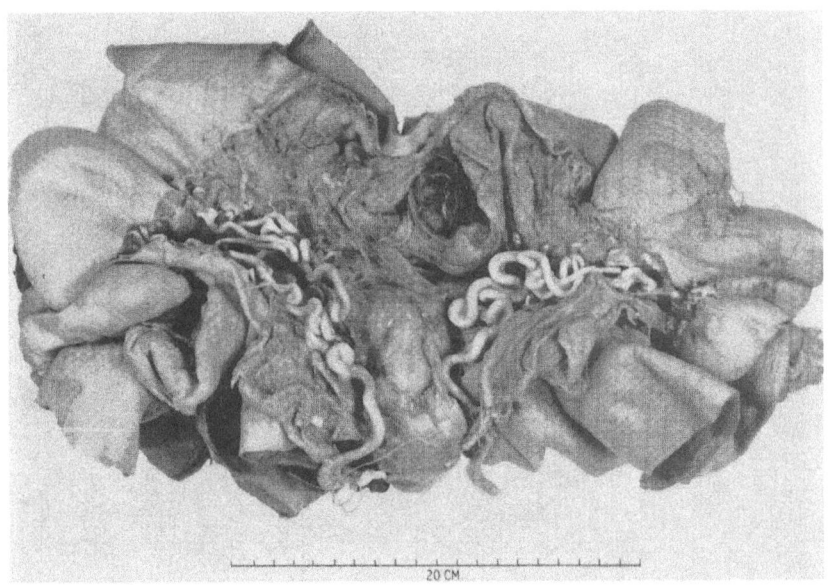

*Fig.* 1. Sheep uterus showing dissected uterine arteries viewed from behind. There is no significant difference in calibre of vessels although right uterine horn (to right of picture) contained a lamb only one third the weight of that in the left.

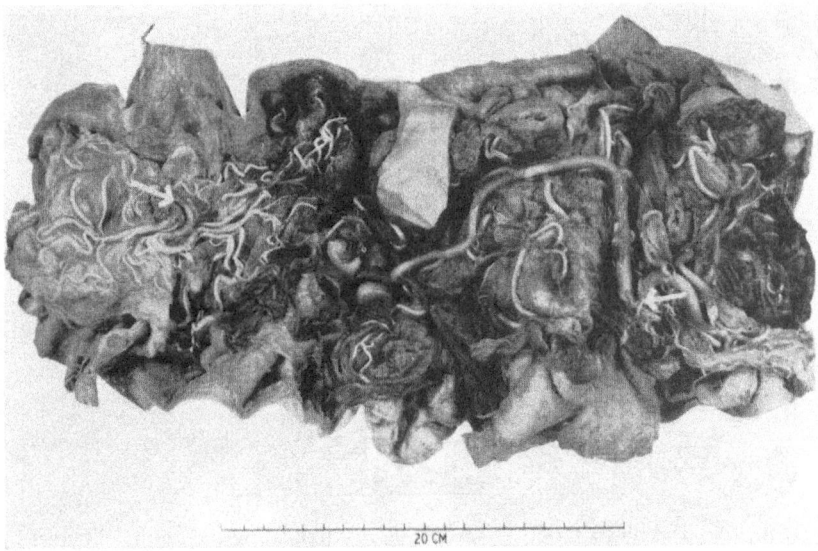

*Fig.* 2. Opened sheep uterus viewed from in front with placentae in situ. Junction between horns is visible upper centre. Placenta of normal lamb (dark area) extends into right uterine horn (to left of picture). Arrows indicate umbilical cords.

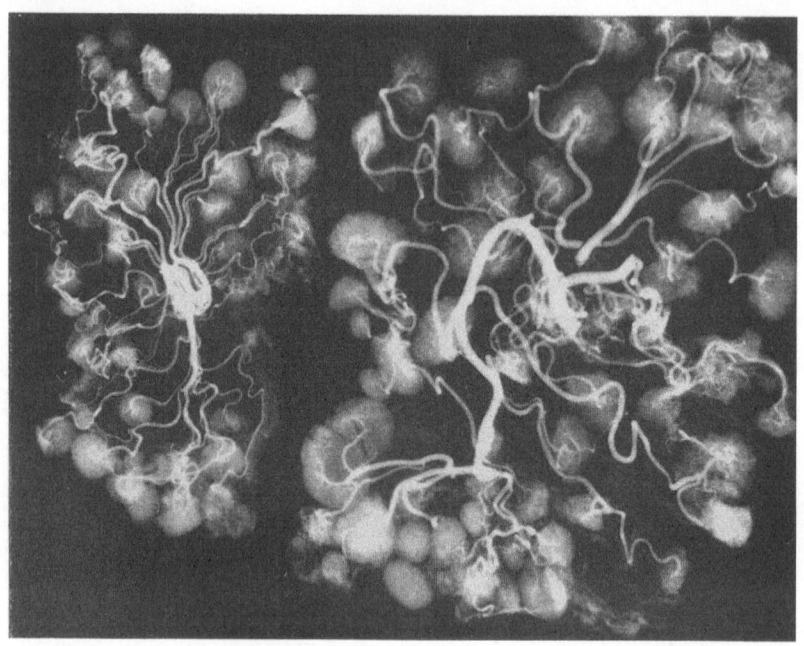

*Fig.* 3.  X-rays of injected lamb placentas after removal from uterus. Placenta of dysmature lamb on left.

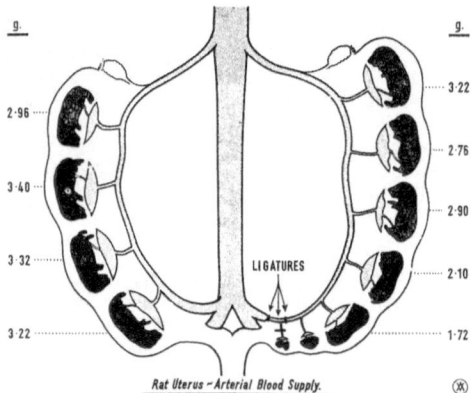

*Fig.* 4.  Arterial blood supply of the rat uterus, indicating the results obtained by the 21st day of pregnancy and five days after experimental production of ischaemia. Figures indicate weights (g) of individual foetuses in a typical experiment.

(Reproduced with permission from the Journal of Pathology and Bacteriology)

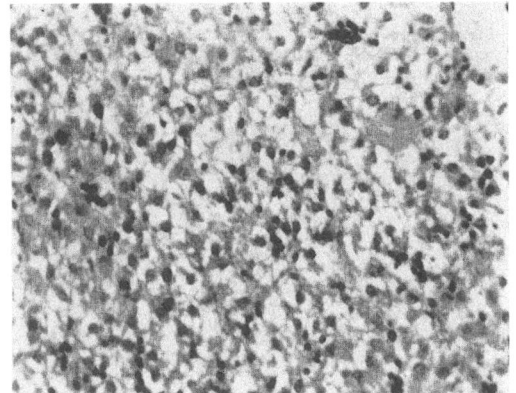

*Fig.* 6.   Liver from foetus in control horn day 21. Normal glycogenic vacuolation of liver cells. H & E x 165.

(Reproduced with permission from the Journal of Pathology and Bacteriology)

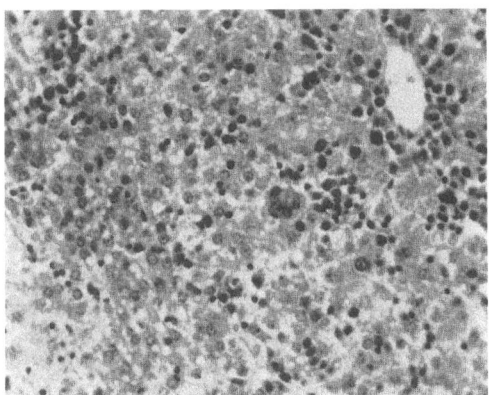

*Fig.* 7.   Liver from stunted foetus in experimental horn day 21. Little glycogenic vacuolation. H & E x 165.

(Reproduced with permission from the Journal of Pathology and Bacteriology)

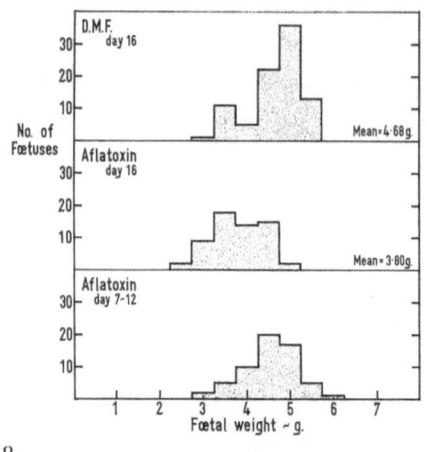

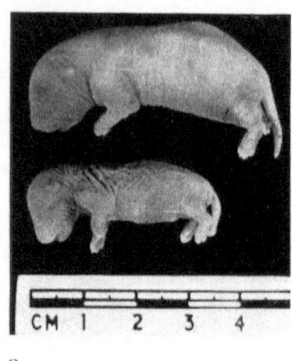

8

9

*Fig.* 8.   Foetal weight distribution at term in different treatment groups of rats. (Reproduced with permission from the Journal of Pathology and Bacteriology)

*Fig.* 9.   Dysmature foetus of rat dosed with Aflatoxin on day 16 (bottom) compared with normal foetus from control rat. Both rats killed on day 21. Note the large head and wrinkled skin of the dysmature foetus.

(Reproduced with permission from the Journal of Pathology and Bacteriology)

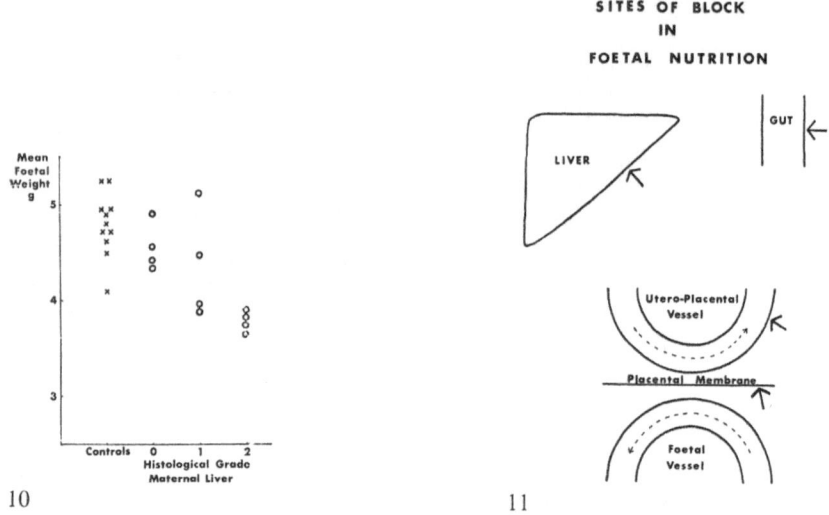

10

11

*Fig.* 10.   Relationship between severity of maternal liver damage according to arbitrary grading and mean foetal weight in rats dosed with Aflatoxin on day 16 of pregnancy.

*Fig.* 11.   Possible sites of block in foetal nutrition which may lead to dysmaturity in animals.

Table 1. *Mean values of average foetal weight at term in litters of rats with normal maternal liver histology as compared to the mean value for litters of rats with abnormal maternal liver histology*

| Liver histology | Mean foetal weight | Standard error |
|---|---|---|
| Normal | 4.86 g | ± 0.04 |
| Abnormal | 4.35 g | ± 0.12 |
| | $p < 0.01$ | |

mature foetuses, and in this case there was evidence of an endometritis even though the liver was normal.

*Dysmaturity in sheep*

It was shown many years ago by WALLACE (5) that ewes fed on a low plane of nutrition during the last six weeks of pregnancy gave birth to lambs 40 per cent less in weight than those of well nourished ewes. The undersized lambs had relatively large well developed brains and small livers, like dysmature babies. A low plane of nutrition in early pregnancy had little effect on birth weight if nutrition in late pregnancy was adequate. This knowledge is put to practical use by farmers in hill districts of Great Britain, with poor grazing, who give food supplements in the last six weeks of pregnancy so as to improve birth weight and reduce losses at lambing.

In the sheep twins occur very commonly but both are usually of similar weight and should each weigh about 5 kg at birth if nutrition has been adequate. In an animal studied recently by courtesy of Dr. L. B. STRANG there was considerable discrepancy in weight on delivery by Caesarean Section at term. The larger was 5.58 kg in weight and the smaller 1.45 kg. Weight of the brain was similar in the two animals but other organs, particularly the liver, were far smaller in the smaller lamb.

Dissection of the uterine arteries after injection of barium gelatine solution (fig. 1), showed no significant difference in blood supply to the horns of the uterus. Examination of the uterine cavity with placentae in-situ (fig. 2), showed, however, that the placenta of the larger lamb had a far more extensive area of implantation extending into both horns, and X-ray of the placentae (fig. 3), confirmed the difference in placental size with 64 cotyledons in the larger placenta and 40 in the smaller. This puts the cause of growth retardation at foetal placental level and as the sheep placenta ceases to grow by about 90 days (6) the situation must have been determined by that time, although retardation of foetal growth would take place mainly in the last 2 months.

*Experimental growth retardation in the foetal rat*

Foetal growth has been experimentally retarded in the rat by dietary methods (7) (8), and in association with congenital malformations by agents acting directly on the foetus (9). FRANKLIN and BRENT (10) showed that brief clamping of the uterine artery in early pregnancy caused foetal malformation and at a slightly later stage foetal growth retardation. In studies of the effects of chronic uterine ischaemia, WIGGLESWORTH (11) performed ligation of the main uterine vessels to one horn on day 16 of pregnancy. The animals were killed 4 days later, 24 hours before delivery was due. Figure 4 indicates the procedure adopted and the effect on the foetuses. There was considerable

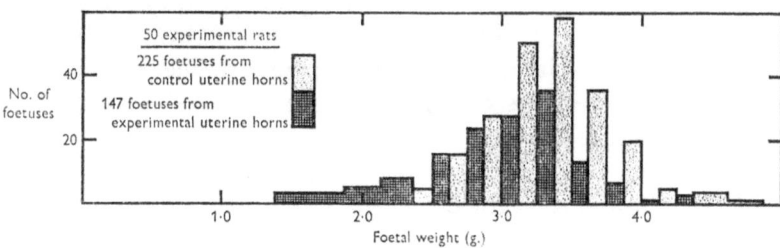

*Fig.* 5. Weight distribution of surviving foetuses from animals killed on the 21st day of pregnancy as compared to those of intact controls.
(Reproduced with permission from the Journal of Pathology and Bacteriology).

stunting of the foetuses towards the vaginal end of the ligated horn where the blood supply was poorest but little or none at the ovarian end. Figure 5 shows the weight distribution of foetuses in the ligated horns as compared to those of foetuses from control horns. There was a wide scatter of foetal weight in the ligated horns due to the mixture of normal and dysmature foetuses.

Further experiments showed that the same situation could be produced in reverse by ligating the ovarian artery and could be induced bilaterally. The brains of dysmature foetuses were relatively large in relation to body weight although smaller than those of littermates of normal weight, and the livers were relatively and absolutely smaller even than those of premature rat foetuses of the same weight. Histology showed maturity of organs as expected for gestation. Figure 6 shows a section from the liver of a control rat foetus with marked glycogenic vacuolation. Figure 7 from a dysmature rat foetus of the same gestation shows however a lack of glycogen. Table 2 indicates the results of chemical estimation of carbohydrate concentration in the livers and hearts of dysmature and control rat foetuses at term using the method of KEMP and KITS VAN HEIJNINGEN (12). Both hepatic and cardiac carbohydrate levels were significantly reduced in the more severely dysmature foetuses.

Table 2. *Total carbohydrate levels in liver and heart of normal and dysmature rat foetuses. Figures given are mean $\pm$ standard error of mean.*

| Foetal weight | Liver carbohydrate mg/g | Heart carbohydrate mg/g |
|---|---|---|
| > 4.45 g (1 SD below mean) | 82.7 $\pm$ 5.04 | 20.3 $\pm$ 0.98 |
| < 3.65 g (3 SD below mean) | 50.56 $\pm$ 6.15 p < 0.01 | 17.0 $\pm$ 1.17 0.01 < p < 0.05 |

A separate series of experiments involved administration of the hepatotoxic agent Aflatoxin $B_1$ to rats at varying stages of pregnancy (13). Aflatoxin $B_1$ is one of a series of substances produced by strains of the mould Aspergillus flavus which is known to bind with nuclear DNA and to cause inhibition of protein synthesis in the liver (14) in addition to being a potent carcinogen. If given in milligram dosage to rats it causes a slowly evolving periportal hepatic parenchymal necrosis with fatty infiltration and bile duct proliferation. Figure 8 shows the foetal weight distribution at term following administration of a single dose of Aflatoxin $B_1$ at different stages in pregnancy as compared to controls and animals given dimethylformamide — (the solvent for the toxin) only.

A single dose given in early pregnancy caused the pregnant rat to become ill with a staring coat for several days but did not cause abortion or malformation of the foetuses and had no significant effect on foetal weight at term. If the toxin was administered on day 16, however, there was considerable reduction in birth weight and entire litters were found to be severely stunted when delivered by Caesarean Section. Figure 9 shows the degree to which individual foetuses might be stunted. The question arose as to whether the foetal growth retardation in this experiment was due to a direct effect on the foetus or an indirect one mediated through some action on the mother. Substances which cause foetal growth retardation by a direct effect on the foetus would be expected to cause abortion or malformation if administered in early pregnancy as is known for antimitotic drugs and irradiation. The failure to produce any ill effects on the foetus by administration in early pregnancy of enough Aflatoxin to make the mother ill strongly favours the view that growth retardation produced by Aflatoxin given later in pregnancy was secondary to some maternal effect.

We could show that Aflatoxin crossed the placenta as we could detect it in the foetal liver by thin-layer chromatography 3—4 hours after administration to the mother, but we found no evidence that it caused damage to any foetal organ.

Examination of the maternal liver showed that there was a very clear relation between the severity of liver necrosis assessed histologically and the extent of reduction in average foetal weight in a particular litter. Figure 10 shows the relation between the severity of maternal liver damage assessed histologically on an arbitrary scale from 0 to 2 and the mean foetal weight of each litter. The histological assessment was carried out 'blind'.

The results of this study taken in conjunction with our findings on natural rat disease indicate that maternal liver damage in late pregnancy in the rat at least can impair foetal growth. As essential stages in the metabolism of proteins and carbohydrates take place in the liver this is perhaps hardly surprising.

Impairment of protein synthesis is an early and prominent feature of the action of Aflatoxin on liver cells so it is tempting to postulate that disordered protein metabolism is the cause of foetal growth retardation after Aflatoxin administration.

From the various investigations discussed in this paper it is possible to indicate a number of sites at which foetal nutrition may be blocked and lead to foetal growth retardation as shown in Figure 11. It is not suggested that this represents a complete list but it does show that a variety of insults to the pregnant animal can have the same final effect of impairing foetal growth. This must surely be true also for man.

CONCLUSIONS

1. Spontaneous runts in rodents may be caused by impairment in local blood supply.
2. Foetal growth retardation in whole litters may result from maternal disease, notably disease of the liver.
3. Impairment of maternal food intake in late pregnancy can cause foetal growth retardation in animals including sheep and rats.
4. In an individual case growth retardation in a lamb was found to be associated with reduction in placental size without impairment of uterine blood supply.
5. Foetal growth retardation can be produced experimentally in the rat by ligation of uterine vessels. The dysmature foetuses from such experiments show organ weight changes and low hepatic and cardiac carbohydrate levels as seen in dysmature babies.
6. The effect of maternal liver disease in retarding foetal growth in rats can be reproduced by administration of Aflatoxin $B_1$ in the second half of pregnancy. It is suggested that impairment of protein metabolism in the maternal liver may play some part in this effect.
7. The variety of insults to the pregnant animal which can cause foetal growth retardation suggests that a similar multiplicity of factors may be involved in causation of foetal growth retardation in man.

REFERENCES

1. HAMMOND, J. (1934) J. Exp. Biol. 11: 140.
2. ECKSTEIN, P., T. MCKEOWN and R. G. RECORD (1955) J. Endocrin. 12: 108.
3. WALTON, A. and J. HAMMOND (1938) Proc. Roy. Soc. B. 125: 311.
4. McLAREN, A. and D. MICHIE (1960) Nature 187: 363.

5. WALLACE, L. R. (1945) *J. Physiol.*, Lond. 104: 34.
6. HAMMOND, J. (1961) In: *Ciba Found. Symp. on Somatic Stability in the Newly Born*, WOLSTENHOLME, G. E. W. and M. O'CONNOR eds., Churchill, London p. 5.
7. BARRY, L. W. (1920) *Contr. Embryol.* 11: 91.
8. CAMPBELL, R. M., I. R. INNES and H. W. KOSTERLITZ (1953) *J. Endocrin.* 9: 68.
9. MURPHY, M. L. (1960) In: *Ciba Found. Symp. on Congenital Malformations*, WOLSTENHOLME, G. E. W. and M. O'CONNOR eds., Churchill, London, p. 78.
10. FRANKLIN, J. B. and R. L. BRENT (1964) *J. Morphol.* 155: 273.
11. WIGGLESWORTH J. S. (1964) *J. Path. Bact.* 88: 1.
12. KEMP, A. and A. J. M. KITS VAN HEIJNINGEN (1954) *Biochem. J.* 56: 646.
13. BUTLER, W. H. and J. S. WIGGLESWORTH (1966) *Brit. J. Exp. Path.* 47: 242.
14. CLIFFORD, J. I. and K. R. REES (1966) *Nature* 209: 312.

# EFFECTS OF PREMATURITY AND DYSMATURITY IN ANIMALS

E. M. WIDDOWSON*

Prematurity and dysmaturity are not the prerogative of the human baby. Animals can be born prematurely, and they can also be born undernourished, small for dates and dysmature. Both prematurity and dysmaturity can occur spontaneously, and they can also be brought about by experimental interference. This paper is concerned with the effects of prematurity and dysmaturity on the anatomical and chemical make-up of newborn animals, and one of its objects is to compare the effects of undernutrition *in utero* with the effects of undernutrition after birth. Secondly, the growth and development of animals that are born undernourished and dysmature will be compared with the progress of animals recovering from undernutrition that has been imposed after birth.

*Prematurity in the guinea pig*

If the mother is well-nourished the size of each of her young at birth depends to a large extent on the number in the uterine horn, the size of the uterus, the blood supply to each particular part of the uterus, and the size of each placenta (1). In the guinea pig, as in man, the length of gestation is progressively reduced by an increase in litter size, and this further limits the size of the individual young at the time of birth. Both the guinea pig and man have a comparatively long gestation period and the young are more highly developed at term than the young of many species. Their bodies already contain a considerable amount of fat — about 16 % in the human baby and 10 % in the guinea pig (2). Looking at it teleologically, one can

* Medical Research Council Infant Nutrition Research Division, Dunn Nutritional Laboratory, University of Cambridge.

perhaps say that they can afford to be born prematurely; even when born prematurely they are more highly developed than the mouse, rat, rabbit, kitten or puppy at term. If these species were born prematurely they would probably never survive at all.

When guinea pigs are born prematurely they generally belong to a litter of six or more. It is thought that the effect of a large litter operates systemically rather than locally, for it is unaffected by the distribution of foetuses between the two uterine horns (3). The small guinea pig born to a well-nourished mother shows all the characteristics of prematurity. The composition of its body and the amounts of fat, water, nitrogen, potassium and chloride in it are appropriate to a single foetus of the same body weight (4). Premature guinea pigs have low concentrations of glycogen in their tissues, which adds to their problems of survival.

## Dysmaturity in the pig

Pigs are not born prematurely, even when the litter is large. In large litters of piglets, however, there is sometimes one that weighs only a half or even a third as much as the others, and this runt piglet provides us with a good example of dysmaturity at birth. In the mouse the foetus in the middle of the uterine horn has the poorest blood supply and smallest placenta (5), and those who remove piglets by Caesarian section say that it is generally the fourth along the uterine horn that is the little runt.

Figure 1 shows the normal growth in weight of a pig foetus, and it also shows the weight of a full term runt. This runt weighed only 433 grams, or about a third as much as the others in the litter, and its weight corresponded to the weight of a normal foetus of 80 days gestation, which is two thirds of the way to term. A pig foetus of this age would certainly not be viable. This runt died too, with hypothermia and hypoglycaemia, but it could have been reared if it had been put at once into a very warm environment and fed. Newborn piglets depend on glycogen in their tissues as their source of energy during the first hours after birth (6). Small dysmature piglets do not have these stores of glycogen, and this is perhaps their greatest handicap. The small piglet is weaker than its littermates, and the shortage of carbohydrate to provide calories, and the consequent low blood sugar, weaken it still further. It loses in the competition for a good suckling position, yet it needs food more urgently than its bigger littermates. Its body temperature falls and it is very likely to die. The mortality rate is always highest in those that have the lowest birth weight within the litter (7).

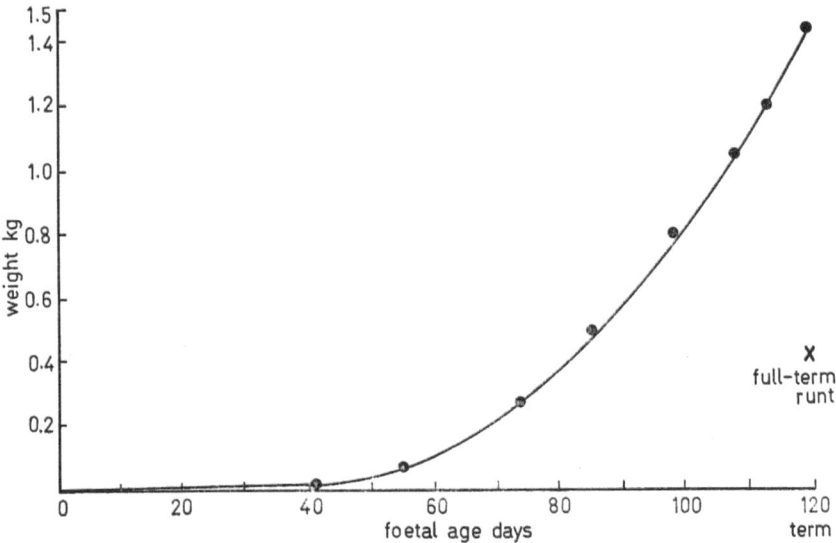

*Fig.* 1.   Growth in weight of foetal pigs.

Table 1 shows the mean weight of the liver, heart, kidneys, brain and quadriceps muscles in the smallest and largest pigs in five litters. The small animals had large brains and small skeletal muscles in proportion to their body weight, and livers, hearts and kidneys that were of similar size in relation to the weight of the animal. This is exactly the same as occurs in pigs undernourished very severely for a year *after* birth (8, 9, 10). The brains were so large that they were considerably heavier than the brain of a normally growing foetal pig of similar body weight (11).

Figure 2 shows the fall in percentage of water in the bodies of pig foetuses growing normally. This reaches about 80 % at term. The runt piglet weighing 433 grams had a little more water, but not much

9

Table 1. *Weights of organs of the smallest and largest newborn pigs in five litters. Mean values*

|  | Smallest | Largest |
|---|---|---|
| Body weight g | 584 | 1553 |
| *Organ weights* | | |
| Liver g | 13.8 | 46.8 |
| % body weight | 2.4 | 2.9 |
| Heart g | 5.1 | 12.9 |
| % body weight | 0.87 | 0.81 |
| Kidneys g | 3.7 | 9.8 |
| % body weight | 0.63 | 0.61 |
| Brain g | 26.2 | 34.0 |
| % body weight | 4.5 | 2.2 |
| Quadriceps muscles g | 3.9 | 12.9 |
| % body weight | 0.66 | 0.83 |

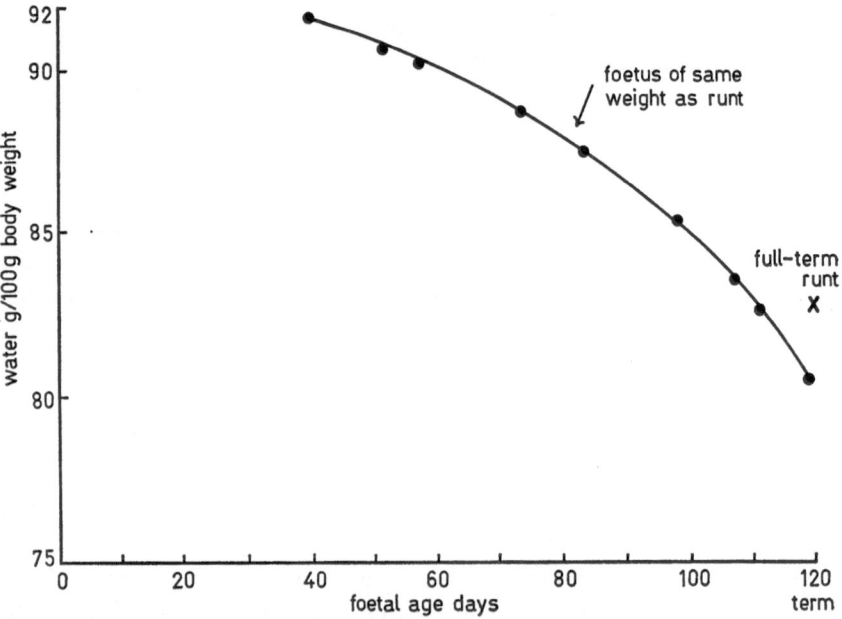

*Fig.* 2. Percentage of water in the bodies of foetal pigs.

more — the percentage in its body was 82.7 — but a well nourished 80 day foetus of the same weight as the runt would have had about 87 % of water. Most of the other slow-changing aspects of body composition confirm the conclusion that a dysmature animal even as small as this is nearer a full-term larger animal than it is to a premature one of the same body weight. Much of the excess water in the body of the dysmature pig is accounted for by extracellular fluid in the muscle and skin, and of all the tissues of the body it is the muscle and skin that suffer most from the effects of the undernutrition. The organs, particularly the brain, and also the heart, always have priority of growth when nutrition is short, whether before or after birth, and apart from the fat, the skeletal muscle and skin are the tissues that are most affected.

We have studied by means of X rays and chemical analysis the skeletal development of the smallest and largest pigs in litters at birth. The dysmature pig has a skeleton which is retarded in development; its ossification centres are somewhat less well calcified and the bones are more cartilagenous than the bones of the large littermate. However, the skeleton is much farther on in development than the skeleton of a normally growing 80 day pig foetus of the same body weight.

*Postmaturity in cattle*

It seems likely that the pig foetus which will become the runt grows slowly and steadily to the size at which it is born, and there is nothing to suggest that it has been heavier and has lost weight. Loss of weight of the foetus due to an ageing and inefficient placenta after full term does, however, occur in some dairy breeds of cattle (12). The postmature newborn calf has a large skeleton, overgrowth of epidermal structures such as hooves and hair and poorly developed muscles. There is some meconium staining and the animals are dehydrated and hypoglycaemic when they are born. The postmature Guernsey calf cannot ventilate its lungs and it dies within a few minutes. The postmature Holstein-Friesian calf breathes but it cannot suck properly, its body temperature falls, it becomes lethargic, its blood sugar falls still lower and it dies with hypoglycaemia in a few hours. Postmature calves rarely survive. It is believed that gestation length within breeds of cattle is influenced by the genetic constitution of the foetus and mother, but the major genetic factor is the foetal genotype.

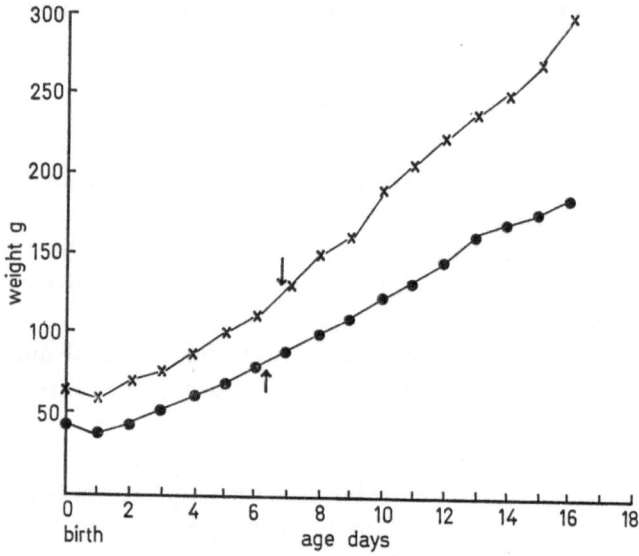

*Fig.* 3.   Gain in weight of two rabbits in the same litter with different birth weights. The arrow indicates the age at which the birth weight was doubled.

### Growth of dysmature animals after birth

Figure 3 shows typical growth curves of two rabbits in the same litter; one weighed 41 grams and the other 64 grams at birth. The small one did not catch up — in fact it fell farther and farther behind. But if we look at the growth of the two rabbits in another way and consider their rates of incremental growth, that is the rate at which the body tissue multiplies itself, then the small animal does not appear to do too badly. It doubles its birth weight between the 6th and 7th day which is just what the big one also achieves, and the small rabbit has just as rapid a rate of incremental growth as the large one. Exactly the same thing is true of pigs. The little runt, if it survives the first hours and days after birth, gains weight more slowly than the big ones in the litter, but it, like the small rabbit, has a rapid rate of incremental growth (fig. 4).

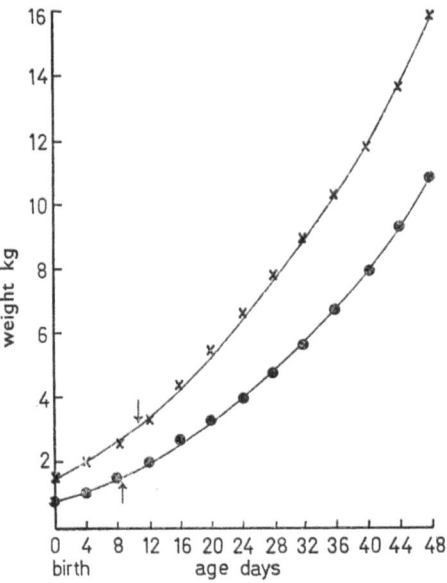

*Fig.* 4.   Gain in weight of two pigs in the same litter with different birth weights. The arrow indicates the age at which the birth weight was doubled.

The slow gain in weight of the small newborn animal in a litter may be partly due to its inability to get all the milk it wants, but not entirely, for the small baby at birth also grows more slowly than the bigger one and here there should be no question of a fight for food.

Poor nutrition of the mother during pregnancy limits the size of the newborn young of some species, and in this case the rate of growth after birth will be further reduced by her poorer ability to lactate. This is illustrated in fig. 5, which shows the effect of feeding female rats from weaning on a diet containing 6 % protein instead of the normal 18 % on the growth of their young. Only a few of the female rats reared on the 6 % protein diet reached sexual maturity, and of these not all became pregnant. However, some did, and figure 5 represents the mean of all those that are available. The young were small at birth. The mothers had very little milk, and the growth rate after birth was exceedingly slow. The young were left with the mothers until they were 6 weeks old, instead of being weaned at the usual 3 weeks, but even so their weight at 6 weeks averaged only 9 grams as compared with 100 grams or so for a normally growing rat. From 6 weeks they were fed on the stock diet containing 18 % protein, but it is clear that this severe growth retardation before and after birth had a permanent effect on the body weight.

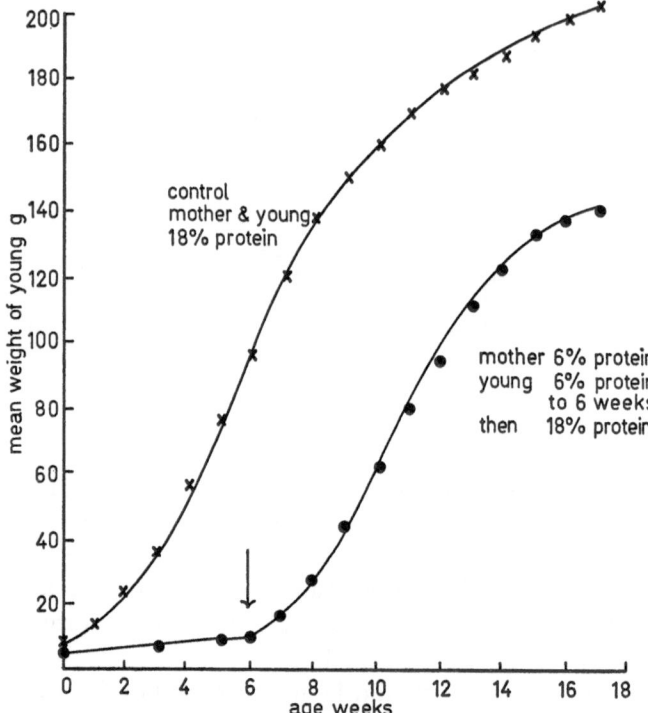

*Fig.* 5.   Growth of young of female rats which had been born and reared on a diet containing 6 % protein.

The size of the guinea pig at birth is influenced by the state of nutrition of the mother. In our laboratory in Cambridge we use a pelleted guinea pig diet (SG 1), while the diet used in the Department of Pathology is based on sugar beet pulp, with additions of bran and oats and 1 % of yeast and 1 % of fishmeal. This diet is much more fibrous and contains less protein than the pelleted diet. LISTER and McCANCE (13) compared the effect of the two diets on the same stock of guinea pigs, and found that the whole trend on the sugar beet diet was towards smaller litters. In spite of this the weight of the individual young of these mothers was low. There was a far higher mortality among the small guinea pigs born of mothers on the poorer sugar beet diet

— 52 % of them died during the first four weeks after birth compared with 21 % of the offspring of mothers on the better 'SG 1' diet. Even when young animals of similar birth weight were compared, mortality was higher in the sugar beet group. Progress after 4 weeks depended on their early nutritional history and on their later diet. Those that were born and reared on the poorer diet grew more slowly than those on the better diet, and they all stopped growing at approximately the same age, so that the slow growing ones became smaller adults. When animals whose mothers had had the poorer diet were given the better diet from 4 weeks they grew better, but they did not catch up to the others.

*Effect of undernourishing rats after birth*

Rats are born in a much less mature state than guinea pigs, and their mature size can be permanently affected by undernourishing them *after* birth. This is easily done by giving one mother a large number, say 15, to suckle and comparing their progress with others suckled in a group of 3. The mother suckling 15 produces more milk than the mother suckling 3, and the total gain in weight of her litter is greater. She cannot produce 5 times as much milk, however, so each of her young gets less, and consequently it grows more slowly. Rats suckled in groups of 3 often weigh 2–3 times as much at weaning as those suckled in groups of 15 or more, and they are of correspondingly greater length (14). As in the newborn pigs undernourished *in utero*, the brain of the rat undernourished for 10 days after birth forms a much higher percentage of the body weight than it ever does in the course of development of a well nourished animal (15).

We have compared skeletal development in the large and small rats and we found that calcification of the centres of ossification in the paws was farther advanced in a rapidly growing animal suckled in a small group than in a smaller slow growing animal suckled in a large group, when animals of the same age were compared, but less advanced when comparison was made between animals of the same body weight. Undernutrition of the rat after birth retards skeletal maturation, but not so much as it retards growth in weight or length, and an animal that has reached a given weight slowly has a more mature skeleton than one which has reached the same weight more rapidly (16).

Thus the same principle holds in a rat undernourished *after* birth as in a pig which is undernourished *in utero*.

CONCLUSIONS

Premature guinea pigs and dysmature pigs born at term are similar in that they are both small; they have a big surface area and they lack glycogen. They both have difficulty in maintaining a normal body temperature if the environmental temperature is low. Their bodies contain a higher percentage of extracellular water than the well nourished full term animal. The runt pig is, however, nearer to the normal animal of the same age in this and other respects than it is to a normal foetus of the same body weight. The premature animal is of normal bodily proportions for its gestational age, which means that its development is farther behind in every way than that of the dysmature animal born at term, and in particular it has a smaller and less highly developed brain. The period of most rapid growth of the brain in the pig is from 50 days before birth until about 40 days after birth (11). In the rat the most rapid growth occurs during the first two weeks after birth. If undernutrition is imposed during this time the gain in weight of the brain is hindered little if at all, and the brain comes to form a higher percentage of the body weight than it does at any stage in the development of a well nourished animal.

Postmaturity is a problem in some breeds of dairy cattle. The postmature calves cannot suck: they become hypothermic and hypoglycaemic and they rarely survive for more than a few hours.

Animals born to a well nourished mother that are smaller than their littermates at birth because of a poor blood supply *in utero* grow slowly after birth in absolute terms, but their rate of incremental growth is just as rapid as that of the larger animals in the litter. If small size at birth is due to malnutrition of the mother, the young are likely to suffer a further handicap because of the mother's poor ability to lactate.

REFERENCES

1. McCance, R. A. (1962) *Lancet* ii: 621.
2. Widdowson, E. M. (1950) *Nature*, Lond. 166: 626.
3. McLaren, A. and D. Michie (1963) *J. Reprod. Fert.* 6, 139.

4. LISTER, D. (1966) *The effects of nutrition before and after birth on adult size and structure*. Ph. D. Thesis. University of Cambridge.
5. McLAREN, A. and D. MICHIE (1960) *Nature*, Lond. 187: 363.
6. McCANCE, R. A. and E. M. WIDDOWSON (1959) *J. Physiol.* 147: 124.
7. POMEROY, R. W. (1960) *J. Agric. Sci.* 54: 1.
8. McCANCE, R. A. (1960) *Brit. J. Nutr.* 14: 59.
9. DICKERSON, J. W. T. and R. A. McCANCE (1964) *Clin. Sci.* 27, 123.
10. DICKERSON, J. W. T., J. DOBBING and R. A. McCANCE (1967) *Proc. Roy. Soc.* B. 166: 396.
11. DICKERSON, J. W. T. and J. DOBBING (1967) *Proc. Roy. Soc.* B. 166: 384.
12. HOLM, L. W. (1966) The gestation period of mammals. In: *Comparative biology of reproduction in mammals*. I. W. Rowlands Ed. Symposia of the Zoological Society of London No. 15 p. 403. Academic Press, London.
13. LISTER, D. and R. A. McCANCE (1965) *Brit. J. Nutr.* 19: 311.
14. WIDDOWSON, E. M. and R. A. McCANCE, (1960) *Proc. Roy. Soc.* B. 152, 188.
15. WIDDOWSON, E. M. (1966) Nutritional deprivation in psychological development: Studies in animals. In: *Deprivation in psychobiological development*. PAHO/WHO Scientific Pub. No. 134.
16. DICKERSON, J. W. T. and E. M. WIDDOWSON (1960) *Proc. Roy. Soc.* B. 152: 207.

# DISCUSSION

## SESSION III

### DISCUSSION PAPERS DR. WIGGLESWORTH AND DR. WIDDOWSON

*Prof. Minkowski* (in the chair): Dr. WIDDOWSON, I like to make a special congratulation not only for the perfect material that you presented, but also for the way you presented it. You are an ideal speaker, you present your material very clearly, very slowly. I don't think anybody here has lost any word of what you have said and I think moreover you explained very well every detail of your slides. Now after this compliment I think I will open the discussion.

*Dr. Gruenwald:* I like to ask Dr. WIDDOWSON whether she has any experiences with rats that were rehabilitated, normally fed, looked normal and then had young. What were they like, compared with the young of entirely normal rats?

*Dr. Widdowson:* Yes, we have made this experiment. Rats that were suckled in large litters, grew slowly during the three weeks suckling. They also grew slowly afterwards, although they then had unlimited food. Sexual development is closely tided to body size, and these rats reached puberty later than others originally suckled in small groups which were continuing to grow rapidly. We mated them as soon as we could, but they became pregnant at a later age than the others. Once they did become pregnant, at about the same bodyweight as fast growing animals, they produced just as many young of similar size, and they were able to lactate just as well. But everything happened a little later.

*Dr. Gruenwald:* The other question concerns the 'praemature' guinea-pig of the large litters. Was there not a combination of praematurity and growth-retardation?

*Dr. Widdowson:* I am glad you asked this. I think this is probably true. It is rather difficult to sort the two out.

*Prof. Minkowski:* I like to add that this is an important question, even in the human. In many studies on human small-for-date infants we are dealing mainly with older infants born after the 37th week. But there is no doubt that there is a rather large material to be studied, in which we are dealing with combined praematurity and dysmaturity.

*Dr. Koldovsky:* Do you think that the effect of aflatoxin $B_1$ on the liver is a quantitative or a qualitative effect? Are you sure that you are really only effecting the liver of the mother? What about a possible effect on the liver of the foetus?

*Dr. Wigglesworth:* We can't say conclusively that we have not affected the foetus. Our only argument was that substances that are known to affect the foetus directly, such as antimitotic drugs, tend to cause either abortion or foetal malformation if given early in pregnancy, in sufficiently large doses to make the mother ill. We have not done any chemical studies on the foetal livers, we studied them histologically, and they appeared normal. But thus abviously remains a possibility. As for the effect on the maternal liver, we thought that this was related quantitatively to the severity of foetal growth-retardation in sofar as we could measure it with our rough histological methods.

*Dr. Koldovsky:* So you have not yet done experiments with partially hepatectomized pregnant females, for example.

*Dr. Wigglesworth:* No, we have not done this. It would be an interesting experiment.

*Dr. Koldovsky:* We have done several years ago experiments where we have studied the growth and several physiological functions of praematurely weaned rats. We compared rats weaned at the third week with rats weaned at the fifth week. We found that the rats weaned at the third week had a retardation of growth and we followed them up compared with the rats weaned at the fifth week. At 90 days both groups were of the same weight and were not different. As far as their general appearance is concerned, on the first view, they look normal. We then have followed some detailed physiological functions until the age of six months or one year. We have found differences in development of condition reflexes between these two groups. And also we have found that their spermatogenesis, their reproduction capacity, was different from that of the normal rat. It was interesting that when we weaned the rats on day 21 and offered them a high fat diet for 41 days, growth-retardation occurred. We fed them later on standard diet. Some of the described differences did not occur after this treatment. So my point is that the weight is sometimes an indication of the damage, but sometimes not.

*Dr. Widdowson:* It is a terrible thought that all our rats are abnormal, because we always wean at three weeks.

*Dr. Sereni:* Do you have any information on the adrenals of your stunted foetuses, which have very low glycogen values in the liver at birth. It is well known that adrenal function is very important for the glycogen deposition in the foetus.

*Dr. Wigglesworth:* We have no information apart from histology which shows no particular abnormality in our animals. I don't know if Dr. Widdowson has any information on this.

*Dr. Widdowson:* No, we have not.

*Dr. Sereni:* I have one comment for Dr. WIDDOWSON. Because to a certain extent I disagree with you. On one slide you showed that in the undernourished newborn rat the brainweight is not different from the well-nourished rat. We have similar data and there were significant differences between undernourished and well-nourished rats at about 45 days of age.

*Dr. Widdowson:* I think this depends on the age at which you make the comparison but I am sure that the brain of an undernourished animal is always large in proportion to the body. The small 'runt' pig had a smaller brain than the big one, but its brain was a higher percentage of its body-weight.

*Dr. Sereni:* My point is different, because we have also data on the human. We made a survey after 6 or 7 years on infants which were very severely undernourished in the first 6 months of life. Their weight

was less than 50 per cent of the average weight of the normal infant.
And in this case, after 6 or 7 years, the head circumferences of the
previously undernourished infants were definitely very much smaller
than the head circumferences of the controls (brothers). So it appears
that in the human undernourishment in the first 6 months of life does
affect indeed the brain development in later periods of life.

*Dr. Räihä:* In relation to Dr. WIDDOWSON's data on these large and
small litters I would like to present some data that we have on biochemical development in rats that were kept in large and small
litters. These studies were done together with Dr. NORMAN KRETCHMER
at Stanford.

Urea synthesis reflects a balance between the intake of protein
on one hand and its utilization for growth on the other hand (fig. 1).
It has been shown in adult animals that if we feed a high protein diet,
the excretion of urea increases and an increase in all the enzymes in
the urea cycle is observed.

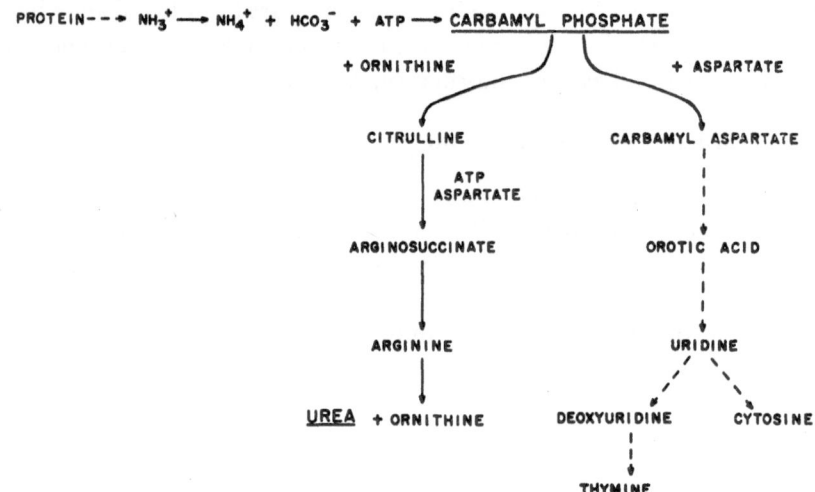

*Fig.* 1.   Relation between urea and pyrimidine synthesis.

In a rapidly growing animal this is different. We studied rats in
small litters and in big litters and on the curve in figure 2 you can see
a difference in weight gain. When we studied the capacity for urea
synthesis in the liver and its change after birth we could see that there

was no difference. This, to us, suggested that in the rapidly growing animal a higher intake of protein could be utilized for growth, better than in an adult animal. We have studied the protein content in the milk; in the mothers that had small and large litters it was the same.

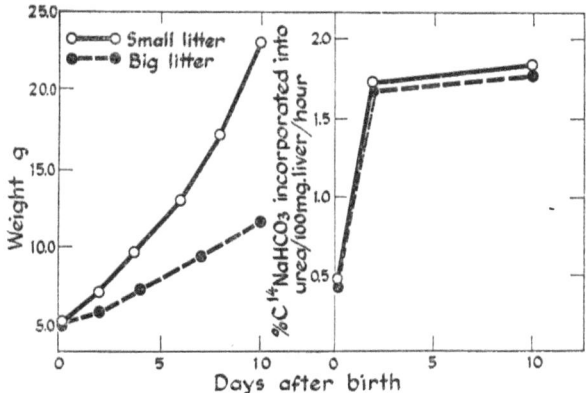

*Fig.* 2.   Urea forming capacity in liver slices of newborn rats nursed in large and small litters.

*Dr. Huber:* We heard this morning Dr. GRUENWALD more or less deny that socio-economic conditions in human pregnant women do effect the birthweight. This afternoon we have heard evidence that there is such an influence definitely. Now, unwillingly more or less, in Indonesia I have experimented with human pregnant women, in so far that they were taken up in the hospital for various lengths of time, sometimes up to 6 weeks before birth. And in due course it became evident that the women who stayed longer in the hospital and consequently were on a better diet and had more rest probably, gave birth to larger babies. And this was, as far as we could ascertain, not related to time of gestation. So I think in the human there is an influence, a shorttime influence, on the birthweight of the babies.

*Dr. Widdowson:* This was the experience after the war from studies in Holland and from studies that Dr. DEAN made in Wuppertal, Germany, that the undernutrition of the mother does have an effect on the birthweight of the babies, but it is a small effect, quantitatively.

*Dr. Wigglesworth:* It is about the same effect as cigaret smoking, isn't it?

*Dr. Widdowson:* Yes.

*Dr. Gruenwald:* I am sorry that I gave this impression, it was not my intention. There is a very large socio-economic difference in the human. In fact, I said that most, if not all, of the difference that had been claimed to exist between negroes and white in America was not racial, but rather socio-economic.

*Prof. De Bruijne:* Could Dr. WIDDOWSON tell us something about the water content of the dysmature animals, because we have so often the impression that our dysmature babies are dehydrated. When I followed your paper well, this was not the case in your dysmature animals. I just wondered if you would have been able to look after the amniotic fluid, because I sometimes hear from my colleagues, the obstetricians, that in the dysmature babies there is sometimes an oligohydramnion. Maybe you have been able to see if there was also not only absolutely but also relatively less amniotic fluid in these small animals.

*Dr. Widdowson:* No, we have not done that, but I am sure that the small dysmature piglet is not dehydrated at birth. But then it is of course not post-mature.

*Prof. Minkowski:* My comment is related to the question of Prof. DE BRUIJNE, about the dehydration of the small rat at least. May I show three slides and ask if you have measured sodium in the plasma. You have mentioned in one of your experiments, that you noticed an increase of body water mainly in the extra-cellular compartment. Is that right?

*Dr. Widdowson:* The small undernourished animal has more extra-cellular fluid per unit body weight, and it has a higher concentration of chloride in its tissues.

*Prof. Minkowski:* I like to show you what happens in the human small for date infants, in which we noticed a special kind of dehydration, and ask to Dr. WIDDOWSON and Dr. WIGGLESWORTH what they think according to their experimental animals. Haematocrite values from the first day to day 13 in dysmature infants are compared with control values. It is obvious that most of the haematocrite values in the dysmature infants are high. The plasma sodium values show two peaks of high values during the first 2 or 3 days of life and values may rise to 160, 170 maeq per liter. One had a concentration of 180 maeq per liter and died in an acute state of convulsion; at the necropsy the only finding was cerebral edema. If you look at the sodium excretion you will find that those children do not excrete at all sodium on a normal mothermilk diet. During a few days they excrete less than 1 maeq/kg/24 hr. So in the human it is obvious that we have a state of high haematocrite value, high plasma sodium concentration and no excretion of sodium in the urine. I would like to know if in some of your animals you or Dr. WIGGLESWORTH have found something which can explain that.

*Dr. Widdowson:* I am afraid we did not measure the haematocrite or serum sodium concentration in our pigs, nor did we collect any urine from them. We will do this next time.

*Prof. Kloosterman:* Could I ask in connection with this at which time you studied these newborn piglets; at the moment immediately after birth or some hours or days after birth.

*Dr. Widdowson:* Immediately after birth. The particular one which I referred, weighing 433 grams, lived for an hour or so, but most of them have been studied immediately after birth.

*Prof. Kloosterman:* I had a possibility to study some monozygotic twins with a third circulation in the common placenta. In these cases often one baby is very big and hydropic, the other baby very small and dehydrated. After birth the small baby sometimes becomes oedematous. In the literature there are such reports about babies who even developed pulmonary oedema after infusion with saline. I tried to explain this as the small babies have also a low protein content of the plasma. According to my experience intra-uterine starvation never gives rise to 'hunger oedema', but to 'hunger dehydration', perhaps because the mother will extract fluid from a baby with a very low protein content in the blood. After birth real hunger oedema can develop in extreme cases.

*Dr. Valaes:* The concept of critical periods during the growth of an individual whereby deprivation is of permanent effect is very important for the clinician. I think in the human there is very little opportunity to collect data on individual cases and to separate one factor

10

out of the mass of possible factors affecting the growth of the individual. Collective data from studies on the influence of socio-economic factors on growth and on birthweight may be more important. The relationship between birthweight and subsequent growth as well as the evidence relating birthweight to socio-economic factors and particularly the social class in which the mother was brought up, point out that if a critical period exists for the human it must be during intra-uterine life. Would you accept this?

*Dr. Widdowson:* It has recently been suggested from work on rats that the effect will be permanent as long as the deprivation is imposed during the period of rapid cell division. It will not be permanent if that period has been passed, and the cells are only growing in size. This is an interesting suggestion and it may be why some organs that develop early, like the heart, are less affected then those that develop late, like the muscle. From what I was hearing about this recently from Dr. DONALD CHEEK in Baltimore, it seems that human muscle cells have not reached their full number at the time of birth as was formerly supposed. Cell division goes on for a long time after birth. I think the idea of a critical period in man is an interesting one, but I think it is a generalization that will be true for all species.

# HEREDITARY AND ENVIRONMENTAL ASPECTS
# OF LOW BIRTHWEIGHT

# FACTORS INFLUENCING FETAL GROWTH

L. O. LUBCHENCO, C. HANSMAN, AND
LEENA BÄCKSTRÖM*

INTRODUCTION

The purpose of this paper is to define patterns of fetal growth which are seen in various maternal and/or fetal diseases or conditions. It is also designed to demonstrate the value of using intrauterine growth charts to detect high-risk newborn infants and to suggest specific morbidities occurring at various positions on the charts.

METHODS AND MATERIALS

Measurements of birth weight, length and head circumference have been tabulated from the medical records of infants with known anomalies or diseases. These measurements have been plotted on the previously described (1, 2) intrauterine growth charts. A median for weight has been obtained for each group of infants for comparison with the intrauterine growth standard. In many instances, it has been possible to determine a median for gestational age as well. Hence, the relative deviation of weight from the standard can be shown and, in some conditions, the gestational age at which most of the infants are born. Infants with specific diseases or conditions were identified from records kept in the Newborn and Premature Infant Center Office. They were born at the University of Colorado Medical Center or transferred to the Newborn and Premature Infant Center during the past 15 years. Those who had congenital anomalies, who were

Newborn and Premature Infant Center, Department of Pediatrics and Child Research Council, University of Colorado Medical Center, Denver, Colorado. Supported in part by grants-in-aid from NIH (HD 373, 601, 675 and HE 6684) and the Children's Bureau in cooperation with the Colorado State Department of Public Health and the University of Colorado Medical Center.

* NIH Research fellow.

10*

products of multiple gestations or whose mothers had diabetes, chronic cardiovascular disease or whose placentas were abnormal were studied.

Additional intrauterine growth material was obtained from the Birth Defects Center Roster and Genetic Counseling Clinic where chromatin studies have been carried out on all newborn infants born at the University of Colorado Medical Center and at General Rose Memorial Hospital in Denver.

Data on intrauterine growth at high altitude were obtained from the records of LICHTY et al. (3) and from IBM data cards of infants born in Leadville, Colorado during the year 1963. These data were coded by personnel in the Newborn and Premature Infant Center.

Finally, larger numbers of infants with anomalies were obtained from the birth certificates of the Colorado State Department of Public Health Bureau of Vital Statistics, since gestational ages and birth weights are recorded. References from the literature to supplement the Colorado data were used freely.

The method used in this study evaluates intrauterine growth at the time of birth and encompasses problems inherent in pre-term delivery and influences on fetal growth other than the conditions under observation. Furthermore, such data from groups of infants will indicate growth trends for those groups, but should not be used to predict growth for the individual.


PRESENTATION

Table 1 presents an outline of conditions which have been associated with aberrant fetal growth and gives the possible related morbidity. The first part lists conditions in which the infant, at birth, is found to be unusually large for gestational age, while the second part details the conditions associated with small-for-gestational-age infants.

Figure 1 presents the data in graphic form. The conditions associated with large-for-gestational-age babies and those noted in small-for-gestational-age infants are boxed in at approximately the birth weight and gestational age at which they are likely to occur.

Data will be presented, when they are available, in the order of the outline to demonstrate the characteristic patterns of fetal growth. Many of the entities listed need additional study, but they are included because the purpose of the outline is to alert one to the morbidities which need to be considered in infants who deviate from the usual intrauterine growth pattern.

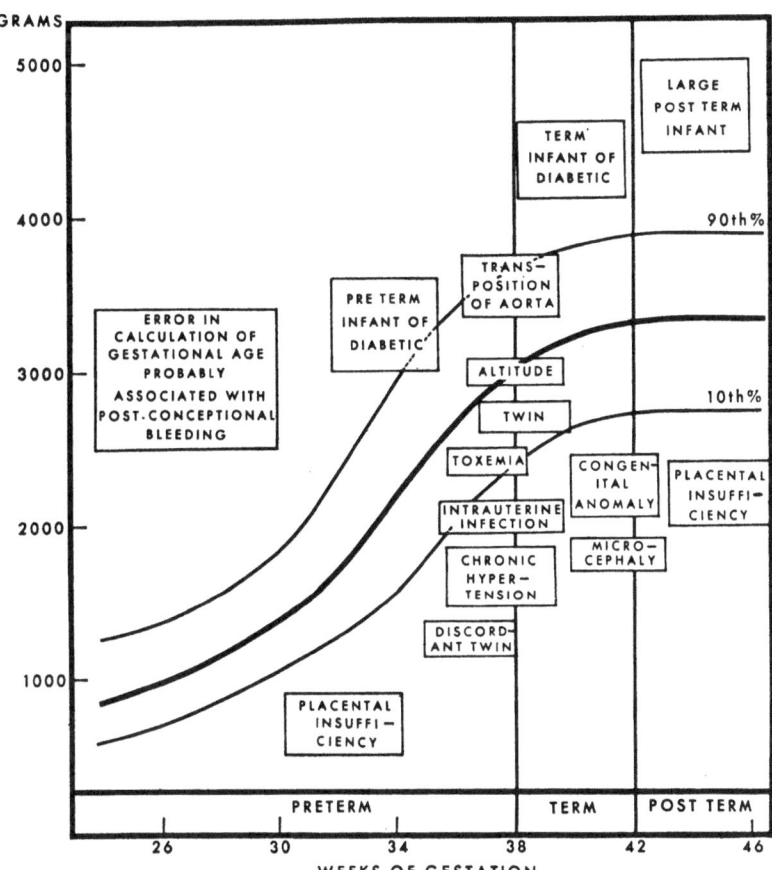

DEVIATIONS OF INTRAUTERINE GROWTH

*Fig.* 1. Graphic representation of conditions associated with deviations of intrauterine growth. The boxes symbolize the approximate birth weight and gestational age at which the condition is likely to occur.

Table 1.  *Conditions associated with deviations of intrauterine growth*

| INFANTS LARGE FOR GESTATION | ANTICIPATED MORBIDITY |
|---|---|
| 1. Large infants of short gestation.<br>   *a.* True pre-term infants. | 1. *a.* Morbidity related to pre-term delivery includes problems in establishing adequate respiration, jaundice, infection, feeding difficulties, hemorrhage, etc. |
|    *b.* Term infants, clinically. Error in calculation of gestational age presumably due to post-conceptional bleeding. |    *b.* There is an increased mortality rate. Cause is not determined. |
| 2. Large infants of long gestation (e.g., infant of 43 weeks gestation who weighs 4500 grams). | 2. Morbidity due to birth trauma. |
| 3. Offspring of diabetic mothers.<br>   *a.* Pre-term delivery.<br>   *b.* Term or post-term delivery. | 3. *a.* Respiratory distress syndrome, hypoglycemia, prematurity.<br>   *b.* Death in utero, birth trauma related to large size, hypoglycemia. |
| 4. Transposition of the aorta. | 4. Cyanosis, heart failure. |

| INFANTS SMALL FOR GESTATION | ANTICIPATED MORBIDITY |
|---|---|
| 1. Intrauterine undernutrition. | 1. Morbidity depends on the gestational age at which rate of growth is retarded, the severity and duration of undernutrition and the underlying cause. |
|    *a.* 'Placental insufficiency' (small, infarcted or aging placenta)<br>     (1) In post-term infant –<br>        There is loss of weight without retardation of growth in length and head circumference. | Morbidity is due to chronic hypoxia in utero leading to passage of meconium. Aspiration of amniotic fluid containing meconium is likely during delivery. There may be feeding problems and hypoglycemia. |
|      (2) In full term or pre-term infants –<br>        Mild undernutrition, or brief period of growth retardation near term. Growth in length and head circumference are not affected. | There may be hypoglycemia, unusual hunger and no loss in weight in the neonatal period. Rapid weight gain. |

INFANTS SMALL FOR GESTATION

Severe growth retardation or prolonged undernutrition occurring early in gestation. The infant, including the discordant twin, is very small for gestation and retardation of growth in length and head circumference may occur.

b. Multiple pregnancies –
There is decreased rate of gain in weight after about 35 weeks of gestation.
c. Hypertensive cardiovascular disease in the mother.
d. Toxemia –
Must be prolonged and severe to affect growth of infant.
e. Other conditions –
High altitude.

Maternal smoking.

2. Infants with congenital abnormalities.
a. Trisomy 21 (Down's syndrome)

b. Trisomy 16—18

c. Trisomy 13—15

d. Silver's syndrome

e. Turner's syndrome

f. de Lange's syndrome

g. Microcephaly
h. Single umbilical artery

i. 'Bird-headed dwarfs' (Seckel's syndrome)
Very small for gestational age – post-term delivery.

ANTICIPATED MORBIDITY

Mortality may be more closely related to birth weight than gestation, Increased incidence of pulmonary hemorrhage. Later physical and mental retardation are likely.

There may be hypoglycemia, etc.

Mortality may be more closely related to birth weight, etc.

Morbidity like mild undernutrition described above.

Probably late gestational growth retardation.

2. Specific morbidity listed below.

a. Hypotonia, feeding problems, heart disease, mental retardation.
b. Physical (?) and mental retardation, congenital heart defects, GU abnormalities.
c. Harelip and cleft palate, mental retardation, congenital heart defects, GU abnormalities.
d. Retarded physical growth, asymmetry, variation in sexual development, mental retardation.
e. Retarded physical growth, sterility, coarctation of aorta.
f. Feeding problems in nursery, physical and mental retardation, questionable deafness and congenital heart defects.
g. Mental and physical retardation.
h. 10 %—50 % associated congenital abnormalities, mainly GI or GU tracts.
i. Physical and mental retardation.

| INFANTS SMALL FOR GESTATION | ANTICIPATED MORBIDITY |
|---|---|
| *j.* Congenital heart disease other than transposition of great vessels. | *j.* Depends on specific defect. |
| *k.* Ostegenesis imperfecta | *k.* Fractures, high infant mortality. |
| 3. Intrauterine infection –<br>   *a.* Extended rubella syndrome | *a.* Purpura, hepatosplenomegaly, congenital cardiac and ocular defects, hearing losses, cerebral palsy and mental retardation. |
|    *b.* Cytomegalic inclusion disease | *b.* Petechiae, ecchymoses, jaundice, hepatosplenomegaly. |
|    *c.* Toxoplasmosis | *c.* Ecchymoses, hepatosplenomegaly, microcephaly, intracranial calcifications, later chorioretinitis. |
|    *d.* Syphilis | *d.* Snuffies, rash, hepatosplenomegaly, jaundice, central nervous system involvement later. |
|    *e.* Listeria | *e.* Meningitis. |

## INFANTS WHO ARE LARGE FOR GESTATIONAL AGE

Two kinds of large infants of short gestation have been identified. The first are true pre-term infants who have grown unusually well up to the time of delivery. These infants after birth have the difficulties associated with pre-term birth in proportion to the degree of prematurity. The second are large-for-gestational-age infants who are much larger than the 90th percentile and who behave like term infants. It is possible, but not definitely known, that the mothers of these babies had menstrual-like bleeding after conception and that the calculated gestational age is in error. These infants nevertheless have a greater mortality rate than do term infants of the same weight (4, 5).

Large infants of long gestation, such as the 4500-gram infants of 43 weeks gestation are seen in pregnancies where growth continues in a linear fashion post-term, presumably because of a large and adequate placenta (6). These infants are at increased risk during the newborn period because of the likelihood of birth trauma.

Mothers who have diabetes are known to produce infants at increased risk. Their intrauterine growth is characteristic and can be seen in figure 2. These infants are heavy for their gestation, they are also long and have large occipitofrontal circumferences. Their weight-

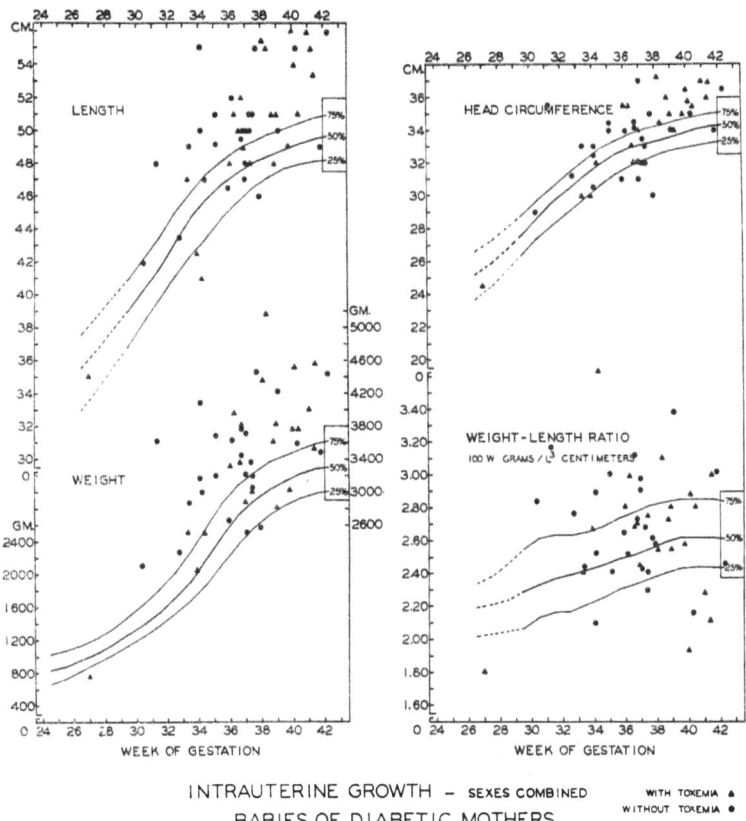

INTRAUTERINE GROWTH – SEXES COMBINED    WITH TOXEMIA ▲
BABIES OF DIABETIC MOTHERS              WITHOUT TOXEMIA ●

*Fig.* 2.   Intrauterine growth of infant of diabetic mothers. Weight, length and
head circumference are large for gestational age. The weight-length ratio indicates
that weight is not consistently excessive for length.

length ratios fall above and below the median, indicating that weight
is not consistently excessive for length.

The babies of diabetic mothers with toxemia of pregnancy were
compared with babies of diabetic mothers without toxemia because
toxemia has been reported to be associated with intrauterine growth
retardation (7). The babies in both groups are large for gestation,
but many of the infants in the toxemic group were delivered later in
pregnancy than the non-toxemic group. The head size of the infants
from toxemic diabetic mothers is larger than from the non-toxemic

group. No exact explanation has been derived for these differences, but since most diabetic mothers at Colorado General Hospital are electively delivered at approximately 37 weeks gestation, it is suggested that prenatal care was less uniform in the toxemic mother.

Two interesting reports show the association of transposition of the aorta with large babies. The average weight of 117 such infants in MEHRIZI's report (8) was 3450 grams, versus 3140 grams for control infants or for infants with other types of congenital heart lesions. NAEYE (9) studied the weights of 36 neonates with complete transposition of the aorta and found them to be large for gestational age.

## INFANTS WHO ARE SMALL FOR GESTATIONAL AGE

Infants who are small for gestational age are divided into three categories for this presentation. The first group is described under the broad term of undernutrition, the second are infants who are born with a variety of congenital anomalies and the third, infants who have acquired chronic intrauterine infections.

The term 'intrauterine undernutrition' is used in a broad sense to include a variety of conditions which result in decreased nutrients to the fetus. It is meant to include infants who are undergrown but are otherwise normal.

Placental insufficiency accompanying postmaturity has been recognized for many years (10) (figure 2a). The nutritional deprivation is brief, though it may be severe. It is late in pregnancy and results in a baby who has continued to grow in length and head circumference. However, weight falls in a much lower percentile zone than do either length or head circumference and the clinical appearance of the baby is that of one who has lost weight. The infant may have hypoglycemia in the newborn period or suffer a variable amount of intrauterine hypoxia.

Placental insufficiency may also occur in term and pre-term infants (figure 2b). In these cases, a small or infarcted placenta is usually seen, Undernutrition in the last month of pregnancy is seen with regularity in multiple births. Figure 3 shows the median growth in weight of twins cared for in Colorado General Hospital. Intrauterine growth retardation begins about 35 weeks of gestation and by 42 weeks the median weight for twins is near the 10th percentile for singletons.

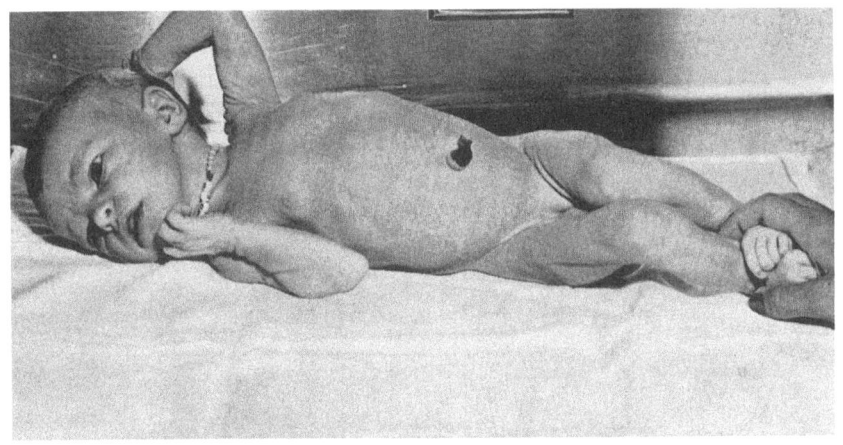

*Fig. 2a.* Post-term infant with placental insufficiency.

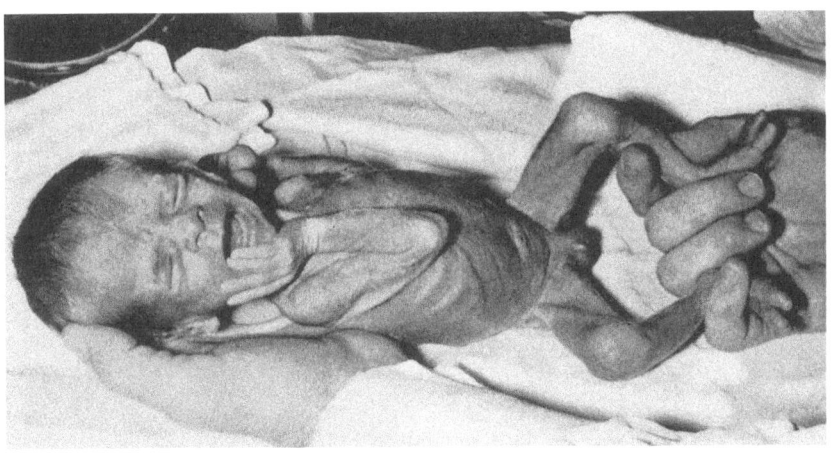

*Fig. 2b.* Pre-term infant with placental insufficiency.

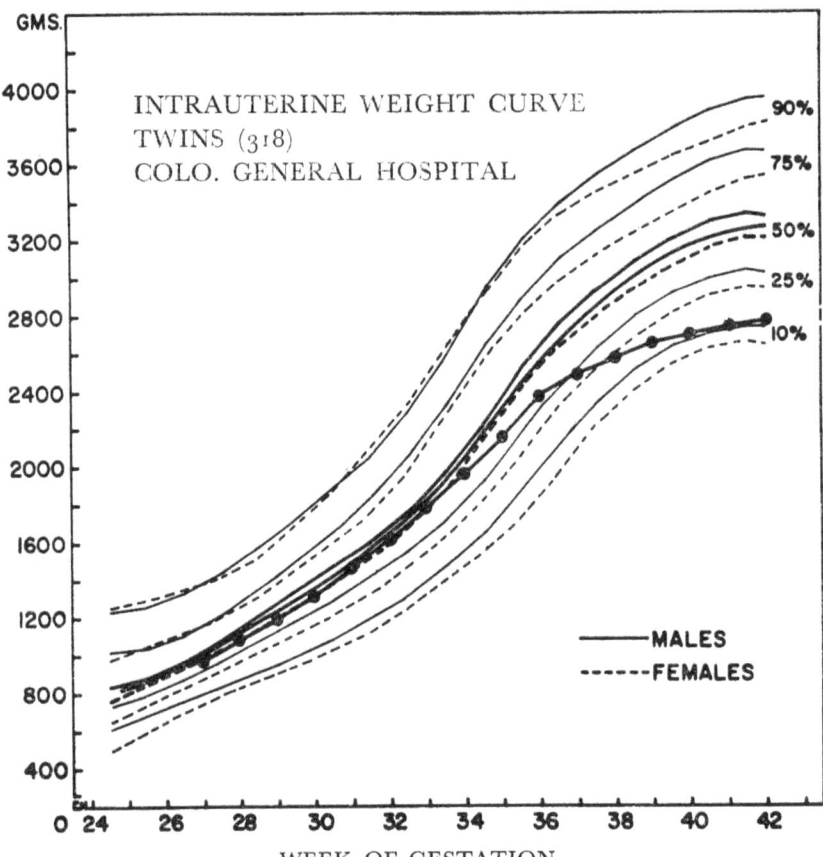

*Fig.* 3. Intrauterine growth of twins. Intrauterine growth retardation begins at about 35 weeks of gestation and by 42 weeks the median weight for twins is near the 10th percentile.

When length, head circumference and weight-length ratio are also examined (figure 4), it can be seen that growth in all dimensions is similar to the singleton prior to 35 weeks gestation. After 35 weeks, the infants of multiple gestation are found to be significantly small in all dimensions.

The sample of twins, as presented, is a mixed group of normally growing infants and infants with true intrauterine growth retardation. To observe the effect on intrauterine growth of severe or prolonged

158          L. O. LUBCHENCO ET AL.

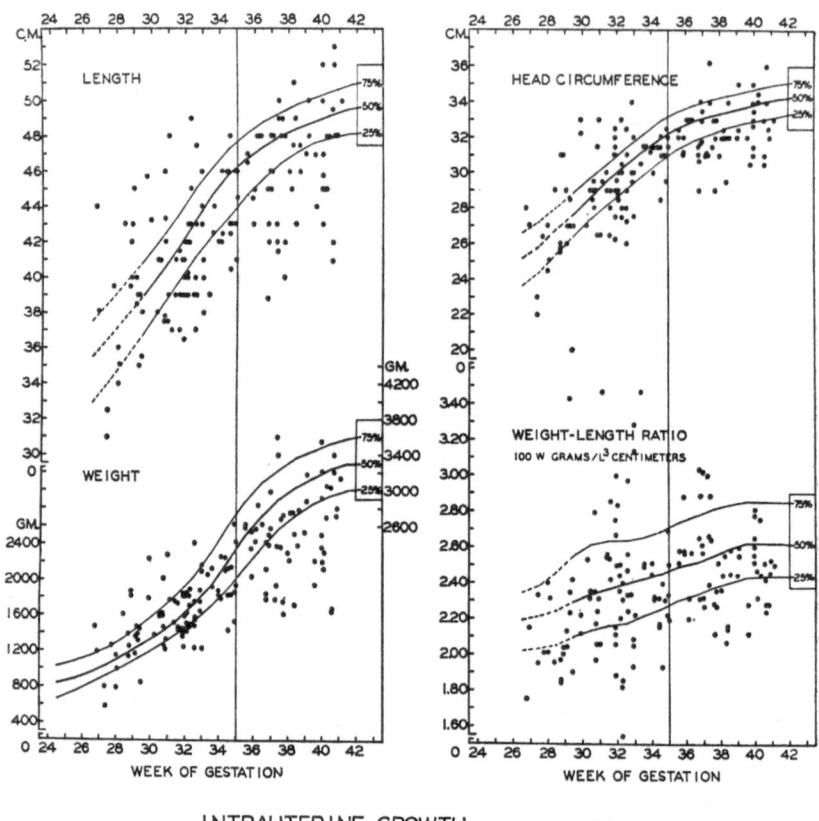

INTRAUTERINE GROWTH – SEXES COMBINED
TWINS

*Fig.* 4.  Intrauterine growth of twins. Growth in weight, length and head circumference are similar to the singleton prior to 35 weeks except for a group of short
babies at 30—32 weeks. After 35 weeks, the twins are significantly small in all
dimensions.

undernutrition, both twins of each pair of discordant twins were
studied. A 20 % difference in weight between the larger and smaller
twin was arbitrarily chosen and 17 such pairs were located among
admissions to Colorado General Hospital in a 17-year period (figure 5).

The larger of the twins was not significantly different from the
singleton, although there was a trend toward decreasing weight after
35 weeks. Length and head circumference were more evenly distributed. The smaller twin, on the other hand, was markedly smaller
in weight, length, head circumference and weight-length ratio.

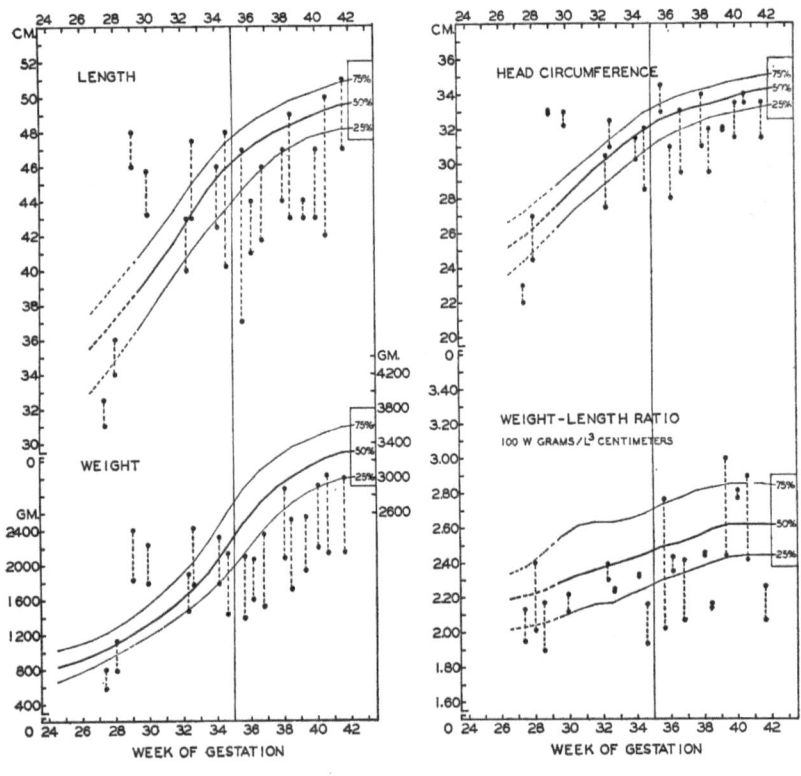

INTRAUTERINE GROWTH – SEXES COMBINED
DISCORDANT TWINS

*Fig. 5.* Intrauterine growth of discordant twins. The larger twin is not significantly different from the singleton, although there is a trend toward decreasing
weight after 35 weeks. The smaller twin is markedly smaller in weight, length and
head circumference.

Chronic cardiovascular disease in the mother results in babies small
for their gestational ages (11). Decreased blood flow to the uterus has
been found in mothers with toxemia as well (12). The size of the baby
has also been correlated with the maternal heart size; the smaller the
heart size, the smaller the baby. (13). These data suggest that the
factor in common in these three conditions is uterine circulation or
blood flow to the placenta and, hence, to the fetus. Figure 6 shows the
intrauterine growth pattern of infants of mothers who have hypertensive cardiovascular disease. Although many are normally growing,

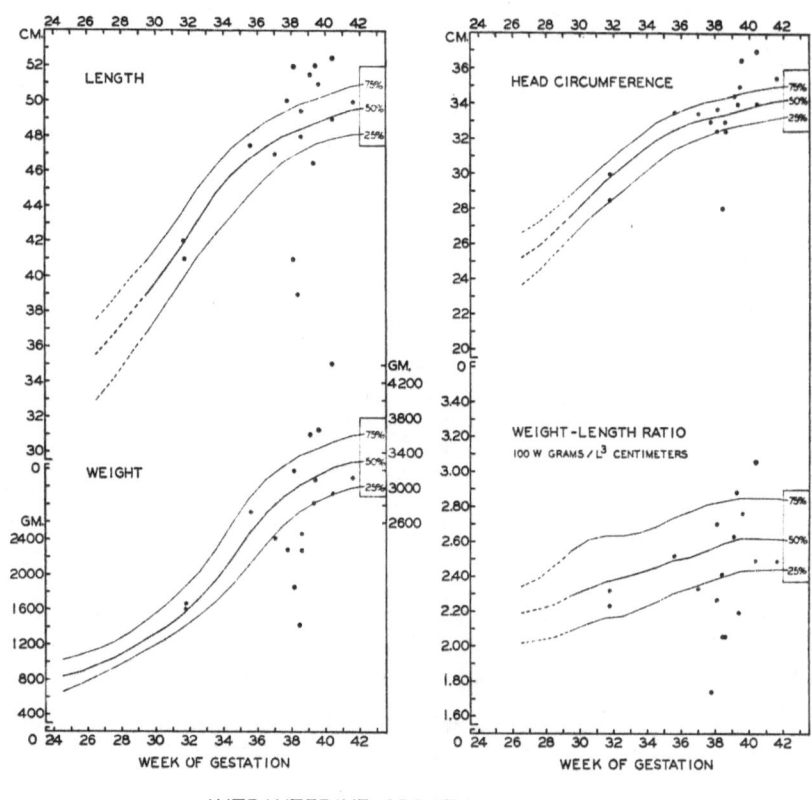

INTRAUTERINE GROWTH - SEXES COMBINED
BABIES OF HYPERTENSIVE MOTHERS

*Fig.* 6.   Intrauterine growth of infants born to mothers with hypertension. Many are normally growing, but one-third of the infants are very light weight for gestation. Fewer have retardation of length and only one shows a small head circumference.

one-third of the infants are very light for gestation. Fewer have retardation of length and only one shows a head circumference below the 10th percentile.

Toxemia has been reported to retard intrauterine growth (7) as has maternal smoking (14).

Still another situation affecting intrauterine growth is high altitude. Figure 7 shows the median weights and lengths of 137 infants born in Leadville, Colorado, a city located at 10,000 feet altitude. Head circumferences are not available for these babies. The weights

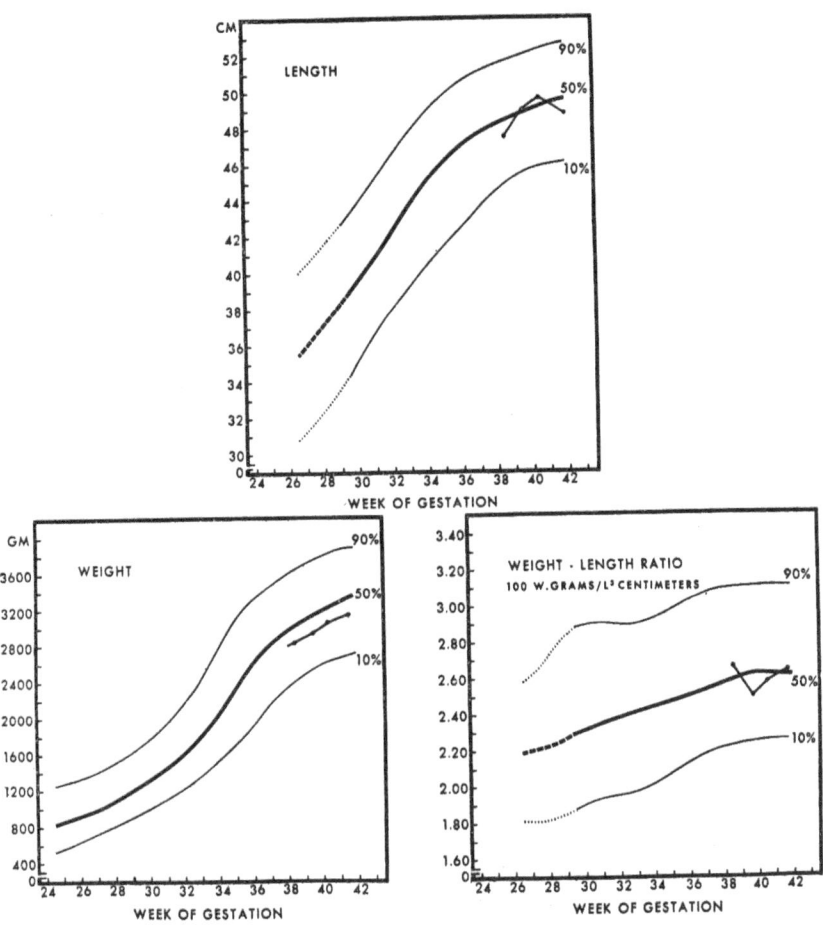

INTRAUTERINE GROWTH - LEADVILLE BABIES

*Fig.* 7. Median weights and lengths of 137 infants born at high altitude (Leadville, Colorado). Altitude has an effect on weight, but not on length.

of Leadville babies are significantly smaller than the singletons born in Denver, while lengths are evenly distributed. The majority of weight-length ratios falls between the 50th and 75th percentiles, suggesting a mixed population with shorter babies also being heavier. The findings indicate that altitude has an effect on weight, but not on length.

The second category of infants who are small for gestational age are

11

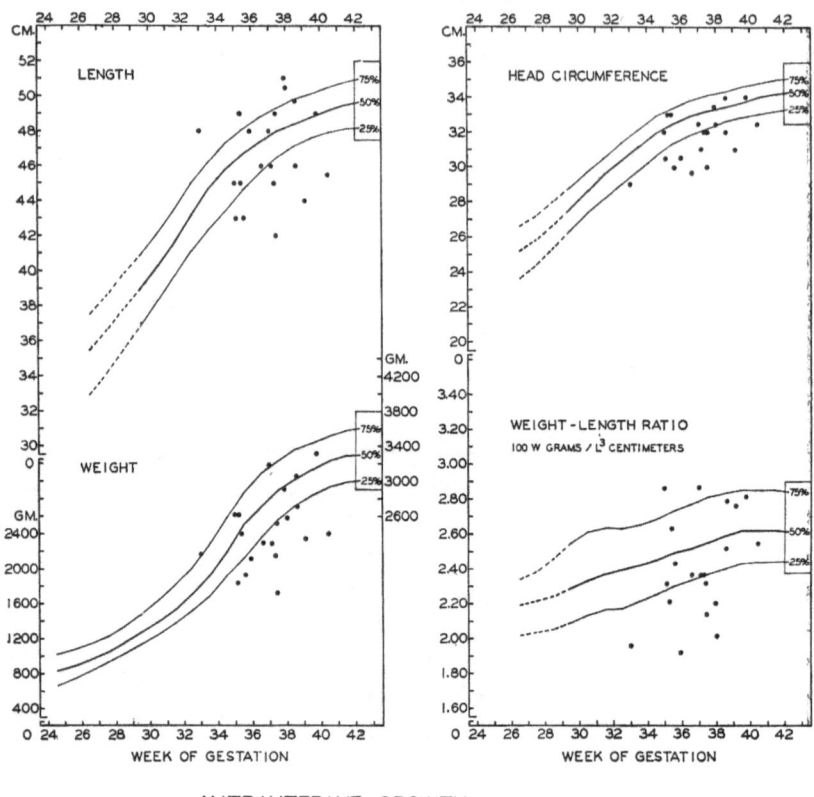

INTRAUTERINE GROWTH – SEXES COMBINED
DOWN'S SYNDROME

*Fig.* 8.   Intrauterine growth of infants with Down's syndrome. The infants are small at all gestational ages. Their lengths are normal, but head sizes are significantly reduced.

infants with congenital anomalies. The majority of these pregnancies progress to term. Gross abnormalities present no particular problem in recognition, but the more subtle syndromes may be quite difficult to identify. The 'funny looking kid' may be a child with Turner's or Silver's syndrome, Down's or other trisomy. Mongoloid babies are known to be small at birth (15); the incidence of low birth weight is approximatelt 20 %. Figure 8 shows the position on the intrauterine growth chart of infants with Down's syndrome. These infants are small at all gestational ages. Their lengths are normal, but head sizes are significantly reduced. Other trisomies, 16—18 and 13—15, also result in infants small for gestational age at birth (16). SILVER (17) describes a syndrome in children who have short stature and congenital hemihypertrophy and who show evidence of intrauterine growth retardation at birth. Other syndromes frequently associated with low birth weight at or near term are TURNER's (18) and DE LANGE's (19).

The group of children whom WARKANY described (20) and who show intrauterine growth retardation also have a high incidence of microcephaly.

The majority of newborn infants with single umbilical arteries are below the 50th percentile (21). They are especially deviant if born before term.

Recently intrauterine growth retardation in 'bird-headed dwarfs' (Seckel's Syndrome) has been described (22).

Two additional examples of intrauterine growth retardation are infants with congenital heart disease other than transposition of the aorta who are noted to be small for gestational age and infants with osteogenesis imperfecta who are strikingly small for gestation and who tend to be born before term. (9).

The list of congenital anomalies associated with intrauterine growth retardation is expected to increase as more studies of intrauterine growth are made.

Intrauterine infections often result in growth retardation in utero. Syphilis has long been related to 'premature' birth. Some babies die in utero and others are born alive in various stages of the disease. Cytomegalic inclusion disease, toxoplasmosis, listeriosis and recently the extended rubella syndrome have been shown to produce infants smaller than average for their gestational ages.

DESMOND (23) has studied the birth weights, lengths and head circumferences of 92 infants with congenital rubella and related them to the Colorado Intrauterine Growth Standards. The mean gestational age of the group is 39.5 weeks, the median weight is below the 10th percentile, median length between the 25th and 50th percentile and median head circumference is between the 10th and 25th percentile.

COMMENT

The foregoing list of conditions found in infants according to their patterns of intrauterine growth is intended to stimulate interest in the detection of high-risk infants by attention to their fetal growth. It is dependent on obtaining gestational age data or estimating length of gestation from the mother's prenatal course or from the examination of the neonate. The unusual history or birth weight for gestation provides a clue to specific morbidity.

Babies large for gestation, other than infants of diabetic mothers, have received little attention until recently (4, 5, 8, 9). Since significant morbidity exists in this group of neonates, their identification becomes increasingly important. As more data become available, their specific morbidities will be clearer.

The detection of infants who show deviations of growth, who are within the appropriate zone for gestational age, presents difficulties. It is anticipated that disproportion in growth between weight, length and head circumference will help identify the individual baby. This expectation is based on studies in early childhood where undernutrition, as a result of insufficient intake of calories or secondary to chronic disease, results in a sequence of slow weight gain or failure to gain and, finally, in severe states, weight loss. The child continues to grow in length for a period of time beyond weight retardation, depending on the severity of the nutritional deprivation. Head circumference continues to enlarge even after growth in length ceases. Animal studies (24) and other data (25) on human infants support the hypothesis that central nervous system growth and development are protected in utero and in the newborn and infant periods of life at the expense of weight and long bone growth. However, if early or prolonged undernutrition in utero occurs, length and head growth are also retarded and there may be a delay in ossification of bones and reduced or absent breast tissue (26) at the usual time of appearance of these signs of maturity.

The infants showing intrauterine growth retardation constitute the largest group of diseases that are identified. Most adverse in utero situations tend to retard the growth of the developing fetus and, therefore, more pathology would be expected in this group. The recognition of abnormality in the baby, versus abnormality in the environment is the first challenge in anticipating specific morbidity.

The diagnosis of placental insufficiency will become even more important and means of defining placental insufficiency are greatly needed. Laboratory support for isolating in utero infection will also be valuable in making definitive diagnoses in infants with infection who are physically retarded at birth.

To detect syndromes and subtle congenital anomalies, the physician is largely dependent upon clinical accumen. As diagnostic procedures such as chromosomal analyses and screening for metabolic abnormalities become more easily available, definitive diagnoses may be made during the neonatal period. Correlation of the defects with intrauterine growth will then become better established. At this time, the birth of a child who is small for gestational age should alert one to the possibility that he may have a congenital anomaly.

## SUMMARY

A list of conditions associated with deviations of intrauterine growth are given. It is meant to be a guide to the detection of high-risk-newborn infants and to suggest specific morbidities in infants with various patterns of fetal growth.

ACKNOWLEDGMENTS

The authors wish to express their appreciation to EDITH BOYD, M.D. for her long-time support and encouragement of the study of fetal growth and for her wise counsel and criticism.

## BIBLIOGRAPHY

1. LUBCHENCO, L. O. et al. (1963) *J. Pediat.* 32: 793.
2. LUBCHENCO, L. O., C. HANSMAN and E. BOYD (1966) *Pediatrics* 37: 403.
3. LICHTY, J. A. et al. (1957) *A.M.A.J. Dis. Child.* 93: 666.
4. BATTAGLIA, F. C., T. M. FRAZIER and A. E. HELLEGERS (1966) *Pediatrics* 37: 417.
5. ERHARDT, C. L. et al. (1964) *Amer. J. Pub. Health* 54: 1841.
6. GRUENWALD, P. (1966) *Am. J. Obst. and Gynec.* 94: 1112.
7. JARVINEN, P. A., P. PANKAMAA and O. KINNUMEN (1958) *Ann. Chir. Gynaec. Fenn.* (Supp. 81) 47: 76.
8. MEHRIZI, A. and A. DRASH (1961) *J. Pediat.* 39: 715.
9. NAEYE,R. L. (1966) Society for Pediatric Research, *36th Annual Meeting*, Atlantic City, New Jersey.
10. CLIFFORD, S. H. (1954) *J. Pediat.* 44: 1.
11. MACGILLIVRAY, I. (1961) *J. Obst. Gynaec. Brit. Commonwealth* 68: 557.

12. Weis, E. B. et al. (1958) *Am. J. Obst. and Gynec.* 76: 340.
13. Raiha, C. E. (1964) *Guys Hosp. Rep.* 113: 96.
14. Abernathy, J. R. et al. (1966) *Amer. J. Pub. Health* 56: 626.
15. Schaffer, A. J. (1960) *Diseases of the Newborn*, W. B. Saunders Co., Philadelphia and London.
16. Schutt, W. (1965) In: *Developmental Medicine*, No. 19, The Lavenham Press Ltd., Lavenham Suffolk, England.
17. Silver, H. K. (1964) *A.M.A.J. Dis. Child.* 107: 495.
18. Lemli, L. and D. W. Smith (1963) *J. Pediat.* 63: 577.
19. Silver, H. K. (1964) *A.M. A.J. Dis. Child.* 108: 523.
20. Warkany, J. et al. (1961) *A.M.A.J. Dis. Child.* 102: 127.
21. Butterfield, L. J. (1964) *Colorado Nurse* 64: 22.
22. Harper, R. G. et al. (1967) *J. Pediat.* 70: 799.
23. Desmond, M. Personal communication.
24. McCance, R. A. (1962) *Lancet* 2: 621 and 671.
25. Jackson, C. M. (1925) *The Effects of Inanition and Malnutrition Upon Growth and Structure* P. Blakiston and Sons, Philadelpia.
26. Silver, H. K. and P. Cunningham (1958) *A.M.A.J. Dis. Child.* 95: 649.

# THE REGULATION OF FOETAL GROWTH

MARGARET OUNSTED*

The velocity at which a human foetus grows is surprisingly variable. At term some healthy infants weigh five times more than others. In the past we have tended to regard the foetus as a quasi-independent and parasitic organism, whose growth is limited by its food supply. I have suggested elsewhere (1, 2, 3) that the matter may be more complex, and in particular that

a. a maternal regulating mechanism constrains trophoblastic invasiveness and foetal growth rate, and

b. that antigenic interaction between the conceptus and the mother may contribute to the variance in foetal growth rate.

In order to ascertain a group of growth-retarded infants a grid is necessary. Professor NEVILLE BUTLER kindly supplied me with a pre-publication copy of the Perinatal Mortality Survey grid (4). This has been employed in all our studies.

*Control series*

A random sample of women attending the ante-natal clinic were interviewed before the 20th week of gestation and followed up to delivery. The sample numbered 225.

*Growth-retarded series*

A growth-retarded infant was defined as one whose birthweight was 2 s.d. or more below the mean for the duration of gestation. This series was derived from mothers who were delivered in the same hospital during the same period of time as the control mothers. There

* Nuffield Department of Obstetrics and Gynaecology, Radcliffe Infirmary, Oxford.

were 90 probands in this series when the data were first analysed. These findings have been reported in detail elsewhere (1).

Comparison of the growth-retarded series with the controls showed that in respect of maternal age, height, abortion and stillbirth rate, ill-health, raised blood pressure, bleeding during pregnancy and duration of proband gestation the two series did not differ significantly. Heavy smokers were over-represented, and Social Class I mothers were under-represented in the growth-retarded series. Neither of these factors made more than a marginal contribution. Examination of data on the duration of previous pregnancies showed that the controls and growth-retarded series were alike. The birth-weight of previous liveborn siblings differed grossly. The mean birthweight of the control mothers' previous babies was 7*lb.* 4*oz.* (3.288 kg). The comparable figure for the growth-retarded series was 5*lb.* 12*oz.* (2.608 kg).

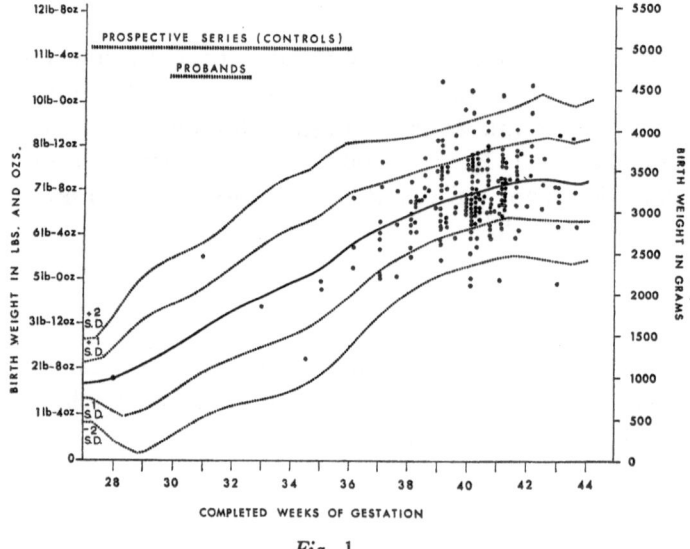

*Fig.* 1.

Figure 1 shows a scattergram of the control probands. The scatter fits well into the Perinatal Mortality Survey grid.

Figure 2 shows the scatter of the liveborn singleton siblings of the controls — again the grid is well fitted.

Figure 3 demonstrates the growth-retarded probands, who by

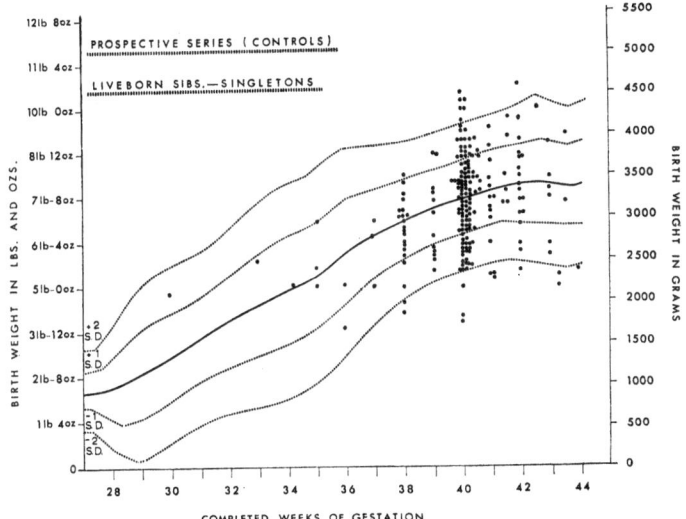

*Fig.* 2.

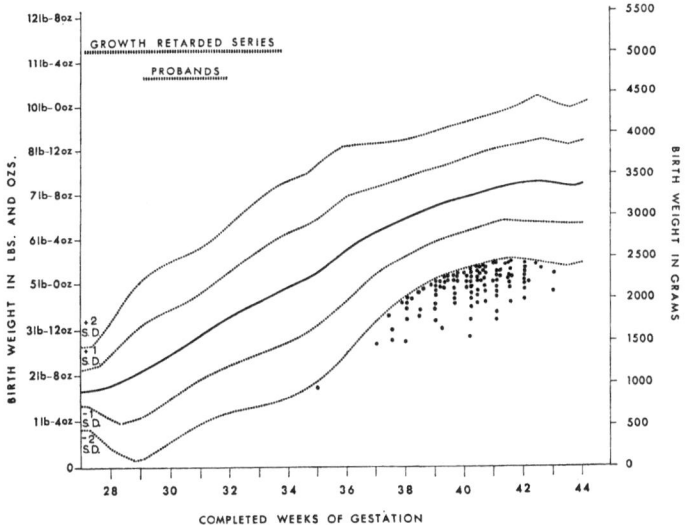

*Fig.* 3.

definition all lay below the second standard deviation. The series numbered 117 probands when the scattergrams were made.

Figure 4 shows the distribution of liveborn singleton siblings in the growth-retarded series. None of these weighed more than 1 s.d. above the mean, and 60 % were themselves growth-retarded by 1 s.d. or more. Thus these mothers appeared regularly to constrain the growth of all their young.

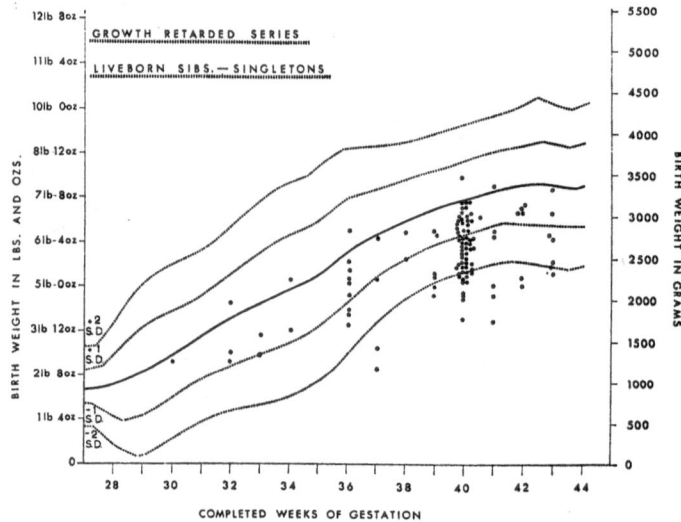

*Fig.* 4.

## Short-gestation prematurity

From a group of 283 consecutive liveborn infants who satisfied the old international definition of prematurity, all those whose birth-weight lay within 1 s.d. of the mean for the lenght of gestation, were taken. They numbered 100. These infants can be regarded as those in whom low birth-weight was determined by the brevity of their gestation. Figure 5 shows the probands.

Figure 6 shows the scatter of the liveborn siblings of these short gestation prematures. Their mean birth-weight was 7*lb*. 0*oz*. (3.175 kg) The distribution is closely similar to that of the controls, and highly

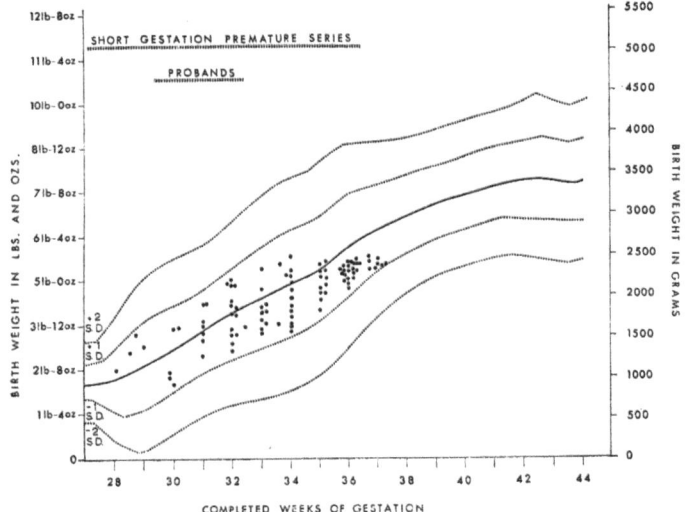

*Fig.* 5.

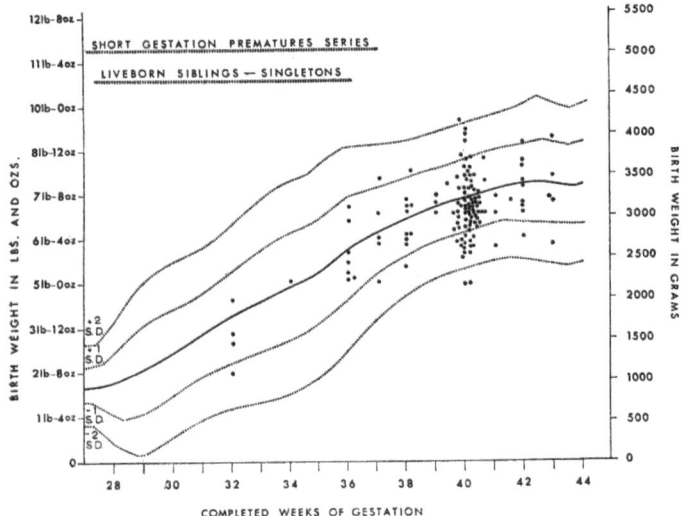

*Fig.* 6.

significantly different from that of the **growth**-retarded series' liveborn
siblings. Thus we see that short-gestation prematurity, unlike growth-
retardation, does not usually repeat itself.

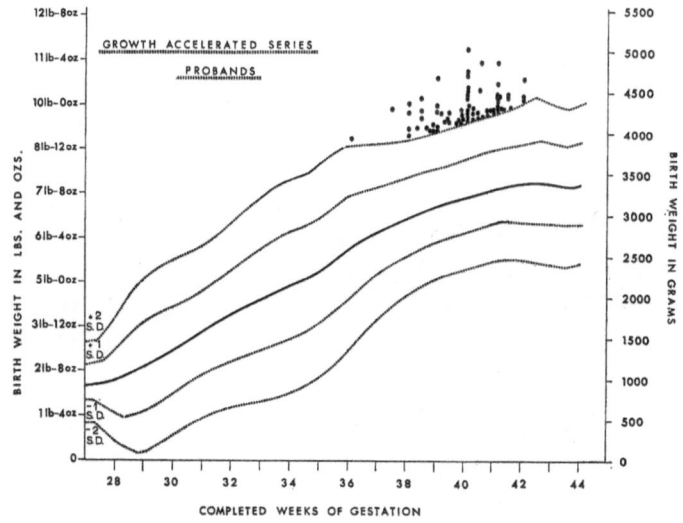

*Fig.* 7.

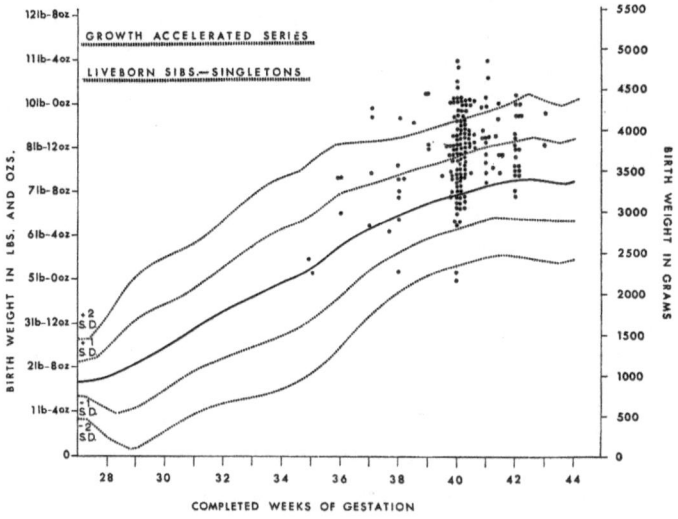

*Fig.* 8.

PERCENTAGES OF LIVEBORN SIBLINGS CLASSIFIED BY STANDARD DEVIATIONS
ABOVE OR BELOW THE MEAN BIRTH WEIGHT FOR THE PERIOD GESTATION

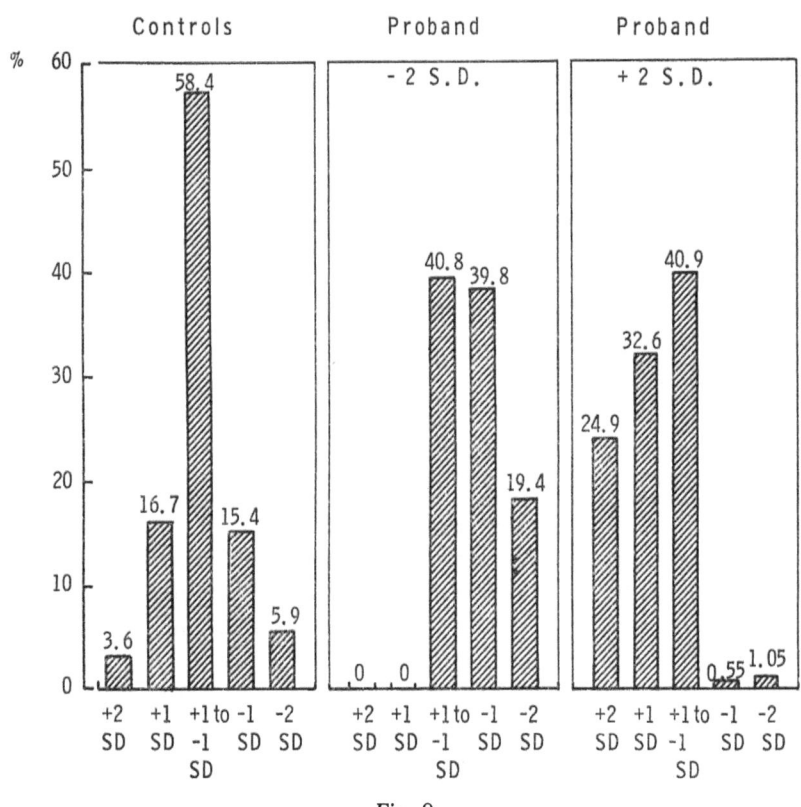

Fig. 9.

*Growth-acceleration*

Next a group of babies who were accelerated in intra-uterine growth
was considered. The operational definition of a growth-accelerated
infant was that its birth-weight lay 2 s.d. or more above the mean for
the duration of gestation. Figure 7 shows these 77 large probands.

In figure 8 the liveborn siblings of this group are shown. They scatter
in the reverse fashion from the siblings of the growth-retarded probands. Their median birth-weight was 8*lb*. 10*oz*. (3.913 kg). Only

three were more than 1 s.d. below the mean. Nearly two-thirds lie above the first standard deviation.

These findings may be condensed into a histogram: figure 9. Here the liveborn siblings in the control, growth-retarded and growth-accelerated series were arranged in standard deviations above or below the mean. This demonstrates that the growth-accelerated and growth-retarded series differed from controls to the same degree but in the opposite sense.

These findings suggest that, in our region, where the population as a whole is healthy and prosperous and where obstetric care is excellent, that socio-economic and pathological factors play only a minor role in controlling the rate of foetal growth in utero at its extremes. The main factor seems to be a biological one of maternal regulation which is fairly constant for any given woman, and quantitative in its action.

## The placenta

The growth of the foetus and placenta go hand in hand. Dr.W. AHERNE (4a) examined morphometrically 20 placentae from our growth-retarded series. He found that they were significantly smaller than normal by weight and on the whole tended to be smaller even than (uninfarcted) placentae from toxaemic patients. The reduction in size (or rather the size deficit) appeared to affect mainly the parenchymal tissue. Non-parenchymal structures such as chorion, decidua, big vessels etc., were less obviously smaller than normal. Histologically the majority of sections showed no clear abnormality, but occasionally one encountered groups of avascular villi as described by GRUENWALD (4b), or intervillous fibrin deposition in excess of the usual amounts. However, the over-riding impression one had was that the main characteristic of these placentae was simply their relatively small quantity of villous tissue. What there was of this usually appeared histologically normal.

## Maternal intrauterine growth rate

Comparison of adult height in the control series and in an enlarged series of 147 mothers who had born growth-retarded infants showed that adult height was the same in both series, the figure at the mean being 5 ft. 3 ins. (1.60 m).

Information about their own weight at birth was sought from the mothers. About two-thirds of the mothers in both series were able to supply this. Figure 10 is a histogram of maternal birth-weight in the two series. Mean birth-weight in the control series was 7*lb.* 2*oz.* (3.22 kg) and in the growth-retarded series it was 6*lb.* 4*oz.* (2.835 kg).

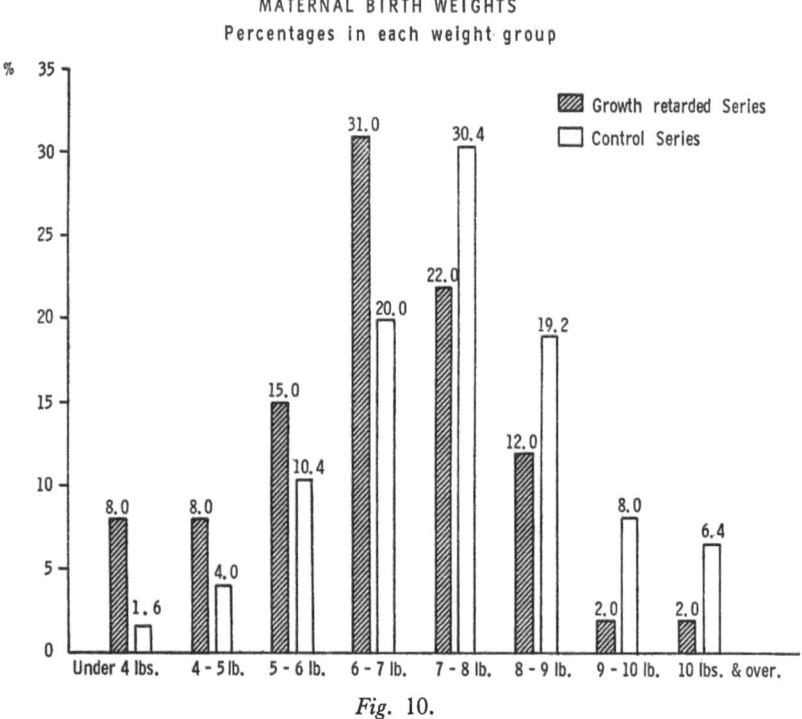

*Fig.* 10.

The histogram suggests a shift of about 1 standard deviation to the left in the distribution of maternal birth-weight in the growth-retarded series. Thus the mothers, like the siblings of growth-retarded probands, seem rather regularly to have been constrained in intrauterine growth.

These data suggest that the factors controlling intrauterine growth are distinct from those factors which govern growth after delivery. They also prompted the suggestion that the quantitative set of the maternal regulator may not simply be determined by the maternal genotype but may also be influenced by the degree of constraint imposed upon the mother when she herself was a foetus.

## The growth-retarded infants

It has been proposed that physiological mechanisms rather than pathological accidents are responsible for most of the growth-retarded infants in our series. This should not be taken to imply that these infants are simply a random sample of the foetal population. One of the main ways in which they differ is that of sex. Table 1a shows

Table 1a. *Sex of probands*

|  | Females | % | Males | % | Total | % |
|---|---|---|---|---|---|---|
| Growth-retarded series | 91 | 62 | 56 | 38 | 147 | 100 |
| Growth-accelerated series | 18 | 23.4 | 59 | 76.6 | 77 | 100 |
| Short gestation prematures | 42 | 42.4 | 57 | 57.6 | 99 | 100 |
| Control series | 101 | 45 | 124 | 55 | 225 | 100 |

that among both controls and short gestation prematures the sex ratios of the probands are very much what one would expect. Controls: 122.8 males per 100 females; short gestation prematures 135.7 males per 100 females. In the growth-accelerated series boys are grossly over-represented: 327 males per 100 females. In the growth-retarded series boys are under-represented: 61.5 males per 100 females. These deviant sex ratios are not altogether unexpected since it is known that boys, in general, grow faster than girls in utero.

The sex ratios among the liveborn siblings were also examined. Table 1b shows that all four groups are alike, and none of them differs significantly from the sex ratio of the general population at birth.

Table 1b. *Sex of liveborn siblings*

|  | Females | % | Males | % | Total | % |
|---|---|---|---|---|---|---|
| Growth-retarded series | 72 | 49.5 | 73 | 50.5 | 145 | 100 |
| Growth-accelerated series | 101 | 55 | 82 | 45 | 183 | 100 |
| Short gestation prematures | 62 | 53 | 55 | 47 | 117 | 100 |
| Control series | 109 | 50 | 109 | 50 | 218 | 100 |

*Labour and delivery*

One might have anticipated that the constraint of intrauterine growth would give growth-retarded infants an advantage in the mechanics of delivery. This was not the case.

Table 2. *Labour and delivery*

2a

| | Control Series | | Growth-retarded Series | | Total |
|---|---|---|---|---|---|
| Onset of Labour: | | | | | |
| Spontaneous | 172 | 76% | 100 | 68% | 272 |
| Induced | 53 | 24% | 47 | 32% | 100 |
| Total | 225 | | 147 | | 372 |

2b

| | Control Series | | Growth-retarded Series | | Total |
|---|---|---|---|---|---|
| Vaginal Deliveries: | | | | | |
| Cephalic | 199 ⎰ 207 | 92% | 121 ⎰ 126 | 86% | 320 ⎰ 333 |
| Breech | 8 ⎱ | | 5 ⎱ | | 13 ⎱ |
| Caesarean Sections | 18 | 8% | 21 | 14% | 39 |
| Total | 225 | | 147 | | 372 |

2c

| | Control Series | | Growth-retarded Series | | Total |
|---|---|---|---|---|---|
| Forceps Delivery | 60 | 29% | 34 | 27% | 94 |
| Unaided Delivery | 147 | 71% | 92 | 73% | 239 |
| Total | 207 | | 126 | | 333 |

12

Table 2a shows that labour was induced equally often in the two series.

Table 2b shows that a slightly higher proportion of growth-retarded infants were delivered by Caesarian section than controls.

Perhaps the most surprising figure appears in Table 2c. Forceps were applied almost as often in the growth-retarded series as in the control series. This fact should be seen in the light of the Perinatal Mortality Survey findings (5) which showed that intra-partum asphyxia was four times more frequent is score minus 2 babies which came to post-mortem, than in score zero cases. The application of forceps in the delivery of a growth-retarded infant may commonly have been prompted by intra-partum foetal distress.

## The infants at birth

Because of difficulty in accurately ascertaining time of death, and therefore length of gestation, macerated foetuses were not included in the growth-retarded series. Table 3 shows that there were no fresh stillbirths in the growth-retarded series, and 3 neonatal deaths compared with 2 in the control series. I should like to emphasize that our obstetric and paediatric teams gave these infants intensive attention, and one should not, I think, generalise from these figures to the fate of growth-retarded infants in the country as a whole.

Table 3. *Infants at birth*

|  | Control Series | Growth-retarded Series | Total |
|---|---|---|---|
| Stillbirths: |  |  |  |
|   Macerated | 1 | — | 1 |
|   Fresh | 0 | 0 | 0 |
| Neonatal Deaths | 2 | 3 | 5 |
| Discharged from |  |  |  |
|   hospital alive | 222 | 144 | 366 |
|                        Total | 225 | 147 | 372 |

*Neonatal deaths*

|  | Control Series | Growth-retarded Series | Total |
|---|---|---|---|
| Intrauterine Asphyxia | 1 | 1 | 2 |
| Extreme Immaturity | 1 | 0 | 1 |
| Bronchopneumonia | 0 | 1 | 1 |
| Multiple Congenital Abnormalities | 0 | 1 | 1 |
| Total | 2 | 3 | 5 |

*Congenital abnormalities*

Some congenital abnormalities, such as the trisomies, are associated with intrauterine growth retardation. Table 4 sets out the facts in our series. It will be seen that congenital abnormality made a negligible contribution to the growth-retarded population as a whole.

Table 4. *Congenital abnormalities*

|  | Control Series (225) | Growth-retarded Series (147) | Total |
|---|---|---|---|
| Down's Syndrome | 1 | 1 | 2 |
| Exomphalos | 1 | 0 | 1 |
| Microcephaly | 1 | 0 | 1 |
| Anencephaly | 1 | 0 | 1 |
| Congenital Heart Disease | 0 | 2 | 2 |
| Osteogenesis Imperfecta | 0 | 1 | 1 |
| Multiple Defects | 0 | 1 | 1 |
| Total | 4 | 5 | 9 |

*Neonatal anxiety*

Although we have suggested that biological mechanisms are prepotent in the regulation of intrauterine growth, this by no means implies that growth-retarded infants are not at risk. The two series were analysed for what I have called severe perinatal anxiety; the criterion

Table 5. *Severe perinatal anxiety*

|  | Control Series | | Growth-retarded Series | | Total |
|---|---|---|---|---|---|
| Severe perinatal anxiety | 13 | 5,8 % | 30 | 20.4 % | 43 |
| The rest | 211 | 94.2 % | 117 | 79.6 % | 328 |
| Total | 224 | | 147 | | 371 |

$x^2 = 18.5$

being whether the infant had established regular respirations within 5 minutes of delivery, or not. The infants were intubated if necessary, in the majority of cases, within a few minutes of delivery. Table 5 shows that a much higher proportion of the growth-retarded series gave rise to severe perinatal anxiety than the control series. The differences are highly significant. Perinatal anxiety was then sub-divided:

*a.* Infants who gave rise to no further anxiety in the neonatal period once regular respirations were established.

*b.* Infants who continued to give rise to anxiety during the first few days of life.

*c.* Neonatal deaths.

The two series were also sub-divided according to the sex of the proband. Table 6 shows the figures. Although boys have the advan-

Table 6. *Severe perinatal anxiety according to sex and kind*

Males

|  |  | Control Series | | Growth-retarded Series | | Total | |
|---|---|---|---|---|---|---|---|
| Severe perinatal anxiety | | | | | | | |
| | A | 5 ⎫ | | 11 ⎫ | | 16 ⎫ | |
| | B | 3 ⎬ 9 | 7.3 % | 3 ⎬ 16 | 28.6 % | 6 ⎬ 25 | |
| | C | 1 ⎭ | | 2 ⎭ | | 3 ⎭ | |
| The rest | | 115 | | 40 | | 155 | |
| | Total | 124 | | 56 | | 180 | |

Females

|  | Control Series | Growth-retarded Series | Total |
|---|---|---|---|
| Severe perinatal anxiety | | | |
| A | 2 ⎫ | 9 ⎫ | 11 ⎫ |
| B | 1 ⎬ 4   4.0 % | 4 ⎬ 14  15.4 % | 5 ⎬ 18 |
| C | 1 ⎭ | 1 ⎭ | 2 ⎭ |
| The rest | 96 | 77 | 173 |
| | — | — | |
| Total | 100 | 91 | 191 |

Males and Females

|  | Control Series | Growth-retarded Series | Total |
|---|---|---|---|
| Total | 224 | 147 | 371 |

tage in growth rate, and hence fewer boys than girls were growth-retarded, yet males were more vulnerable during the neonatal period than females in both series, and there is the same order of difference between the two sexes and between the two series:

1. Female controls 4 %
2. Male controls 7.3 %
3. Female growth-retarded infants 15.4 %
4. Male growth-retarded infants 28.6 %

BUTLER (5) found, for all perinatal deaths, that male mortality is always higher, the difference being minimal at the average weight for gestation, increasing progressively as score minus two is reached. Our findings confirm this for perinatal morbidity, and indicate the necessity of growth-retarded infants being delivered in hospital where skilled resuscitation is to hand.

Among those infants who established regular respirations early, an equal proportion in both series needed attention from the paediatricians during the neonatal period for a variety of other reasons. As before, in both series, the boys were more vulnerable than the girls.

The notion that the constraint or acceleration of intrauterine growth is determined by a maternal regulator stems from the classical studies on the horse which Sir JOHN HAMMOND and his colleagues reported on in 1938 (6). These showed that foals born to Shetland dams of Shire sires were similar in birth weight to pure Shetland foals. Foals of Shire dams by Shetland sires were nearly as large at birth as pure Shire foals. Thus maternal regulation in the horse was prepotent in determining the velocity of intrauterine growth.

Similar experiments have since been reported in several different species of mammal. VENGE (7), working with rabbits, transplanted fertilized ova from large to small breeds and vice versa. He showed marked maternal effects on the growth rate of the foetus which were independent of the foetal genotype. HUNTER (8) demonstrated comparable maternal effects by crossbreeding and egg transplantation experiments in large and small breeds of sheep. We have suggested (3) that in women a maternal regulator operates; that it is set within fairly narrow limits and that it may receive part of its set from the intrauterine experience of the mother.

One way of testing these notions is to look at the quantitative likeness in birth weight in different classes of relative. MORTON studied this in detail (9), and here his findings are rearranged and eight classes of relative arrayed in order of the size of the intraclass correlation between them. The sequence from the largest to the smallest is as follows:

|      |                                                          |        |
| ---- | -------------------------------------------------------- | ------ |
| I.   | Opposite-sexed twins                                     | 0.655  |
| II.  | Maternal half-siblings                                   | 0.581  |
| III. | Like-sexed twins                                         | 0.557  |
| IV.  | Full siblings adjacent in birth rank (unrelated parents) | 0.523  |
| V.   | Full siblings adjacent in birth rank (first cousin parents) | 0.481 |
| VI.  | Full siblings with one sibling intervening               | 0.425  |
| VII. | Full siblings with two siblings intervening              | 0.363  |
| VIII.| Paternal half-siblings                                   | 0.102  |

There is not time to expand on this fascinating sequence. I would like, however, to draw attention to the high correlation between half-siblings related through a common mother, and the low correlation between half-siblings related through a common father. ROBSON's study (10) showed similarly that the correlation between the birth weights of *maternal* first cousins was positive, whereas the correlation in birth weight between *paternal* and *mixed* first cousins was very small, and could not be shown to depart significantly from zero. The simplest interpretation of these studies is that maternal regulation accounts for much of the variance.

Another factor which contributed at the extremes of growth rate in our series was the sex of the foetus. There was a marked increase in girls among the growth-retarded, and an even more notable increase in boys among the growth-accelerated infants. It may be that the male advantage in growth rate in utero is not simply due to the inherent XY constitution of males. An interactional process between the XY system of the conceptus and the maternal system, which is necessarily XX, is another possibility.

Although the sex ratios among the probands in both the growth-retarded and growth-accelerated series were grossly deviant, the sex ratios among the siblings did not differ in any of the groups studied.

My husband showed (11), and HEWITT and his colleagues confirmed (12), that though the frequencies of all-female sibships and mixed sibships of all types can be explained by chance, there exists within the general population an excess of women who generate all-male single-sexed sibships. Some women, in a word, only bear sons. The normal sex ratio found among the siblings of both growth-retarded and growth-accelerated probands suggests that this phenomenon of all-male single-sexed sibships, though biologically interesting, is not relevent to our present problem.

Other foetal factors which affect the rate of intrauterine growth seem to be relatively uncommon. SCHUTT (13) has suggested that many infants with chromosomal aberrations are retarded in their intra-uterine growth. Severe connective tissue disease such as osteo-genesis imperfecta congenita reduces intra-uterine growth rate, but hereditary skeletal tissue disease, like achondroplasia, does not do so. Intra-uterine dwarfs such as the bird-headed and Russel-Silver types should be mentioned. In general, abnormalities of the foetus appeared to make little contribution in the present study.

In a series of elegant experiments, KIRBY and his colleagues have

shown that the velocity of placental growth depends in part on immunological factors. BILLINGTON (14), working with mice, has shown that
the antigenic dissimilarity of mother and foetus is quantitatively
related to the size of the placenta: the greater the antigenic difference,
the larger the placenta. Placental size depends upon the extent of
trophoblastic invasion of the maternal decidual tissue. This invasion
is more extensive when the trophoblast is antigenically dissimilar
from the decidua than when it is similar. JAMES (15) confirmed these
findings and has shown that the immunological sensitivity of the
mother to foetal antigens can be manipulated to demonstrate that the
greater the mother's sensitivity the larger the placenta. KIRBY (16)
has shown that trophoblast transplanted into other tissues of the body
will rampantly invade them. In the uterus the invasion of the trophoblast is constrained by the decidua. Quantitative constraint of the
trophoblast in mice is probably exercised by a chemical specific to
the decidua. Thus there exists a possible mechanism for the modul-
ation of foetal growth rate. It may be of interest here to note that
SCIARRA and his colleagues (17) have shown that a growth promoting
hormone is to be found in the syncytial cytoplasm of the villous
trophoblast. This substance has been identified in human placentae
as early as the twelfth week. We may speculate that, if the quantity
of growth hormone produced were a function of trophoblastic exube-
rance, then a mechanism underlying the rules governing foetal
growth might emerge.

I have not been able to find much literature on antigenic relationships
between the foetus and the human mother. MORTON (18) did however,
show that consanguineous unions between first cousins reduced birth
weight. They also reduced the postnatal dimensions of such infants
at the age of 8 months in respect of height and chest girth but not,
interestingly enough, in respect of skull circumference. These findings
are quite compatible with the experimental data I have mentioned.
It is possible also that the differing velocities of intrauterine growth
in the two sexes may have an antigenic explanation. Sons plainly
differ from their mother more than daughters do.

It has been suggested (1) that prospective physiological studies
should be made in women who have borne growth-accelerated and
growth-retarded infants when they are again pregnant, since we know
that we are rather likely to be monitoring another such pregnancy.

But here one would like to sound a note of caution. If we should find a correlation between the urinary output, say, of a particular hormone, and the rate of foetal growth we should not assume a causal relationship. For example, FRANDSEN (19) showed that there was a very close correlation between the birth weight of the infant and the urinary output of oestriol by the mother. Oestriol is probably generated by a complex interaction between the placenta and the foetal zone of the foetus' adrenal gland. The foetal adrenal is thought to produce a steroid precursor which is aromatized in the placenta to produce oestrogens. This might suggest that oestriol and its related compounds were involved in the regulation of the growth of the conceptus. But in anencephalic monsters the foetal zone of the adrenal is usually absent and their mothers' oestriol excretion is much reduced. Nevertheless the somatic growth rate of the anencephalus is normal and so is that of her placenta. It seems likely that the high correlation between birth-weight and the level of oestriol excretion is not causal but simply a reflection of the well-known relationship between placental capacity and foetal growth rate.

The theoretical notions in this paper may be briefly summarized. We propose that two main variables external to the foetal genotype control the rate of intrauterine growth: the antigenic dissimilarity of the mother and the foetus and the predetermined set of the maternal regulator which operates by the decidual constraint of trophoblastic invasiveness. The rate of growth of a foetus, it is suggested, is a reflection of the relative potency of each of these factors. Within a sibship maternal constraint will be relatively constant but the velocity of growth will be conditional on the antigenic interactions of the mother and each individual foetus. Thus infants within a sibship will vary in birth-weight but will tend to cluster together when due correction is made for their length of gestation. These theories are proposed with heuristic, rather than explanatory intent.

One method of studying the problem further might be by means of egg transplantation experiments in mammals followed through several generations. In human work we can seldom arrange marriages to suit our convenience, but our theories predict certain relationships in birth-weight between different kinds of kin. For example, one would expect to find that first cousins of growth-retarded probands through maternal uncles did not differ in birth-weight from controls.

First cousins through maternal aunts should, if our notions have any strength, show constraint in the velocity of their intrauterine growth. The pedigrees which I have so far been able to examine do not conflict with this prediction.

## SUMMARY

1. A series of growth-retarded infants was compared with a control series for maternal factors. Maternal age, height, abortion rate, ill-health, raised blood pressure and bleeding during pregnancy did not differ between the two series.

2. The durations of proband gestations were comparable in the two series.

3. Heavy smokers were over-represented in the growth-retarded series, and Social Class I mothers were under-represented. Neither of these two factors made more than a marginal contribution.

4. The durations of previous pregnancies were alike in the two series.

5. Birth-weights of previous liveborn siblings differed grossly. The mothers of growth-retarded infants had had no large young.

6. A series of short-gestation premature infants was examined. The distributions both of lengths of previous gestations and birth-weights of liveborn siblings were similar to controls.

7. The pattern of birth-weights among the siblings in a series of growth-accelerated probands differed from controls in a way similar to that of the growth-retarded series, but in the opposite sense.

8. The placentae of growth-retarded infants appeared small but otherwise healthy.

9. The birth-weights of mothers of growth-retarded infants were reduced by about one standard deviation.

10. Boys were grossly over-represented in the growth-accelerated series.

11. Girls were over-represented in the growth-retarded series.

12. No deviation from the expected sex ratio was found among the siblings of any of the series.

13. The growth-retarded series did not differ from controls in:
a. The mode of presentation of the foetus
b. The frequency of induced labours
c. The frequency of instrumental delivery
d. The frequency of Caesarean section.

14. Congenital abnormality was not markedly increased among the infants in the growth-retarded series.

15. Failure to establish regular respirations within 5 minutes of birth occurred with the following frequency:
a. Female controls 4 %
b. Male controls 7.3 %
c. Female growth-retarded 15.4 %
d. Male growth-retarded 28.6 %

16. Other forms of neonatal anxiety, in those infants who established regular respirations within 5 minutes of birth did not differ in the two series, boys again being more at risk than girls.

17. The findings of this paper are discussed in the light of the literature. It is suggested that two parameters may control the velocity of intrauterine growth: the predetermined set of the maternal regulator, and the degree of antigenic dissimilarity between the conceptus and the mother.

18. A speculative sketch of the possible physiological mechanisms is tentatively outlined.

### REFERENCES

1. OUNSTED, M. (1965) *Develop. Med. Child Neurol.* 7: 479.
2. OUNSTED, M. (1966) *Develop. Med. Child Neurol.* 8: 3.
3. OUNSTED, M. and C. OUNSTED (1966) *Nature* 212: 5066, 995.
4. BUTLER, N. R. , *Perinatal Mortality*, Vol. II (in the press).
4a.AHERNE, W. (1966) Personal communication.
4b.GRUENWALD, P. (1963) Biol. Neonat. 5: 215.
5. BUTLER, N. (1965) in Gestational Age, Size and Maturity *Clinics in Developmental Medicine*, No. 19, W. Heinemann, Ltd., London, pp. 74—82.

6. WALTON, A. and J. HAMMOND (1938) *Proc. Roy. Soc. B.* 125: 311.
7. VENGE, O. (1950) *Acta Zoologica* 31: 1, 1.
8. HUNTER, G. L. (1965) *J. Agric. Sci.* 48: 36.
9. MORTON, N. E. (1955) *Ann. Hum. Genet.* 20: 125.
10. ROBSON, E. B. (1955) *Ann. Hum. Genet.* 19: 262.
11. OUNSTED, C. (1953) *J. Neurol. Neurosurg. Psychiat.* 16: 267.
12. HEWITT, D., J. W. WEBB, A. M. STEWART (1955) *Ann. Hum. Genet.* 20: 155.
13. SCHUTT, W. (1965) in Gestational Age, Size and Maturity, *Clinics in Developmental Medicine*, No. 19, W. Heinemann, Ltd., London, pp. 1—7.
14. BILLINGTON, W. D. (1964) *Nature* 202: 317.
15. JAMES, D. A. (1965) *Nature* 205: 613.
16. KIRBY, D. R. S. (1965) in the Early Conceptus, Normal and Abnormal (edit. by PARK, W. W.), Livingstone, London, pp. 68—73.
17. SCIARRA, J. J., S. L. KAPLAN, M. M. GRUMBACH (1963) *Nature* 199: 1006.
18. MORTON, N. E. (1958) *Amer. J. Hum. Genet.* 10: 344.
19. FRANDSEN, V. A. (1965) *Europ. Rev. Endocrin.* 1: 227.

ACKNOWLEDGMENTS

I am grateful to Professor J. CHASSAR MOIR and Dr. VICTORIA SMALLPEICE for jointly sponsoring this work. Mr. JOHN STALLWORTHY, Mr. MOSTYN EMBREY, the late Mr. WILLIAM HAWSKWORTH, Mr. ARTHUR WILLIAMS, Dr. HUGH ELLIS and Dr. BRIAN BOWER kindly gave me access to their patients. I am grateful to Professor NEVILLE BUTLER for providing me with a pre-publication copy of the Perinatal Mortality Survey grid and Dr. W. AHERNE for his examination of the placentae. I should also like to thank my husband Dr. CHRISTOPHER OUNSTED, who plays a major role in all my work.

# DISCUSSION

DISCUSSION PAPER DR. LUBCHENCO

*Dr. Widdowson* (in the chair): Thank you very much, Dr. LUBCHENCO, for the clear presentation of your data. This paper is open for fiscussion.

*Dr. Drillien:* I should like to comment on the group of babies in which Dr. LUBCHENCO thought there was an error in calculation of the gestation period. These large babies were said to be praematurely born appeared to be perfectly normal, except that they had a higher mortality rate. If as Dr. LUBCHENCO suggested there was postconceptional bleeding, in other words threatened abortion, you would of course expect a higher mortality rate. There is a higher mortality rate in all babies with a history of threatened abortion. So this seems to bear out that these are babies who are in fact not praemature but full-term and who, in early pregnancy, threatened to abort. This is why they have a higher mortality rate.

*Dr. Gruenwald:* I would also like to say a word about the same group of babies. Of course there is a possibility that some of them are large for their gestational age or immature for their weight. As I think, it was brought out yesterday in the discussion, some of them may be the result of undetected diabetes during pregnancy, and that would explain the higher mortality rate.

I would like to say a word about the 38-week limit of the full-term infant. Some people object to it and would rather see a 37-week limit. I used to defend the 37-week limit. Studying the mortality rate of various conditions for weeks of gestation I have found that there is in many pathologic conditions a conspicuous drop in incidence between 37 and 38 weeks. So I think that there is a biological justification for the 38 rather than the 37-week limit.

Finally I would like to comment on the two forms of placental insufficiency which Dr. LUBCHENCO showed in her beautiful table, one before term and one after term. These two groups correspond probably to some extend to what I showed you yesterday as chronic and sub-acute foetal distress. In the first place I am sure that Dr. LUBCHENCO will agree that what she calls placental insufficiency is not necessarily insufficiency, but is an inadequate supply-line. And in the second place I would make a plea for distinguishing these two groups, because it may, very well, turn out that the late sequelae are different and that the infant that is growth-retarded and deprived for a long time may in the future show more growth-retardation and more brain damage than the one who was just deprived for a few days and has lost some weight. When we plan follow-up studies it might be nice to develop some criteria to keep these groups as far apart as we possibly can.

*Dr. Wigglesworth:* I would like to draw attention to another grouping of two types of small babies that Dr. LUBCHENCO has mentioned. These are the ones that have relatively normal head circumference and the ones that have low head circumference. In general I think that the babies who had the normal head circumference were the infants of the mothers with hypertension. These are probably the most pure examples of foetal malnutrition that we have. The ones with the low head circumference were those with congenital anomalies, tri-somic syndromes and congenital rubella. I think that these groups fit in very well with NAEYE's hypothesis (NAEYE, R. L. (1965), Amer. J. Pathol. 47: 905), which he has some experimental evidence for, that there is a group that has primarily reduced cell-mass being the intrauterine malnutrition babies, and a group that has a reduced cell population of the varying organs. I would think it might be of considerable importance as far as prognosis for cerebral development is concerned to seperate these groups. If a low head circumference at birth is associated with a low cell population in the brain this would certainly carry a very poor prognosis and I would imagine that these babies would do worse in the long run.

*Dr. Lubchenco:* It is true that the head circumference was not retarded in the group with hypertension.

*Dr. Nicolopoulos:* I have two questions. Does Dr. LUBCHENCO have any information about the placentas of these babies born at high altitude in Leadville? There was a report from Peru describing the placentas of infants born there as very large ones, and I would like to know if this is confirmed. And the second one is, what is Dr. LUBCHENCO's experience with the criteria described by USHER et al. estimating morphologically the gestational age of praematures.

*Dr. Lubchenco:* We did study the weight of placentas at high altitude and I am embarrassed to say that our placental studies were not very good, but I will tell you what we found. In Leadville the placenta was weighed after the cord was cut off, and the membranes left on. I compared the median weight of Leadville placentas with those at Colorado General Hospital where nothing was removed. They just weighed them. Then, I compared these medians with Dr. GRUEN-WALD's, who very carefully prepared and weighed them. Now, when you compared these median weights, the lowest median was Dr. GRUENWALD's; then came the Leadville values and, finally, the Colorado General ones; I believe this means that they were probably the same size. This was the conclusion we drew although we recognized that these were poor data. Now, the other question concerns the use of USHER's criteria. We are delighted with them and are finding them very helpful. We have added, maybe half a dozen, items to them.

*Dr. Valaes:* May I make a plea that we pass no judgement, for the moment, for the group of babies which are very large for dates.

We know that they have a higher mortality rate than expected from their weight and a lower than the mean of their gestational age. But as we don't know from what causes they die this information is insufficient and the hypothesis, that this group represents errors in the calculation of the length of pregnancy, because of postconceptional bleeding, to which the high mortality should be ascribed, cannot be considered proved.

Nobody has yet presented evidence on the maturity of these infants at birth using morphological and neurological criteria. This is crucial information because we cannot exclude another explanation for this group. It is not illogical to postulate that if there is a group with advanced rate of growth, these babies, as we know from twins, will be born praematurily, because, as Dr. GRUENWALD has pointed out, the uterus cannot support well more than a certain weight. So, although I myself believe that in the great majority there are errors in the calculation of the length of gestation, still I think we have not sufficient evidence to pass a judgement about this group.

*Dr. Lubchenco:* Thank you for these very good words. I quite agree.

*Dr. Widdowson:* Could I ask what do you suppose is the reason for the low birthweight at high altitude? I was very interested in this. I presume the mothers are climatized to the high altitude.

*Dr. Lubchenco:* I just don't know.

DISCUSSION PAPER DR. OUNSTED

*Dr. Widdowson* (in the chair): The paper of Dr. OUNSTED is now open for discussion. Bur I believe Dr. DRILLIEN likes to show us a few slides. So may I ask her to do this first.

*Dr. Drillien:* When Dr. OUNSTED's paper about maternal constraint came out 18 months ago I'm sure many other people started looking at the birthweights of sibs of low-weight or growth-retarded infants and so did I. I would like to show you the findings of my study (fig. 1). The difference between my group and Dr. OUNSTED's group is that all these babies were 2000 grams or less. Of her series of 90 growth-retarded infants only 12 were of this very low birthweight. Using Dr. LUBCHENCO's percentiles one part of my group was poorly grown and one part was well grown. At least the majority of them was also praemature.

I looked at the mean birthweight of the sibs of the poorly grown and of the well grown low-birthweight infants. The mean birthweight of all sibs was rather lower than the mean birthweight of all children in the population. But in social grades 1, 2 and 3 there was very little difference. There was however a much bigger difference in the mean birthweight of siblings born to women in the poorest social class (grade 4).

Then I looked at the proportion of siblings who had been 2500 grams or less at birth. Although there were more here compared with the general population, there was very little difference between the sibs of the poorly grown and the sibs of the more adequately grown infants in social grades 1, 2 and 3. But there was a very great difference in the siblings of the women in the lowest social class (grade 4) who had had low birthweight infants.

The other thing I have got here is the proportion of short mothers:

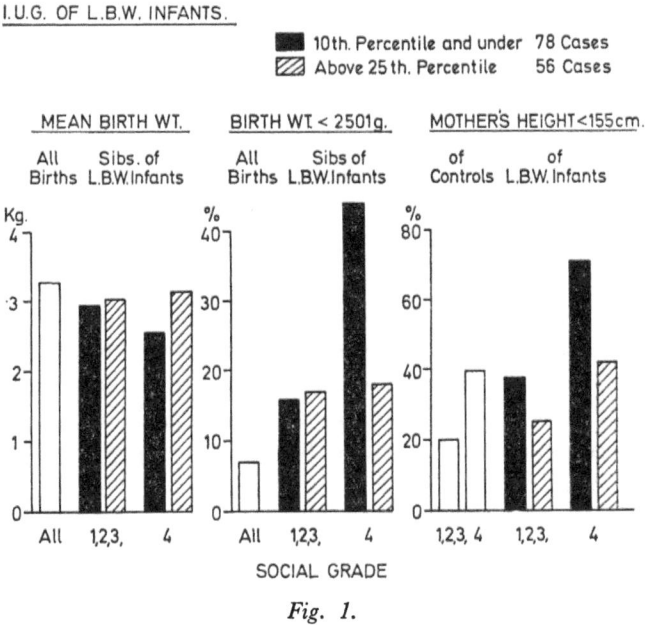

*Fig. 1.*

mothers who were less than 5 feet 2 inches. Here we noticed quite a difference among the poorly grown infants. There were significantly more short mothers in all social classes, but particularly the mothers in the lower social grade.

So my findings in these low birthweight infants agree entirely with Dr. OUNSTED's for women from the lowest social grade but do not seem to agree for women from the better social grades. I have no explanation for this. I'm hoping Dr. OUNSTED will be able to tell me why.

13

*Dr. Ounsted:* Well, I think the main explanation is that we studied very different problems. All your babies weighed 2000 g or less, and also were below the 10th percentile. Most of my babies weighed between 2000 g and 2500 g and were below the 2nd standard deviation which is equivalent, roughly, to the 2.5th percentile. Thus your babies were smaller than mine, most of them of short gestation, and much less growth-retarded. The picture they give is of praematurity combined with a much milder form of growth-retardation. Our probands were different, and we would not expect the same findings. I think your series shows all the factors of small effect, which we all know are there to a slight degree, especially in the so-called lower social classes, and which add up to this picture.

*Dr. Valaes:* In your series mean maternal height was the same between your controls and your growth-retarded infants. Have you got any information on paternal height in your series?

I was very intrigued that the mothers of your growth-retarded group were also growth-retarded in utero themselves. Later on they achieved normal height. This is of course opposite to the animal experience you have just mentioned. I wonder if you have any information on the age of menarche of the mothers of your series, because this might be an explanation. I think that your group probably includes what in the postnatal period is called slow growing children: they follow the lowest end of the normal percentile and yet they might achieve average normal height in the end. Perhaps what you have shown is that the mothers and their children were belonging to this group. Have you any data on the later growth of your retarded group?

*Dr. Ounsted:* Unfortunately I have not yet any data on the growth of my retarded group but they are being followed up and we hope to have them in a few years. I did take the information about the age of menarche but I have not analysed these data and I cannot give you any answer.*

I agree that the data about the maternal heights were surprising. In the original 90 there was not a significant difference but there was

---

* I was most grateful to Dr. VALAES for this penetrating question. I have now looked at the age of menarche in the controls and growth-retarded series. The two means coincide precisely at 13.1 years.

some difference in the means. But when the figures were increased in fact they came to exactly the same means for heights. I think the answer is that the mothers were growth-retarded but not as growth-retarded as their infants. They had a tendency to growth-retardation. I think we must learn from this that intra-uterine growth and extra-uterine growth are controlled by very different factors, although I agree that we don't know what is going to happen with these growth-retarded infants themselves in adult life.

*Dr. Wigglesworth:* First I should like to ask if there are any data — perhaps I missed this — on the status of the mother of the growth-accelerated group in relation to possible diabetes or pre-diabetes.

*Dr. Ounsted:* I should emphasize that in these series the control-group and the growth-retarded group were personally collected by me. The growth-accelerated group and the short gestation series shown in the scattergrams were from the hospital notes and I didn't see the mothers myself or examine the babies. In the growth-accelerated group there were two frank diabetics and in the control group there was one frank diabetic. Of the mothers who have produced large babies some had glucose tolerance tests done. One was very slightly abnormal. But they have not all been checked.

*Dr. Wigglesworth:* Secondly I would like to comment on your paper. You suggested that the retardation of the mother's own growth in utero might be related to subsequent constraint of her foetus' growth. Now I would think that this explanation, possibly extending into the postnatal period, would go far to explain a lot of the growth-retardation found in races who are in poor nutritional status. It is in the earliest part of life that inadequate nutrition is most likely to cause permanent reduction in stature with, I suspect, a corresponding small uterus, and this in turn will impair foetal growth in the next generation. This effect may be more important than that of food intake during pregnancy. All the nutritionists who have studied nutrition of the mother during pregnancy in relation to the growth of the foetuses and the birthweight of the babies have been twenty years too late. They should have studied the nutritional status of the mother shortly after birth.

*Dr. Ounsted:* I'm not sure whether I have quite followed you. I agree that everyone knows that starvation in the human mother does reduce birhtweight. I have no specific explanation for the reason why the mothers of these babies were growth-retarded. I should like to hear anyone ideas on this subject. I do agree with the fact that this might explain the change in birthweight in generations in a population.

*Dr. Gruenwald:* I think we should congratulate Dr. OUNSTED on this beautiful work. One comment I should like to make is on the placental growth hormone. It is my impression, and I'm sure there are people present who know more about this, that the placental growth hormone does not reach the foetus but only the mother. Also in the British Perinatal Mortality Survey there was a difference in maternal height correlating with growth of the foetus. I wonder whether, if you had a large number of cases, this might again appear.

*Dr. Ounsted:* Yes, in the survey there was a difference. Did they actually take one or two standard deviations in the maternal height measure? I'm not sure about that. I think we are studying a specific population in Oxford. That allows for these biological factors to appear where they might have been covered up by excessive pathological factors in a less prosperous population.

*Prof. R. Schwartz:* I wonder if you could tell me again what the total sample is from which you obtained your 90 low birthweight infants who were studied. I know that you have a control series of 225 but I'm not sure that I understand what the total sample is.

*Dr. Ounsted:* They were consecutive births of growth-retarded infants.

*Prof. R. Schwartz:* How many deliveries did occur during the same time interval?

*Dr. Ounsted:* About 5000 deliveries. This gives a slightly low incidence for growth-retardation as defined, but patients in whom the length of gestation was at all questionable were ruthlessly excluded, and a few were missed when I was away.

*Prof. R. Schwartz:* What is the mortality rate in your series of large infants?

*Dr. Ounsted:* We have not yet data on the mortality rate of large infants. I'm now personally collecting a large for date series in the same way as I did the small for date series. But it is not large enough to give you any reliable figures yet.

*Dr. Rappaport:* Is there any study on bone maturation in these children of low birthweight? Is there any correlation between bone age and gestational age?

*Dr. Ounsted:* We have not done this investigation. Someone has done X-rays to study ossification in this group. I think it is USHER*. He found that the ossification was related to the bodyweight of the baby and not to the maturity.

*Prof. François:* Have you done any measurement on the blood glucose and blood calcium in the newborn with severe perinatal anxiety?

*Dr. Ounsted:* We did not check blood calcium. In some of them we did blood glucose. In fact it was interesting that we had only one infant in this series of 147 that gave symptoms of hypoglycaemia and had to be treated. Some of the others were routinely checked and were not hypoglycaemic. The very low incidence of hypoglycaemia in our severely growth-retarded infants is, we think, due to the regime of early feeding with undiluted breast milk which has been used in our praemature baby nursery for the last 4 years (SMALLPEICE, V., DAVIES, P. A., (1964) Lancet 2, 1349).

* SCOTT, K. E., USHER, R., (1964) New Eng. J. Med., 270, 822.

# ADAPTATION OF THE LOW BIRTHWEIGHT INFANT TO EXTRA-UTERINE LIFE

# THE METABOLIC RATE IN PRAEMATURE, DYSMATURE AND SICK INFANTS IN RELATION TO ENVIRONMENTAL TEMPERATURE

J. H. P. JONXIS, J. J. VAN DER VLUGT, C. J. DE GROOT,
E. R. BOERSMA AND E. D. K. MEIJERS*

Much has been published recently about the metabolic rate of normal and praemature infants in their first days of life. The data on dysmature infants are less abundant. Most workers have limited their measurements to the determination of the oxygen uptake and only relatively few investigations have been made on respiratory quotient (R.Q.). In the passed year we have tried to fill up partly these gaps.

The neutral temperature of the full-term infant amounts from 32° C to 33° C shortly after birth. At this temperature at a humidity of 50 per cent the oxygen uptake is on an average of 4.7 ml/kg/min. In the next fortnight the neutral temperature drops and the oxygen consumption rises to about 6.5 ml/kg/min. In the praemature infant the neutral temperature is higher, reaching levels of 35° C to 36° C in praematures with a birth-weight of less than 1300 g. In these infants the neutral temperature does not drop appreciably during the first weeks of life. The oxygen consumption which is initially 4 ml/kg/min rises gradually to about 6 to 7 ml/kg/min. In the dysmature infants the neutral temperature is higher than in the normal full-term infants and drops more slowly. Their oxygen consumption which is initially 4.7 ml/kg/min rises to 6.8 ml/kg/min during the first 10 days of life. At that moment it is higher than that of the normal full-term infant. This is likely due to their small amount of fat and their greater cell-mass.

Our measurements were made with a diaferometer (Kipp). This instrument enables us to measure $O_2$ uptake and $CO_2$ production simultaneously. Environmental temperature was kept constant by placing the metabolic box in a waterbath of a constant temperature. The neutral temperature was determined by rising gradually the environmental temperature till the oxygen consumption did not drop any longer.

* Department of Paediatrics, State University, Groningen.

Measurements were only taken when the infant had been practically motionless or asleep for a quarter of an hour. Skin and oesophageal
temperatures were measured with a thermocouple. We did our investigations in three groups of children, namely: (1) normal children of

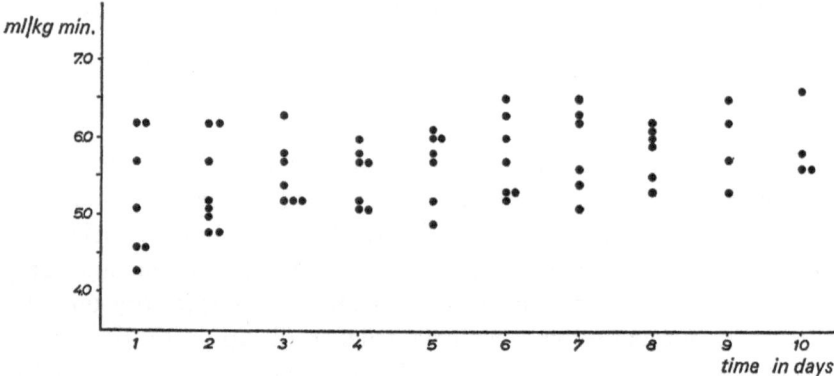

*Fig.* 1.   Oxygen consumption in ml/kg/min at neutral temperature of normal
babies (group 1).

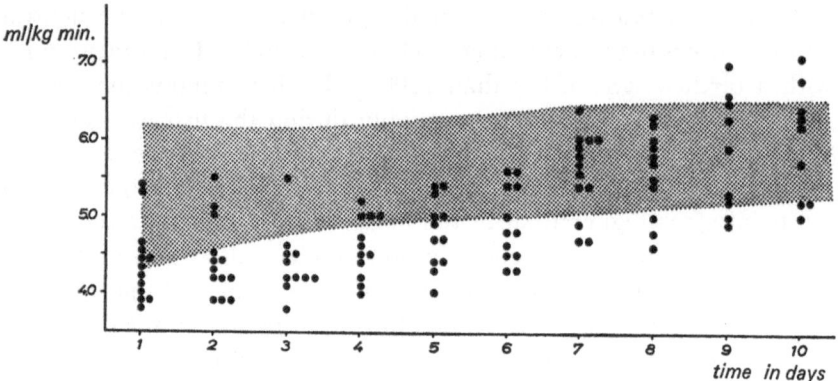

*Fig.* 2.   Oxygen consumption in ml/kg/min at neutral temperature of praematurs
(group 2). The shaded zone gives the values for normal babies.

an average birthweight of 3500 g, (2) praematures of a gestational
age of less than 36 weeks and a birthweight that was normal for the
gestational age (average birthweight in this group 1750 g), and (3)
dysmatures of a gestational age of more than 36 weeks and an average
birthweight of 1890 g. Each group consisted of 9 to 12 children. Daily

during the first 10 days of life oxygen uptake and $CO_2$ production were measured at neutral temperature and at an environmental temperature of 26° C. Blood glycerol and glucose levels were determined daily at both temperatures. All children were on a formula of a humanized milk, Almiron $M_2$, which contains 1.5 % of protein, 7.3 % of lactose and 3.4 % of vegetable oil. Feeding was started on the second day of life, so that at the tenth day of life the child was receiving 100 cal/kg bodyweight daily. Figures 1, 2, 3 give the oxygen uptake in these three groups of children, figures 4, 5, 6 the respiratory

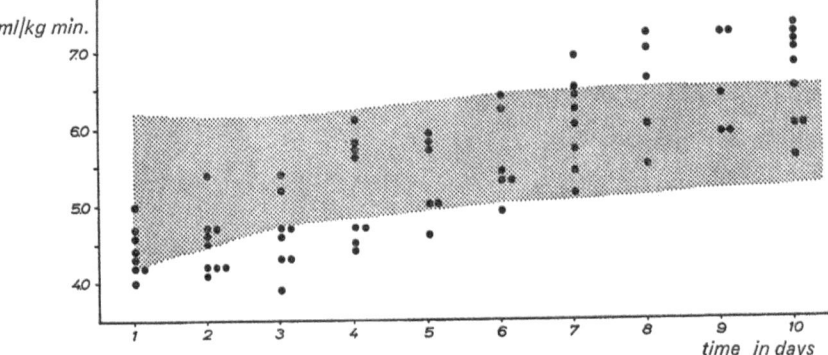

*Fig.* 3. Oxygen consumption in ml/kg/min at neutral temperature of small for date babies (group 3). The shaded zone gives the values for normal babies.

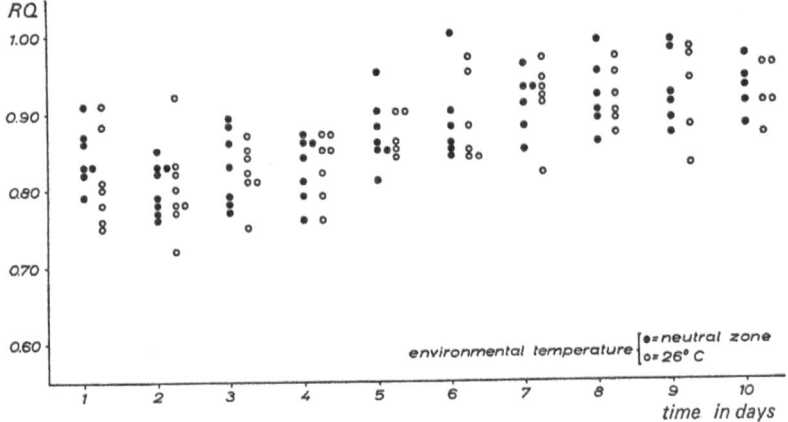

*Fig.* 4. Respiratory quotient of normal babies (group 1) at different temperatures.

quotient, figures 7, 8, 9 the deep-body temperature. Our results are in agreement with those mentioned in literature. In the full-term infant at the age of 24 hours the average oxygen uptake amounted to 5.26 ml/kg/min at neutral temperature.

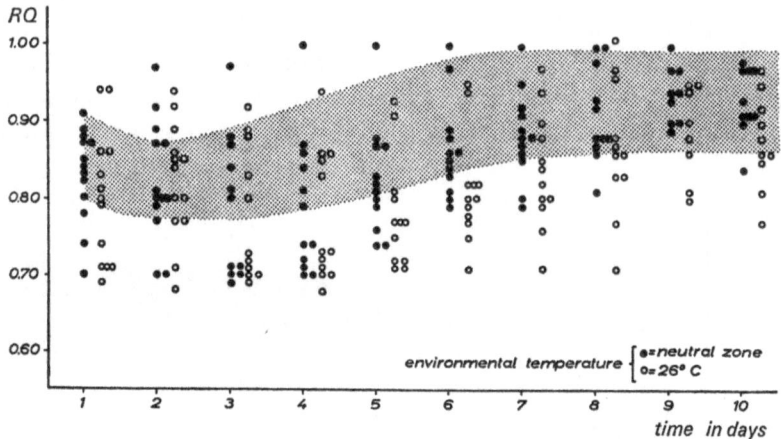

*Fig.* 5.   Respiratory quotient of praemature babies (group 2) at different temperatures. The shaded zone gives the values for normal babies at neutral temperature.

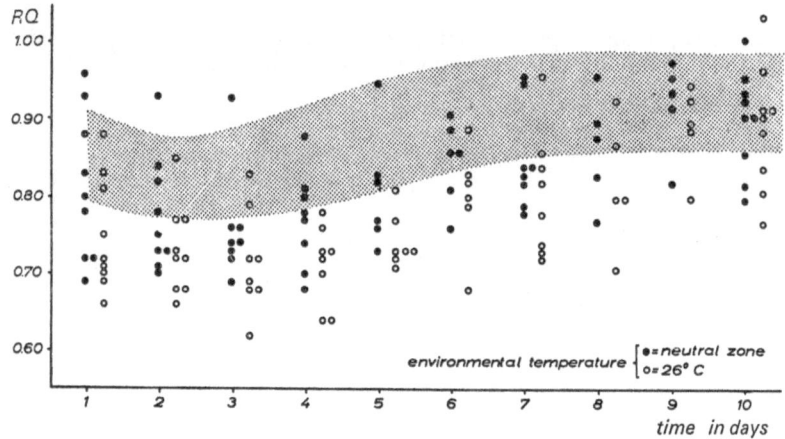

*Fig.* 6.   Respiratory quotient of small for date babies (group 3). The shaded zone gives values for normal babies at neutral temperature.

In a few cases the measurement was repeated at a humidity of 80 per cent. The oxygen consumption dropped about 20 per cent in some infants whose basal oxygen consumption was rather high at a humidity of 50 %. For praematures at the end of their first day of life we obtained the average value of 4.16 ml/kg/min; for dysmatures of 4.43. At an environmental temperature of 26° C their values were respectively 6.96, 6.46 and 7.08; that means a rise of resp. 32 %, 55 % and 59 %.

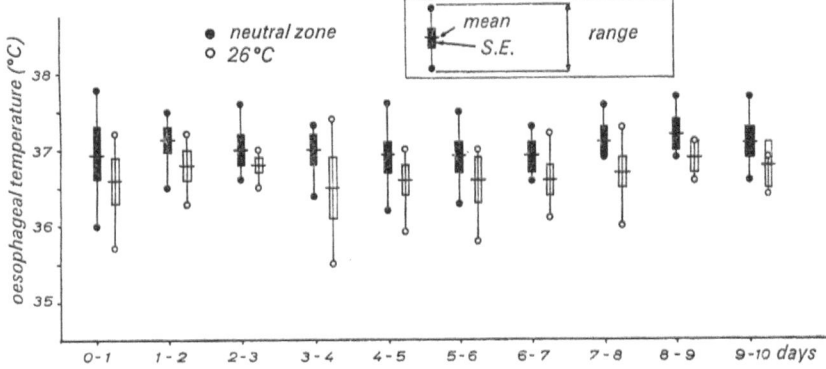

*Fig.* 7.   Deep body temperatures of normal babies (group 1) at different environmental temperatures.

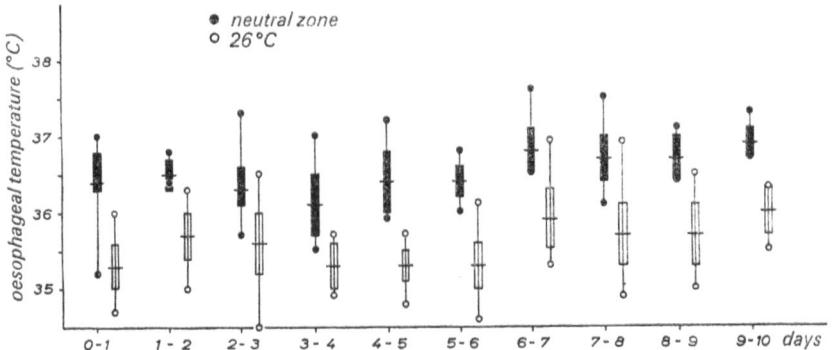

*Fig.* 8.   Deep body temperatures of praemature babies (group 2) at different environmental temperatures.

In the dysmature the rise is the most marked one. In all three groups exposure to 26° C caused a drop in deep-body temperature. This drop was most marked in the praemature (resp. 0.3° C, 1.1° C, 0.7° C). When we take into account this drop in deep-body tempera-

ture the metabolic response of the praemature is the smallest one and
of the full-term infant the largest. In the praemature infant the marked
drop in body-temperature will tend to lower the metabolic rate, what
might explain the more limited response in the praemature.

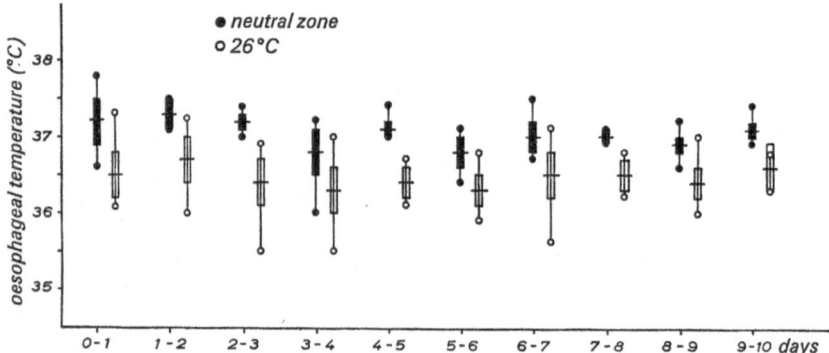

*Fig.* 9.   Deep body temperatures of small for date babies (group 3) at different
environmental temperatures.

At the eighth day of life the average oxygen uptake at neutral temperature of the three groups was resp. 6.2, 5.8 and 6.5 ml/kg/min.
At the environmental temperature of 26° C these values amounted
to resp. 8.54, 8.83 and 9.36; thus a rise of 37 %, 52 % and 44 % resp.

The deep-body temperature dropped in the three groups, 0.3° C,
1.2° C, and 0.5° C resp. At that moment the differences between the
full-term infant and the dysmature infant have become less pronounced. The oxygen uptake of the dysmature infants at their eighth day of
life is higher than that of the two other groups. This is likely caused by
their greater cell-mass, the drop in deep-body temperature in the praemature and its metabolic response still being the same.

In all three groups the respiratory quotient drops during the first
days of life and rises again from the third day onward. At the third
day of life the R.Q. is resp. 0.8, 0.78 and 0.75. Especially in the dysmature child values near 0.7 occur. In all groups the R.Q. rises when
larger quantities of food are given. At the ninth day of life the average
values are resp. 0.94, 0.93 and 0.90. It is however noteworthy that
even then the R.Q. of the dysmature child remains the lowest one,
although half of the caloric value of its food consists of carbohydrate.
In full-term infants the R.Q. does not drop appreciably during expo-

sure to cold, but in many dysmature children there is a marked drop in the R.Q. during exposure to low temperatures. The average R.Q. of the latter groups drops from 0.75 to 0.72 (fourth day of life).

The blood sugar values of all three groups are rising gradually during the first ten days of life, those of the dysmature being lowest, although no cases of hypoglycaemia occurred in our children. Blood glycerol levels were high during the first day of life to drop thereafter. During exposure to an environmental temperature of 26° C there is a marked rise in the blood glycerol levels of each group. This is an indication of an increased mobilisation of fat and of the metabolism of fatty acids. In the full-term infants this is not accompanied by a drop in R.Q. In the praemature and especially in the dysmature infants, however, the R.Q. tends to drop markedly. In the full-term infants there is a rise in the blood sugar level, in the two other groups the blood sugar levels remaining about the same. One might ask what is the meaning of the drop in R.Q. to a value of 0.7 and sometimes even lower in the dysmature infant? The only source of energy practically used must be the fatty acids. One wonders however, why carbohydrate metabolism has been reduced so much, although the blood-sugar levels were not especially low in the infants under investigation. Might it be that in the dysmature infant the utilisation of glucose is limited by a high turnover of fatty acids? At the third or fourth day of life when the drop in R.Q. is deepest the infants were receiving already on the average four grams of lactose pro kg bodyweight daily. The drop in R.Q. in praemature and dysmature infants exposed to environmental temperatures lower than their neutral temperatures may form an indication that it is desirable to keep these infants at their neutral temperatures during their first 10 days of life. When the infant is getting older, the drop in R.Q. diminishes. Whether this depends on the increased food intake is uncertain.

My friend, the late Professor HESSEL DE VRIES, was kind enough to build a balance for us which makes it possible to weigh a moving infant with an accuracy of 20 mg. This balance allows measuring the perspiratio insensibilis of the child. We started our work along this line only a few months ago, but we like to give you some preliminary results. At neutral temperature at a humidity of 40 % an infant of about one week old is losing on the average 25 mg/kg/min. At a humidity of 80 % this loss drops to 15 mg. By covering the infant with a layer of absorbing tissue and an outerlayer of plastic we have tried to measure the losses by respiration ($H_2O$ and $CO_2$). At a humidity of 40 % these losses are about 9 mg. These values agree with those obtained by other workers by indirect methods.

The energy necessary for the evaporation of these amounts of water counts to 14 calories/kg/min at a humidity of 40 % and 8 calories at a humidity of 80 %, the total caloric production of the infant being about 34 calories/kg/min. Therefore 40 % of the calories produced by metabolism are lost by evaporation at a humidity of 40 %, and 25 % at a humidity of 80 %. The other forms of heat loss, mainly radiation, therefore increase sharply with the rise of the humidity.

Fever caused by inflammation causes a rise, in many cases larger than 50 %, of the oxygen uptake (SCOPES, 1966). We have studied a few infants with fever (temperature between 38.2° and 38.8° C), caused by dehydration and hyperelectrolytaemia in their first days of life. We found a normal oxygen consumption of between 5.2 and 6.1 ml/kg/min and a normal R.Q. A rise in body temperature of 1° C increases the rate of metabolic reactions with about 10 per cent and should therefore influence basal metabolism in a positive way. There-fore other factors must counteract the tendency to a rise in metabolism in these infants. The dehydration fever is not caused by an increased heat production, but must be due to a decreased heat release. This is in agreement with the fact that the skin temperatures of these infants were found to be within the normal range, although their deep-body temperatures were about two degrees elevated.

Infants with high serum bilirubin levels are often lethargic and are slow in feeding. In a few cases which we were able to study we found a moderately decreased oxygen uptake with a R.Q. that was normal for infants of that age-group. These results are in agreement with those of SCOPES. As the depression of the oxygen uptake is not very constant, it is not likely that this effect is due to a direct action of the bilirubin on the energy production sites in the cell (mitochondria). In very high concentrations bilirubin blocks the phosphorilation and increases the oxygen consumption. The decreased oxygen uptake is therefore more likely to be indirectly related to the hyperbilirubinaemia. Kern-icterus in many of these children might be the cause of a total depres-sion of metabolism.

Which practical conclusions might be drawn from these studies?

In the normal young infant exposure to cold causes a sharp rise in metabolism. Although this may be a stimulus when the exposure time is short, it seems preferable to avoid this over a longer period and to keep the child at its neutral temperature, especially as long as its food intake is insufficient, to cover its caloric needs. Neutral temperature may be reached either by clothing or by placing the child in temperature controled surroundings.

In the praemature and dysmature infant these arguments are even more pronounced, since their energy balance tends more to the negative side. Praemature and dysmature infants differ from the full-term infant by a marked drop in R.Q. during exposure to lower temperatures. This is an additional argument to keep them at their neutral temperatures.

Fever in dehydrated newborn infants is due to a decreased heat-transport through the skin.

## REFERENCES

1. ADAMSON, K. (1966) *Pediat. Clin. N. Am.* 13: 3.
2. BRÜCK, K. (1961) *Biol. Neonat.* 3: 65.
3. BRÜCK, K., A. H. PARMELEE, M. BRÜCK (1962) *Biol. Neonat.* 4: 32.
4. CERUTI, E. (1966) *Pediatrics* 37: 556.
5. CROSS, K. W., J. P. M. TIZARD, D. A. H. THRYTHALL (1958) *Acta Paediat.* 47: 217.
6. CROSS, K. W., D. M. FLYNN (1966) *Pediatrics* 37: 565.
7. HILL, J. R. K. A. RAHIMTULLA (1965) *J. Physiol.* 180: 239.
8. KARLBERG, P. (1960) *Acta Paediat.* 49: suppl. 122.
9. NOVAK, M., V. MELICHAR, P. HARN (1965) *Biol. Neonat.* 8: 253.
10. PARMELEE, A. H., K. BRÜCK, M. BRÜCK (1962) *Biol. Neonat.* 4: 317.
11. PRIBYLOVA, H. (1963) *Ann. paediat.* 201: 399.
12. SCOPES, J. W., I. AHMED (1966) *Arch. Dis. Child.* 41: 407.
13. SCOPES, J. W., I. AHMED (1966) *Arch. Dis. Childh.* 41: 417.
14. VAN DER VLUGT, J. J. (1967) *Studies on metabolic rate in low birthweight infants.* Thesis, State University Groningen.

# GLUCOSE CONTROL IN THE NEWBORN INFANT*

ROBERT SCHWARTZ, PETER A. J. ADAM**, KATHERINE KING
AND DAVID KORNHAUSER

The newborn infant at term has rapid changes in metabolism over the initial hours and days of life. During this phase, although his blood glucose is lowered to one-half to two-thirds of the adult level, he manages to sustain cerebral metabolism in most instances.

In contrast, the low birth weight infant has a larger range of glucose values, sustains a glucose concentration less well and is more susceptible to extremely low blood sugar levels (1). In fact, symptomatic hypoglycemia is often found in dysmature infants (2). Figure 1 demonstrates that infants with symptomatic hypoglycemia tend to be of low birth weight for gestational age, using the LUBCHENCO grid as a reference standard. This is similar to data reported by others (3, 4, 5).

Since the liver is the major if not sole source of glucose to the body in the post absorptive state, measurement of hepatic glucose output is of importance in understanding normal physiological control of blood glucose. If the arterial concentration is constant and there is no glycosuria, then net hepatic glucose output must equal non-hepatic or peripheral glucose uptake. Ideally, this is accomplished by the triple cannulated preparation in which portal, hepatic vein and arterial bloods and flows are analyzed. Since this is impractical in man and technically difficult in animals, indirect techniques have been used. One method involves measurement of glucose A-V differences across the splanchnic bed using hepatic vein catheterization and estimation

* Department of Pediatrics, Western Reserve University School of Medicine at Cleveland Metropolitan General Hospital, Cleveland, Ohio. Aided by U.S. Public Health Service research grant ≠AM 06795 and training grant ≠5-T1-AM 5356 from the National Institute of Arthritis and Metabolic Diseases and by grant ≠FR-00210, Perinatal General Clinical Research Center of the Division of Research Facilities and Resources.
** Trainee in pediatric metabolism, U.S. Public Health Service.

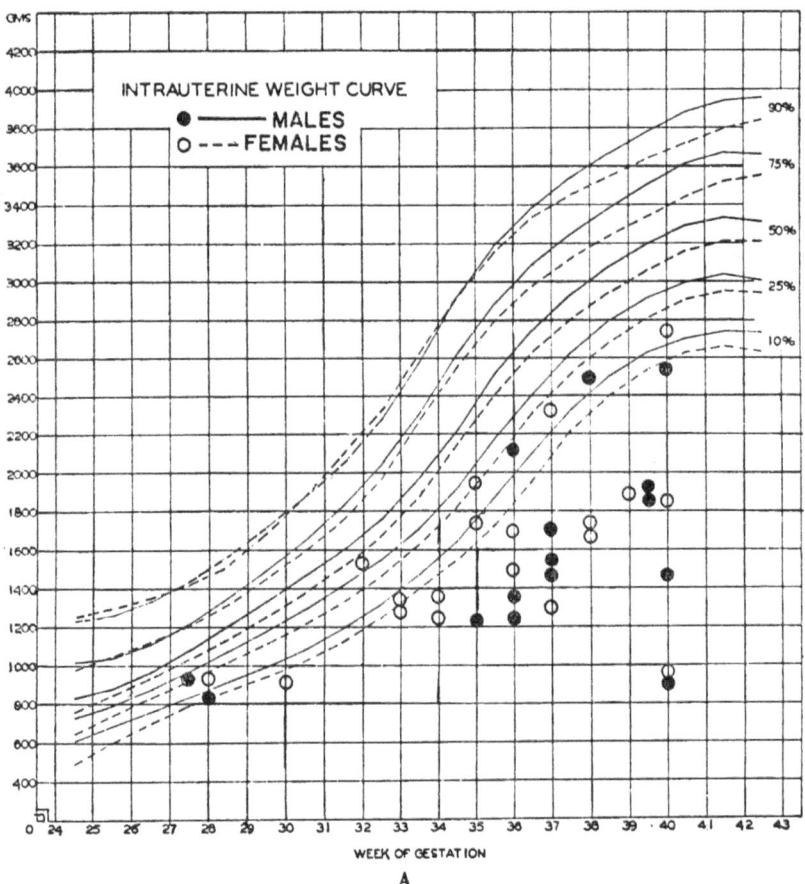

*Fig.* 1.   (Taken from reference (1) p. 85, by permission). Weights at birth of 34
infants with transient neonatal hypoglycemia plotted against weeks of gestation
(using Denver reference grid of Lubchenco).

of splanchnic blood flow using extraction of BSP. The other technique
depends upon isotope dilution with $C^{14}$-glucose. Although neither technique has been used in the newborn, the former has been used in
adult man and in animals. In normal man, net splanchnic glucose
production is virtually all net hepatic glucose output. MYERS (6)
found mean basal values of 2 mg/kg/min while BONDY (7) found values
of 3.5 mg/kg/min. SOSKIN (8) originally showed in the dog that a slow
infusion of glucose of a magnitude to balance the hepatic glucose

output abolished net glucose release. Similar observations in adult man were found by MYERS (6). For example, an infusion at 1 mg/kg/min only raised the arterial glucose concentration by 5 mg per 100 ml with no effect on hepatic A-V difference; however a rate of 3 mg/kg/min resulted in an increment of 17 mg per 100 ml and a negative A-V difference indicating that net hepatic uptake instead of release occurred. On the premise then that an increment rise in blood glucose would be associated with cessation of net hepatic output, studies of steady state glucose infusion in normal adults and infants were under-

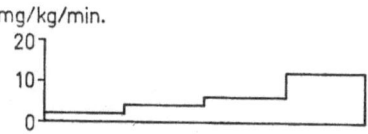

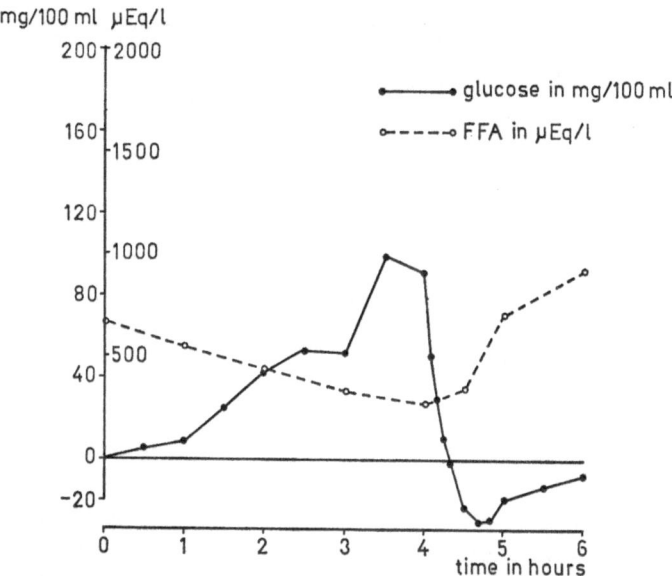

*Fig.* 2. Relationship between increment in blood glucose concentration above fasting and plasma free fatty acids (FFA) in a normal fasting adult given glucose by constant infusion at 2—12 mg/kg/min for successive hours.

taken (9). The minimal rate at which a rise in blood glucose concentration occurs during glucose infusion may then represent an estimate of both basal hepatic glucose output as well as peripheral glucose uptake. Furthermore, in order to study hypoglycemic conditions in a steady state, continuous infusion of glucose may be necessary for therapeutic reasons.

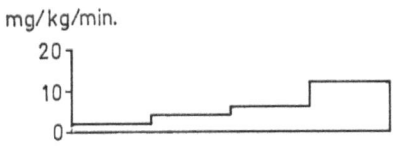

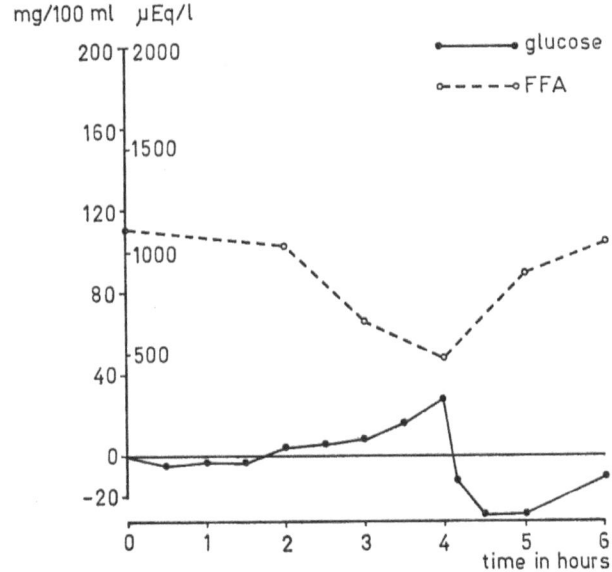

*Fig.* 3.   Similar relationship to fig. 2 in infants of the first year of life.

Figure 2 shows the response for an adult to stepwise steady state glucose infusion; altogether nine normal subjects were studied. After an overnight fast, indwelling infusion and sampling needles were inserted in peripheral vein sites. Following a control blood sample, glucose was administered by a constant infusion pump for one hour at 2 mg/kg/min. The mean increment of 19 mg per 100 ml was observed. During the second hour at 4 mg/kg/min, a very definite rise of 31 mg per 100 ml was noted. Similarly at 6 mg/kg/min an increment of 49 mg per 100 ml while at the final rate of 12 mg/kg/min a rise of 91 mg per 100 ml above fasting was observed. During this time, plasma free fatty acids which were elevated initially were suppressed to low levels. Plasma insulin rose successively at the end of each infusion rate from 3 μ U/ml to 38 μ U/ml at the highest rate. When the infusion was abruptly stopped after the fourth rate, glucose fell precipitously to levels well below the control value within an hour, but stabilized toward base-line during the last hour. Insulin levels were at basal values within thirty minutes; however FFA remained suppressed. During the second hour following the hypoglycemic phase, FFA rose to levels well above the initial fasting value.

Similar observations were made on four normal infants, age 1 day to 13 months (fig. 3). When glucose was infused at identical rates on a weight basis, no rise in blood glucose level was achieved until a rate of 6 mg/kg/min was administered. As indicated there was no fall in plasma FFA and the plasma insulin level was not different from the control level below 4 mg/kg/min. At 6 mg/kg/min of infused glucose, an increment of 8 mg/100 ml was achieved while at 12 mg/kg/min a rise of 28 mg/100 ml was found. This was comparable to the effects of one-third the rate in the adult. At the highest rates FFA were suppressed, and returned to fasting levels post infusion. Although the incremental rise was not as great as in the adult, nevertheless, significant hypoglycemia was found in the post infusion phase. Again rebound counter-regulation was achieved by two hours.

Since we were carrying out simultaneous observations on newborn infants of diabetic mothers, we extended similar observations to normal infants in the first 3-4 hours of life. We administered glucose at higher rates to give comparable data for our infants of diabetic mothers who dispose of an acute load very rapidly, in contrast to normal infants whose tissues remove an acute load slowly. The full term newborn, at 3-4 hours of life, as shown in figure 4, responds to 12 mg/kg/min similarly to the adult, while at twice this rate he achieves remarkable levels of 260 mg per 100 ml above fasting. He suppresses FFA at these levels of blood glucose and develops a post infusion hypoglycemia although his initial level is somewhat low. His rebound is surprisingly effective to this stimulus yet the rate of fall is not rapid. Even with these high rates, there is no glycosuria so that all glucose disposal is by tissue uptake, including liver.

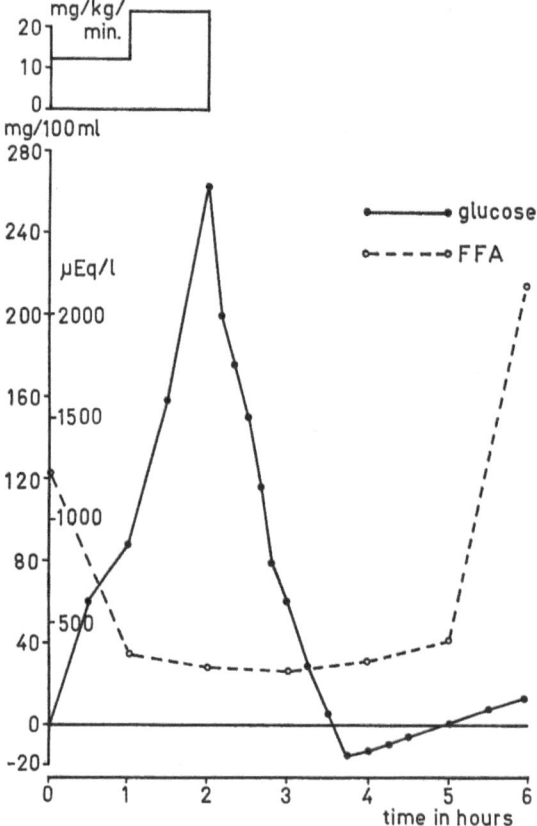

*Fig.* 4. Relationship of blood glucose and plasma FFA in newborn, aged 3—4 hrs given glucose by constant infusion at high rates (12—24 mg/kg/min).

The data in the newborn cannot be interpreted with reference to minimal glucose output or utilization; however in the adult and older infant, if one assumes no change in peripheral uptake and a prompt cessation of hepatic output as the blood glucose level is raised; then the minimal rate at which an incremental change occurs could be considered the rate of hepatic glucose output under these steady state conditions. Thus the adult raises his blood sugar at 2-4 mg/kg/min

while the older infant does so at above 6 mg/kg/min. One could speculate that the newborn at term in the first hours of life would have a
rate closer to the adult values.

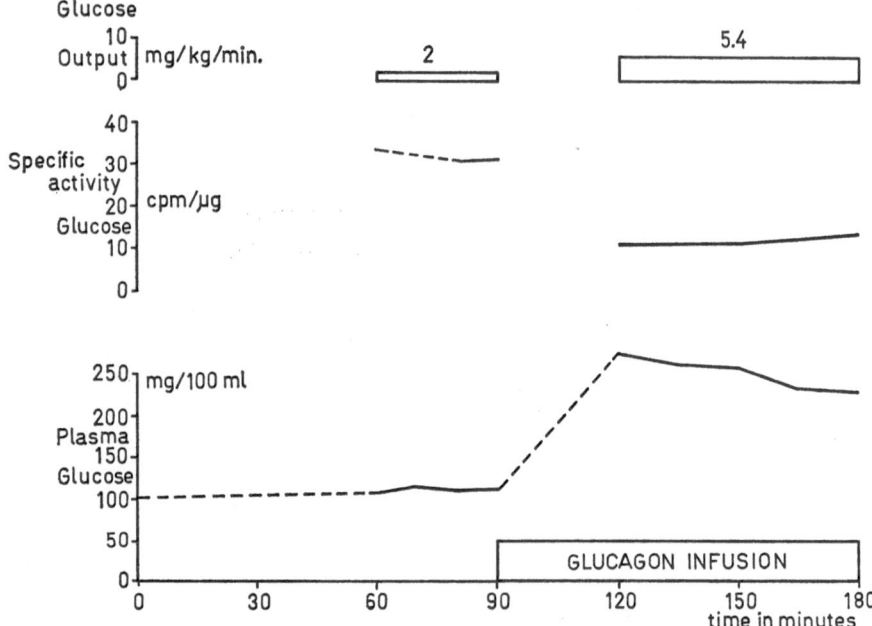

*Fig. 5.* The effects of glucagon on basal glucose output in an adult dog during
constant infusion of tracer radioglucose.

In order to obtain more direct information of glucose output and
utilization, we turned to the steady state infusion of C¹⁴- radio-glucose
to the adult dog and puppy (fig. 5). Using a technique similar to
that of DEBODO and STEELE (10) in which a priming dose of radio-
glucose is followed by a sustaining infusion, a steady level of glucose
specific activity and glucose concentration is found after 60 minutes.
Plasma glucose was measured by glucose oxidase, and C¹⁴-glucose
was separated by thin layer chromatography after addition of an
internal standard of tritiated glucose. Both C¹⁴ and H³ were counted
by liquid scintillation. As seen in figure 5, during the control period
after an overnight fast, the adult dog had a calculated hepatic new
glucose output of 2 mg/kg/min when his plasma glucose level was
about 110 mg per 100 ml. He was then given a glucagon infusion while

continuing the radio-glucose infusion until a new steady state was reached. At this time, his output was 5.4 mg/kg/min. Although the latter data may be somewhat invalid due to recirculation of labeled glucose precursor, they represent minimal levels of new glucose released.

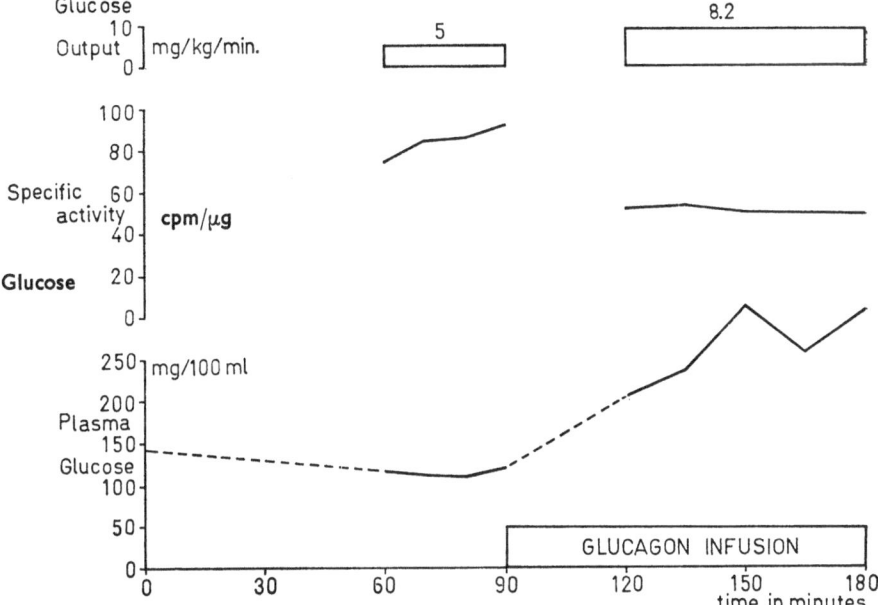

*Fig.* 6.   Similar data to fig. 5 in a 2 day old puppy.

Under comparable conditions, several puppies have been studied after a four hour fast. Figure 6 shows the data for a 2 day old puppy. Basal new glucose output was 5 mg/kg/min while a glucagon infusion raised this to 8.2 mg/kg/min. In the group of puppies ages 1 to 4 days, basal glucose output varied from 4.1 tot 7.3 mg/kg/min compared to two adult dogs with values of 2-2.2 mg/kg/min. After glucagon stimulation, the adult increased his glucose output to 4.8-5.4 while the puppy was 5.5 to 10 mg/kg/min. The puppy then appears to release and utilize glucose at 2-3 times the adult level on a weight basis. This is similar in magnitude to the data in man with exogenous glucose infusion.

If the liver of the newborn has this large capacity for providing glucose under minimal conditions of environmental stress, and can respond to acute stimulation by glucagon, what then are the limitations?

At the previous symposium NELIGAN (11) has commented on some of these. May I remind you of the changes in glycogen in the liver during gestation and post-natally. SHELLEY's (12) original summary (fig. 7, 8) for several species pointed out the increase in the last trimester and the rapid fall post-natally. She (13) extended these observations to stillbirths and infants who died in the perinatal phase. Again although these data may represent minimal values of glycogen due to anoxia or postmortem change, nevertheless a similar trend is observed in the human. She also studied some small for dates infants who had very low levels; however hypoxia may explain some of this.

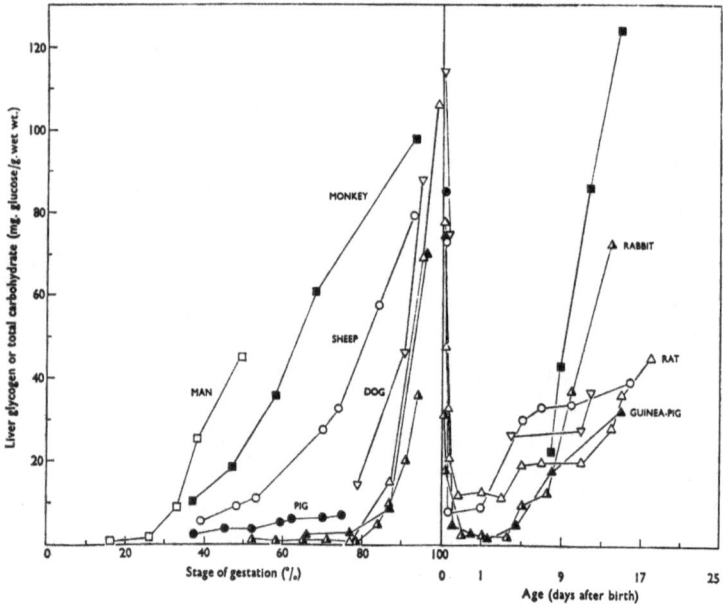

*Fig. 7.* Liver glycogen in different species before and after birth. (Taken from reference (12) p. 138, by permission).

We (14) have studied the puppy extensively in this regard and have confirmed Shelly's observations in this species. In addition we have performed glucagon tests at various ages (fig. 9). Spontaneous hypoglycemia was not observed, but the response to glucagon correlated with the decrease in liver glycogen with age.

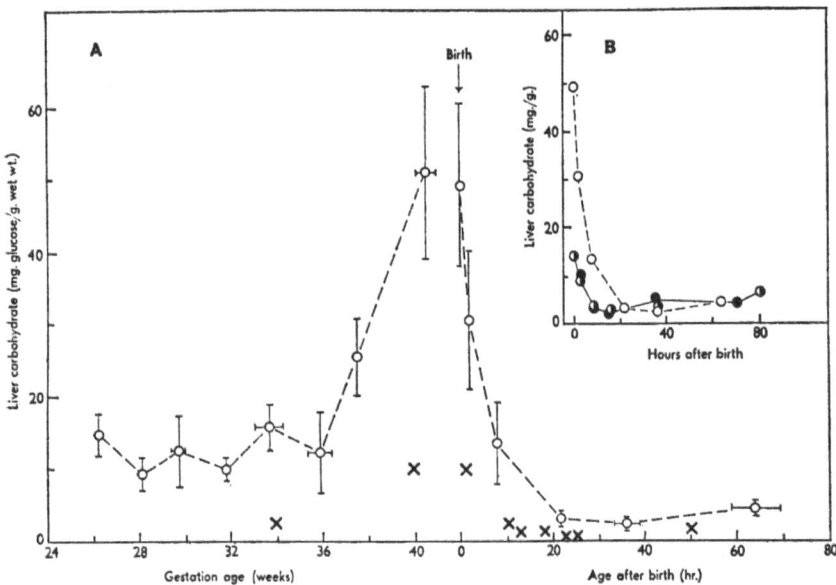

*Fig.* 8.  Liver glycogen in man before and after birth. (Taken from reference (13), p. 36, by permission).

It is apparent from these observations that the acute responses to increased metabolic demands for glucose are likely to be determined by the gestational age at birth as well as by the post-natal age as regards availability of glucose from glycogen. These comments apply to the pre-term infant especially.

To what extent does maternal nutrition influence this? DAWKINS (15) has commended on the production of intrauterine malnutrition in the sheep by restriction of maternal food intake in the latter half of gestation. He stated the fetus is underweight with low levels of glucogen in liver, cardiac and skeletal muscle. The production of hypoglycemia in the sheep has been related also to the number of fetuses when food intake is limited (16).

In our studies of the dog, we followed maternal blood sugar levels before and after delivery. In one instance, significant hypoglycemia was observed in the mother prior to delivery (fig. 10). She also had mild diarrhea so that no conclusions could be drawn concerning her intake which appeared grossly adequate. She had a large litter of ten

pups spontaneously; however she was only required to nourish a few
animals post delivery so that no extensive demands were made of her
nutritionally. As figure 10 indicates, the hypoglycemia observed
before delivery subsided after delivery. The normal dog D had a
litter with six pups at about the same time. The litter of ten pups

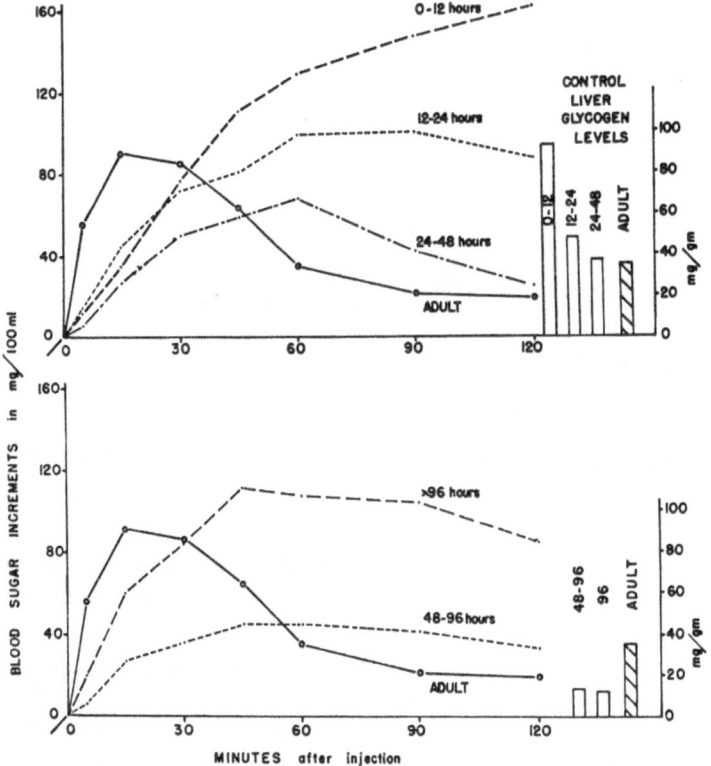

*Fig.* 9.   Relationship between glucagon response on blood glucose increment and
liver glycogen in puppies of various ages after birth (modified from reference (14), by
permission).

from the hypoglycemic mother had three stillborn. Of the remaining
seven, liver glycogen stores were normal in three pups at 4-5 hours
of age (45, 108, 111 mg/g liver), but were markedly reduced in the
remaining four at 18-28 hours (0.25, 0.34, 1.3 and 18 mg/g liver).
Two of the abnormal puppies were tested for glucagon responsiveness
(fig. 11). The responses were blunted or absent in pups C5, C6 at
18-21.5 hours. In one case a minimal rise of 14 mg per 100 ml was

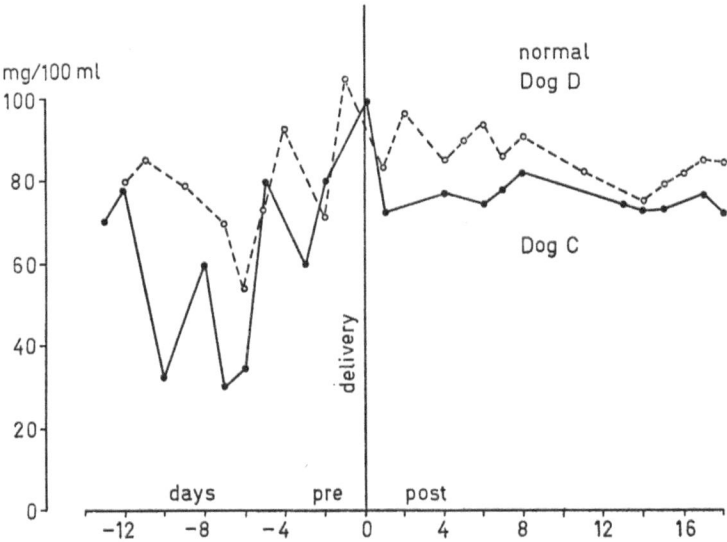

*Fig.* 10. Fasting blood glucose concentrations in two pregnant dogs, pre-and post delivery. Both were treated with same diet and environmental conditions.

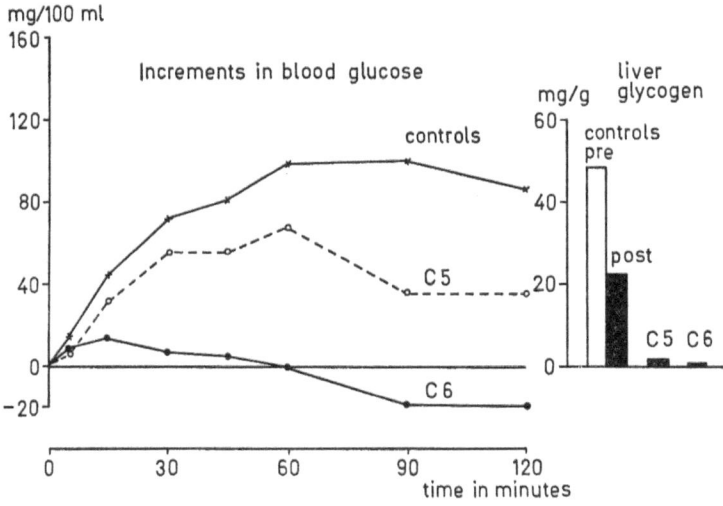

*Fig.* 11. Glucagon responses of two puppies with low liver glycogen at 12—24 hrs of age compared to mean control values (ref. 14).

followed by a fall of -19 mg per 100 ml to hypoglycemic level of 34 mg per 100 ml. Whether these represent the effects of maternal nutritional inadequacy pre-natally, or post-natally (i.e. inadequate lactation and milk feedings) cannot be determined from these observations; however they suggest that this species may serve as another useful model for evaluating the effects of maternal hypoglycemia in 'intrauterine malnutrition'.

The effects of maturation and post-natal feeding have been of renewed interest to many neonatologists in recent years. During the course of observations on the effects of early feeding on bilirubin levels (17), initial studies were begun on blood glucose and glucagon responses. Since then, several reports have appeared (18, 19); however I wish to illustrate these effects with our data.

In order to minimize interpretation and speculation, our observations were limited to larger low birth weight infants who had no significant problems in the initial hours of life. Matched infants were either fed early at 4-6 hours of age and every 3 hours thereafter or starved for the initial forty-eight hours. The starved infants in some instances received distilled water only. The fed infants received either 70 ml per kilogram per day of formula consisting of 5 per cent glucose in 0.45 per cent sodium chloride, or an equicaloric solution of 15 per cent glucose in water at 23 ml/kg/day. Two groups only are considered, one with no glucose intake, the other with 3.5 g/kg/day of glucose, a mere 14 calories/kg/day. No differences in blood glucose level were observed prior to 48 hours. At that time suggestive differences were observed with mean glucose levels of 54 mg per 100 ml in fed group in contrast to 34 mg per 100 ml in starved group. Of equal interest are the glucagon responses at 48-60 hours in the paired infants. As a group, the fed infants had slightly higher responses than the starved group. More importantly, however, when separated by weight a spectrum of response was noted. The larger infants had greater responses as a group than the smaller infants. The fed infants at each level had greater responses. These are evident in figures 12a,b, c,d. Increment above fasting is shown, as is body weight, the percentile for gestational age using the Lubchenco grid, and the fasting blood sugar level. The degree of maturity as judged grossly by weight appears to be as important as early feeding as regards glucagon responsiveness.

In addition to the influence of maternal nutrition, placental

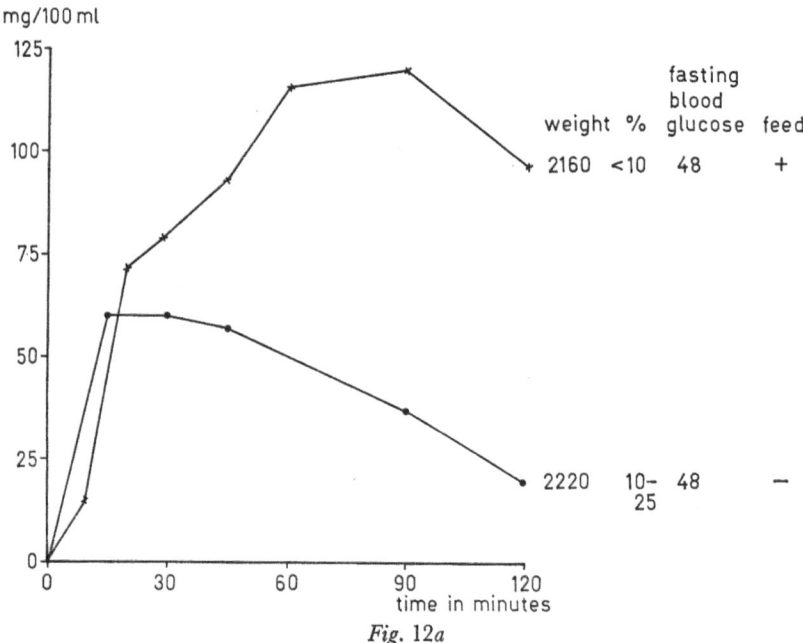

*Fig.* 12a

*Fig.* 12a—d. The effects of glucagon in infants either starved for 48 hrs. or fed small amounts of glucose beginning at 6 hrs. Weight groups are separated. % refers to percentile of weight for gestational age (estimated from Lubchenco).

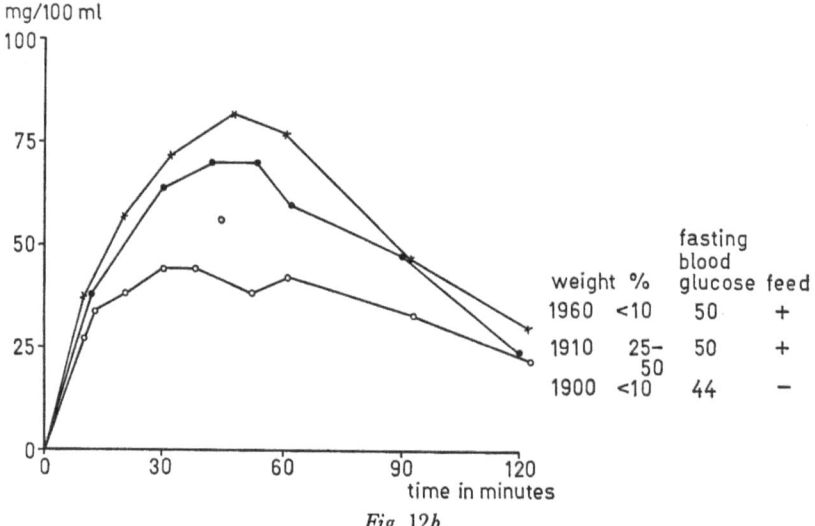

*Fig.* 12b

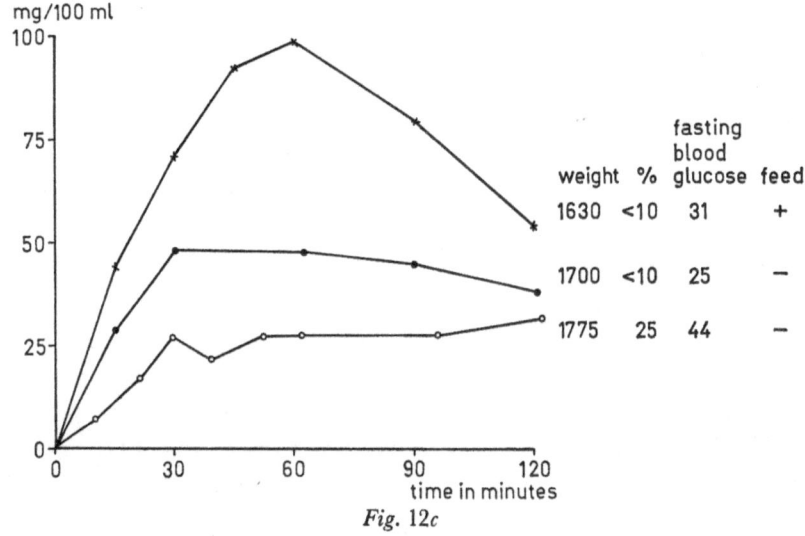

Fig. 12c

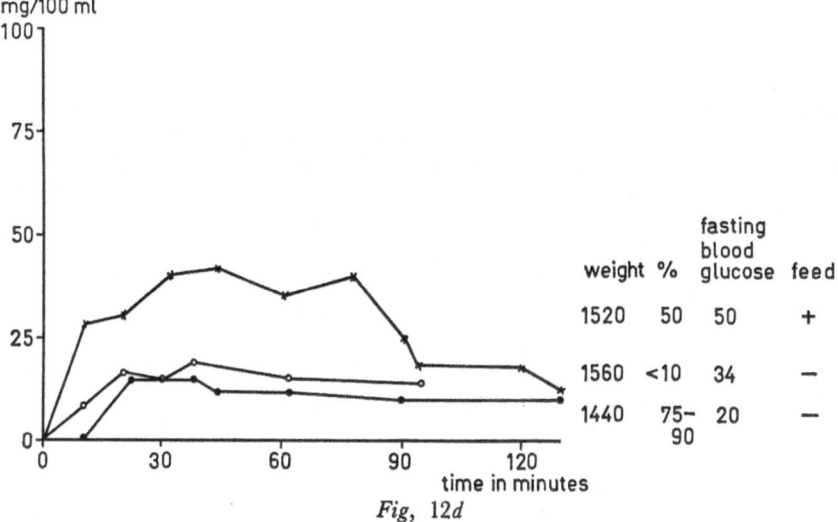

Fig, 12d

transport, maturity and post-natal feeding on glycogen stores and glucose control, energy consumption may also be important. Since oxygen consumption increases from the theoretical fetal value of 3.6 ml/kg/min to the immediate post-natal value of about 4.5 ml/kg/min and finally to levels of 7.0 for the older newborn infant (20), the rate of glucose metabolism would be expected to rise.

Furthermore, the requirement immediately after delivery when the RQ is close to 1 would be different from that later when the RQ approaches 0.80. The infant with a minimal oxygen consumption of 5-7 ml/kg/min with an RQ of 1, deriving all his calories from glucose would consume 6-8.5 mg/kg/min. If the RQ were 0.8 only one-third of the calories would be from carbohydrate and his glucose needs would be 1.9-2.7 mg/kg/min. If he is hypermetabolic then higher consumption of glucose may also occur.

For comparison, KETY (21) found the adult brain to consume 46 ml $O_2$ per minute with a blood flow of 750 ml/min and a glucose consumption of 76 mg/min. The oxygen consumption in the adult is twenty per cent of basal oxygen requirement of body as a whole. The glucose requirement is approximately 1 mg/kg/min, while resting hepatic glucose output in the adult is about 2-3 mg/kg/min, so that cerebral metabolism requires one-third to one-half hepatic output in the adult. Similar data are not available for the infant.

Since the dysmature infant may be found at various stages of development, consideration must be given not only to the usual level for gestational age of glycogen stores, but to the superimposed *in utero* nutritional restriction which results in depleted glycogen supply. The role of gluconeogenesis in sustaining the glucose level in the human normal infant as well as the dysmature infant has not been defined. Whether immature enzyme systems limit glucose production is also unknown in the human. The data (20) on temperature control and oxygen consumption indicate that minimal oxygen consumption in 'small for dates' infants does not rise until about 4 days of age; later a larger rise occurs so that hypermetabolism is noted after 7 days. It is during the early phase, however, of relatively lower oxygen consumption that such infants often exhibit hypoglycemia. SCOPES' (20) interesting observations of infants with hypoglycemia are of further note because they suggest that the low oxygen consumption is related to the hypoglycemia.

Whether hormonal factors are deficient in maintaining blood glucose is not adequately known. STERN and associates (22) have recently studied catecholamine excretion in five infants with neonatal hypoglycemia. They could not demonstrate a rise in urinary excretion and postulated a defective adrenal medullary response. CORNBLATH (1, 2) has reported a few tolerance tests in such infants. Rapid intravenous

15

glucose tolerance tests did not indicate a rapid tissue uptake. Leucine and tolbutamide suggested increased sensitivity since hypoglycemia tended to be greater and more prolonged than in normal infants. The most striking responses, however, were the diminished glucagon tolerance tests. Thus defective glycogen stores appear to be a major factor in the genesis of hypoglycemia observed in dysmature infants.

## SUMMARY

The normal infant and puppy have high rates of basal glucose output and utilization compared to the adult on a weight basis, even though glycogen stores may be lower in the older newborn.

In newborn puppies, however, hepatic glycogen concentration and glucagon responsiveness are directly related and both decrease during the first few days of life.

Low birth weight and dysmature infants have decreased glucagon responses. Dysmature infants may be hypoglycemic as well. The hypoglycemia is presumably related to inadequate hepatic glucose output.

## REFERENCES

1. CORNBLATH, M and R. SCHWARTZ (1966) *Disorders of Carbohydrate Metabolism in Infancy*, Vol. III in Major Problems in Clinical Pediatrics, W. B. Saunders Co., Philadelphia, Pa., p. 85.
2. CORNBLATH, M., S. H. WYBREGT, G. S. BAENS and R. I. KLEIN (1964) *Pediatrics* 33: 388.
3. BROWN, R. J. K. and P. G. WALLIS (1963) *Lancet* 1: 1278.
4. NELIGAN, G. A., E. ROBSON and J. WATSON (1963) *Lancet* 1: 1282.
5. CHANCE, G. W. and B. D. BOWER (1966) *Arch. Dis. Childh.* 41: 279.
6. MYERS, J. D., (1950) *J. Clin. Invest.* 29: 1421.
7. BONDY, P. K., D. F. JAMES and B. W. FARRAR, (1949) *J. Clin. Invest.* 28: 238.
8. SOSKIN, S., H. E. ESSEX, J. F. HERRICK and F. C. MANN (1938) *Am. J. Physiol.* 124: 558.
9. ADAM, P. A. J., K. KING and R. SCHWARTZ (1967) submitted for publication.
10. DEBODO, R. C., R. STEELE, N. ALTSZULER, A. DUNN and J. S. BISHOP (1963) *Recent Prog. Hormone Res. XIX*: 445.
11. NELIGAN, G. (1964) in Nutricia Symposium on *The Adaptation of the Newborn Infant to Extra-uterine Life*. H. E. Stenfert Kroese N.V., Leiden, Holland, p. 42.
12. SHELLEY, H. J. (1961) *Brit. Med. Bull.* 17: 137.

13. SHELLEY, H. J. and G. A. NELIGAN (1966) *Brit. Med. Bull.* 22: 34.
14. ALLEN, D. T., D. KORNHAUSER and R. SCHWARTZ (1966), *Am. J. Dis. Child.* 112: 343.
15. DAWKINS, M. (1963) in Panel Discussion reported in *The Sinai Hospital Journal* 11: 60—61.
16. REID, R. L. and J. P. HOGAN (1959) *Australian J. of Agricultural Research* 10: 81—96.
17. WENNBERG, R. P., R. SCHWARTZ and A. Y. SWEET (1966) *J. Pediat.* 68: 860.
18. HAWORTH, J. C. and J. D. FORD (1963) *Arch. Dis. Childh.* 38: 328.
19. BEARD, A. G., T. C. PANOS, B. V. MARASIGAN, J. EMINANS, H. F. KENNEDY and J. LAMB (1966) *J. Pediat.* 68: 329.
20. SCOPES, J. W. and I. AHMED (1966) *Arch. Dis. Childh.* 41: 407.
21. KETY, S. (1962) in *Neurochemistry*, Ed.ELLIOTT, PAGE and QUASTEL. Charles Thomas, Publisher, p. 113.
22. STERN, L., T. L. SOURKES and N. RÄIHÄ (1967) *Am. Ped. Soc. Seventy-seventh Annual Meeting April* 26—29, Atlantic City, New Jersey, U.S.A., p. 3.

# NEUROPATHOLOGICAL FINDINGS IN SEVERE NEONATAL HYPOGLYCAEMIA WITH REMARKS CONCERNING LESIONS DUE TO HYPOXIA

SABINA J. STRICH*

It is now well known, though it was not ten years ago, that the babies under discussion, that is the very premature and the malnourished, are liable to suffer from severe and prolonged hypoglycaemia in the first few days of extrauterine life (1, 2). It has also become clear that the most important cause of severe hypoglycaemia in the newborn is lack of liver glycogen which is the main source of circulating glucose until feeding is fully established. Liver glycogen is laid down in the last 3 months of intrauterine life and it is thus the very prematurely born infants who may be unable to maintain an adequate blood glucose level. In babies who are underweight for their gestational age the lack of liver glycogen is due to the fact that the liver is disproportionately small and, furthermore, contains less glycogen/unit weight than that of the normal newborn infant (2). In dysmature babies the tendency to become hypoglycaemic is aggravated because the brain is only slightly affected by the growth retardation (3) and its glucose consumption is the same as that of a baby of normal birth weight (For other causes of neonatal hypoglycaemia see CORNBLATH and REISNER (4)).

The tissue most likely to suffer because of hypoglycaemia is that of the nervous system since its major, possibly its only exogenous source of energy is blood glucose (5). There have indeed been several clinical accounts of brain damage following neonatal hypoglycaemia (6, 7, 8), though there have been no necropsy reports of such cases. This communication presents pathological evidence that neonatal hypoglycaemia can damage the brain and that such damage can be prevented by timely treatment.

Our experience is based on the necropsy findings in 6 patients, of whom 5 died in the neonatal period and one died aged 6 months

* Institute of Psychiatry, de Crespigny Park, London S.E. 5. This work was supported by a generous grant from the Nuffield Foundation.

(These cases have been reported in detail (9)). Clinical and pathological data are summarised in the table. In 5 patients one or more glucose estimations were less than 20 mg/100 ml and in four of these patients an intravenous glucose tolerance test was done. In each case this showed an abnormally rapid disappearance of glucose from the blood — confirmation that the tissue demands for glucose outstripped the supply. In one case (case 3) the diagnosis of severe hypoglycaemia was not made during life, although the very low levels of tissue glycogen and lactate found immediately after death by SHELLEY (10) strongly suggested that blood glucose had been low for some time before death. Three infants were thought to have died from hypoglycaemia and they all showed severe degeneration of the nervous system. In three patients the hypoglycaemia was successfully treated but the infants died of unrelated causes later. The nervous system in these babies appeared normal, or nearly so.

Two infants were of less than 30 weeks gestation and 4 were malnourished or dysmature. The question of the clinical recognition of dysmaturity arises here. In case 1 the diagnosis of hypoglycaemia was not considered until it was too late because the infant's birth weight was within normal limits for his gestational age (39 weeks). At post mortem, however, the liver only weighed 96 g (normal 143 $\pm$ 35 g (3) ) whereas the brain was rather large weighing 430 g (normal 400 $\pm$ 50 g (3) ) so that the ratio of brain weight to liver weight was 4.4 (normal 3 or less (11) ) indicating that this baby had been somewhat malnourished.

Before presenting the pathological findings I should like to give the clinical history of just one of these patients.

Case 2, R. B. (Maudsley no. 3187). Male aged 46 hours. This infant was born at 32 weeks gestation weighing 1000 g (normal 2000-2500 g (12)). He breathed immediately and was of good colour, but he was thin and had the appearance typical of severe intrauterine malnutrition. At 3 hours there was slight respiratory irregularity and a catheter was inserted into the umbilical artery. During the next 40 hours repeated $pO_2$ and pH measurements were within normal limits, but despite frequent milk feeds 5 out of 7 blood glucose determinations were below 20 mg/100 ml. Of the other two readings one was 21 mg/100 ml and one, at 30 hours, was 56 mg/100 ml. It was probably this reading which misled the clinicians so that the diagnosis of severe hypoglycaemia was not made until later. The infant was awake most of the time, hyperactive and irritable; there was no respiratory distress. At 41 hours he became limp and cyanosed and from this time there were apnoeic episodes of increasing length. Blood glucose was 8 mg/ 100 ml and an intravenous glucose tolerance test showed a very rapid disappearance of glucose (the rate constant (K) for glucose disappearance was 13.8, normal 0.5 $\pm$ 0.19 (13)). At 45 hours the arterial $pO_2$ was 59 mm Hg and the pH was 7.09 — the lowest values recorded. Intravenous administration of glucose resulted in slight improvement in the infant's condition but this deteriorated again and he died aged 46 hours. At post mortem the mesenteric artery was thrombosed and there was infarction of the gut with peritonitis.

Histologically there was severe degeneration of nerve cells and glial cells throughout the neuraxis in cases 1 and 2 and somewhat less widespread changes in case 3. In *small nerve cells* there was clumping of chromatin and the nuclear membrane had disappeared. Chromatin fragments had aggregated into a beaded, densely staining mass or lay scattered in the cytoplasm (fig. 1). This change was seen wherever there are small neurones e.g. in the cerebral cortex, the caudate nucleus and the putamen, and in the internal granular layer of the cerebellum. The cells in the griseum pontis were surprisingly unaffected and cells in the germinative zones and in the external granular layer of the cerebellum appeared normal. In the cerebral cortex damaged nerve cells were seen in all layers and the cortex at the bottom of sulci or at the arterial boundary zones was not more severely involved than that elsewhere; the occipital lobes were most affected and the temporal lobes, Including the hippocampus, least. *Large neurones* showed chromatolysis, and swelling and granularity of the cytoplasm (fig. 2). Their nuclei were shrunken and dense or faintly staining and were often surrounded by a clear zone. These changes were seen in the globus pallidus, in the thalamus and in the brainstem (the motor nuclei of the cranial nerves and most of the main sensory nuclei were severely affected) as well as in the anterior horn cells of the spinal cord. Purkinje cells in the cerebellum were also affected. Glial cells throughout the nervous system had small pyknotic nuclei in cases 1 and 2. In case 1 there were a few sharply demarcated areas of periventricular leukomalacia in which the nerve fibres were swollen and

Table 1.  *Summary of clinical and pathological findings*

| Case | Sex | Ge-station weeks | Age at death | First symptoms at | Approx. duration of hypoglycaemia | Other features | Brain wt/ liver wt. ratio* | K | Brain damage Macro-scopic | Brain damage Micro-scopic |
|------|-----|------|------|------|------|------|------|------|------|------|
| 1 (No. 3301) | M | 39 | 55½ hrs | 17 hrs | 38 hrs | malnourished convulsions | 4.4 | — | normal | ++++ |
| 2 (No. 3187) | M | 32 | 45½ hrs | 3 hrs | 40 hrs | malnourished peritonitis apnoeic episodes hypoxic | 7.0 | 13.8 | normal | ++++ |
| 3 (No. 2016) | F | 28 | 45½ hrs | 7 hrs | 38 hrs | | 3.5 | — | i.v.h. | +++ |
| 4 (No. 3487) | M | 25 | 7½ days | none | 37 hrs intermittent | | 2.7 | 2.5 | i.v.h. | + |
| 5 (No. 3299) | M | 33 | 64 hrs | none | 9 hrs | malnourished malformed heart | 6.8 | 2.1 | normal | + |
| 6 (No. 3699) | M | 38 | 6 months | 16 hrs | 18 hrs intermittent | malnourished smaller twin | — | 1.8 | normal small | O |

i.v.h. — intraventricular haemorrhage   *normal less than 3 (11)   K = rate constant for glucose disappearance, normal 0.5 ± 0.19 (13)   ++++ = very severe;   +++ = severe;   + = slight;   O = none eosinophilic. Except for a few foci of microglial cells there was no mesodermal or glial reaction in the sections examined.

Neither the cytological changes nor the distribution of the lesions just described are specific for hypoglycaemia. They are also found in perinatal hypoxia, though uniformly devastating histological changes are rare in this condition and are only seen in what one might irreverently call 'resuscitated still births'. The more usual findings in hypoxia (in adults as well as in babies) include the so-called ischaemic nerve cell change (fig. 3) in which the cytoplasm becomes eosinophilic and the nucleus small, pyknotic and irregular in outline. After hypoxia (unless extremely severe) or ischaemia the lesions in the nervous system in adults (14) and almost certainly in babies (personal observations) are not diffuse and uniform as in neonatal hypoglycaemia but are localised in certain areas which are determined either by vascular factors or by the fact that some nerve cells are more sensitive to abnormal conditions than others. Examples of this 'selective vulnerability' are the necrosis of the globus pallidus in carbon monoxide poisoning; or the necrosis of Sommer's sector (H I) of the hippocampus and the 3rd layer of the cerebral cortex especially at the bottom of sulci after anoxia. The only hint that some parts of the nervous system of the newborn may be more sensitive to hypoglycaemia than others comes from our case 3 in which nerve cells were affected but glial cells were not, and in which the basal ganglia and the cerebellum were more severely affected than the cerebral cortex while the lower brainstem and cervical spinal cord were almost spared.

Evidence of 'selective vulnerability' is often seen in the brain after temporary cardiac arrest or in post-epileptic brain damage (14). Interestingly enough 'selective vulnerability' is rarely spoken of when discussing the pathogenesis of lesions in the nervous system of older children with cerebral palsy due to 'birth trauma'. Here the lesions are patchy and focal (15, 16, 17) and the emphasis is on circulatory disturbances — arterial, venous or both, depending on the outlook of the investigator. (There is very little information about the pathology of cerebral hypoxia in infants dying in the neonatal period). Lesions in the regions where the branches of the main cerebral arteries anastomose with each other either on the surface or within the nervous system are also seen. The arterial boundary zones are weak points in the cerebral circulation and tissue in such regions is the first

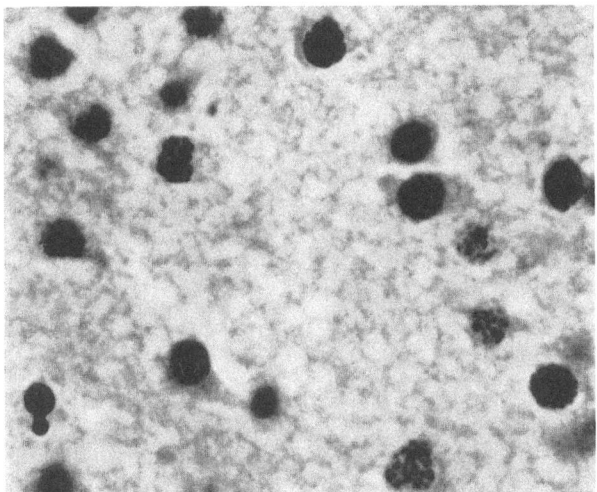

*Fig.* 1 *a.* Cerebral cortex of case 1. Nuclei of nerve cells are fragmented or pyknotic and beaded. Compare with fig. 1 *b.*

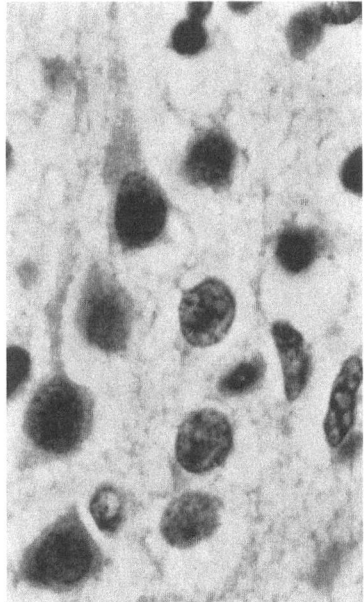

*Fig.* 1 *b.* Normal cerebral cortex from a full term infant. The nuclei of the nerve cells have a well defined nuclear membrane and a delicate chromatin network.

Haematoxylin and eosin x 1200

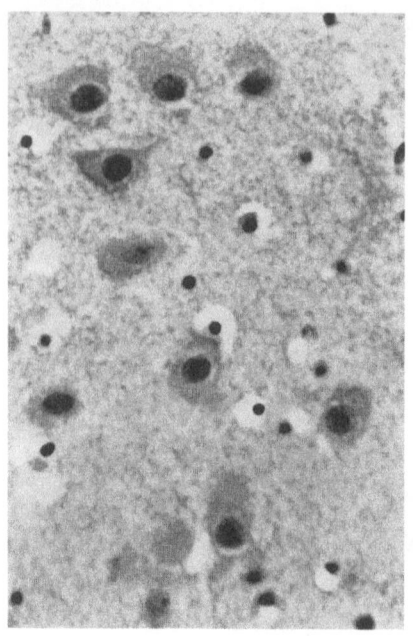

*Fig.* 2 *a.*　　Thalamus of case 1. The outline of the nerve cells is indistinct and there are no Nissl bodies in the cytoplasm which looks granular. The nuclei are small and dense. Compare with fig. 2 *b.*

Haematoxylin and eosin x 450

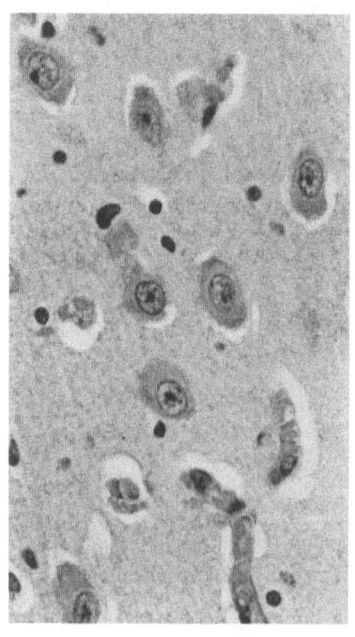

*Fig.* 2. *b.* Normal thalamus from a full term infant. The nerve cells have pale nuclei with a well marked nuclear membrane. Nissl bodies can be seen at the periphery of the cell body.

Haematoxylin and eosin x 450

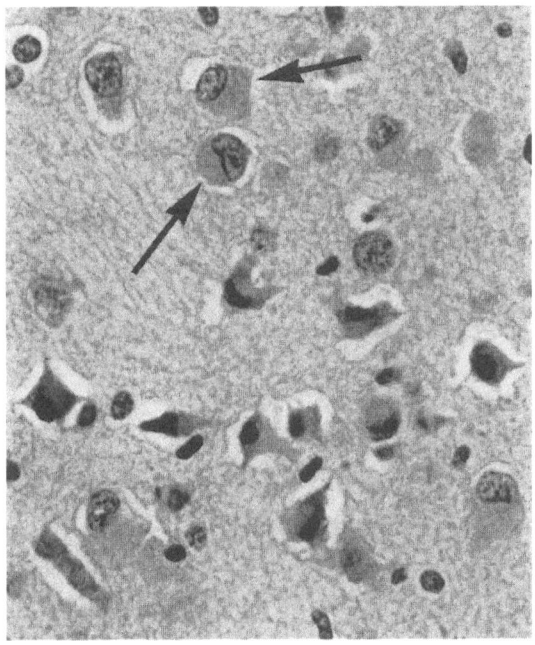

*Fig.* 3.   Nerve cells in the griseum pontis of an infant who had been severely hypoxic. Many nerve cells show 'ischaemic cell change' that is, their cytoplasm is eosinophilic and the nucleus is shrunken, dense and irregular in outline. Normal nerve cells are also seen (arrows).

Haematoxylin and eosin x 480

to show damage after episodes of systemic hypotension (18, 19).

There were practically no lesions which could be related to circulatory disturbances in our cases of hypoglycaemia. The only focal lesions were small areas of periventricular leukomalacia in case 1 such as have been discussed by BANKER and LARROCHE (20), see also SCHWARTZ (16).) That the brain damage due to hypoglycaemia in the first week of life is so much more severe, widespread and diffuse than that due to presumed perinatal hypoxia may be related to the way in which these two conditions affect the heart. Heart muscle is as dependent on oxygen as is nervous tissue. In fact an infant may die because the heart fails, before very extensive brain damage has had time to develop. In any case, circulatory disturbances are likely to play an important role in the pathogenesis of brain lesions in hypoxia. On the other hand the heart is probably not particularly sensitive to lack of circulating glucose, partly because it has a large store of glycogen (10), partly because heart muscle can use exogenous substrates other than glucose for its energy supply. Since nervous tissue is very sensitive to hypoglycaemia severe and diffuse brain damage unrelated to vascular disturbances is likely to be seen in this condition.

Of the three patients in whom the hypoglycaemia was treated one died of intraventricular haemorrhage having been hypoxic and acidaemic for 4 days before death. One patient died of congenital heart disease. The only microscopic abnormalities in these two cases were a few 'ischaemic nerve cells' in the thalamus and brainstem. Patient 6 appeared to be a normal baby until he died of bronchopneumonia aged 6 months. The brain was small (600 g, normal 760 $\pm$ 70 g) but showed no obvious histological abnormalities.

It is clear from looking at our cases of neonatal hypoglycaemia that nervous tissue can survive very low blood glucose levels for many hours (see table), especially if the hypoglycaemia is intermittent. Although glucose is the chief *exogenous* source of energy for nervous tissue, this can of course utilise *endogenous* substrates other than glucose e.g. amino acids, lipids and ribonucleic acid as has been shown experimentally by various workers (21, 22, 23). The oxidation of cell components which cannot be replaced in the absence of glucose is likely eventually to lead to irreversible cell damage such as was seen in our untreated patients.

234                                S. J. STRICH

## REFERENCES

1. CORNBLATH, M., G. B. ODELL and E. T. LEVIN (1959) *J. Pediat.* 55: 545.
2. SHELLEY, H. J. and G. A. NELIGAN (1966) *Brit. med. Bull.* 22: 34.
3. GRUENWALD, P. (1963) *Biol. Neonat.* (Basel) 5: 215.
4. CORNBLATH, M. and S. H. REISNER (1965) *New Engl. J. Med.* 273: 378.
5. McILWAIN, H. (1966) *Biochemistry and the central nervous system.* Churchill, London, p. 6.
6. BROWN, R. J. K. and P. G. WALLIS (1963) *Lancet* 1: 1278.
7. CORNBLATH, M., S. H. WYBREGT, G. S. BAENS and R. I. KLEIN (1964) *Pediatrics* 33: 388.
8. HAWORTH, J. C. and K. N. McRAE (1965) *Canad. med. Ass. J.* 92: 861.
9. ANDERSON, J. M., R. D. G. MILNER and S. J. STRICH (1967) *J. Neurol. Neurosurg. Psychiat.* 30: 295.
10. SHELLEY, H. J. (1964) *Brit. med. J.* 1: 273.
11. DAWKINS, M. J. R. (1964) *Proc. roy. Soc. Med.* 57: 1063.
12. BUTLER, N. R. and D. G. BONHAM, (1963) *Perinatal Mortality.* Livingstone, Edinburgh.
13. BAIRD, J. D. and J. W. FARQUHAR (1962) *Lancet* 1: 71.
14. MEYER, A. (1963) in *Greenfield's Neuropathology* ed. 2. Arnold, London p. 255.
15. NORMAN, R. M., H. URICH and W. H. McMENEMEY (1957) *Brain* 80: 49.
16. SCHWARTZ, P. (1961) *Birth injuries of the newborn.* Karger, New York.
17. MALAMUD, N. (1963) in *Selective vulnerability of the brain in hypoxaemia.* SCHADÉ and McMENEMEY eds. Blackwell, Oxford. p. 211.
18. MEYER, J. E. (1953) *Arch. Psychiat. Nervenkr.* 190: 328.
19. ADAMS, J. H., J. B. BRIERLEY, R. C. R. CONNOR and C. S. TREIP (1966) *Brain* 89: 235.
20. BANKER, B. Q., and J. C. LARROCHE (1962) *Arch. Neurol.* (Chic.) 7: 386.
21. GEIGER, A. (1958) *Physiol. Rev.* 38: 1.
22. VRBA, R. (1962) *Nature* (Lond.) 195: 663.
23. BARBATO, I. W. M. and L. BARBATO (1965) *J. Neurochem.* 12: 60.

# HYPERBILIRUBINAEMIA IN DYSMATURE
# VERSUS PREMATURE INFANTS

J. I. DE BRUIJNE*

In the many articles on dysmaturity which appeared in the last years, little is said about hyperbilirubinaemia. For a long time it is known that premature infants have higher serum bilirubin levels than full-term infants and that the hyperbilirubinaemia is of longer duration. The risk of kernicterus is probably correlated as well with the height of the bilirubin level as with the duration of the high bilirubin levels above 18–24 mg/100 ml, according to different authors.

However, in an infant, for example, born 6 weeks before term, the hyperbilirubinaemia persists only a few days longer than in full-term infants and not 6 weeks longer as one could expect. This fact points in the direction of the role which adaptation to extra-uterine life plays, in activation of the enzyme glucuronyltransferase. It is known from experiments in newborn rats that the activity of the liverenzymes concerned with coupling of bilirubin is very low immediately after birth, but increases daily. From all clinical experience it is probable that in the human newborn the same process of maturation occurs in the first few days of extra-uterine life and that, though premature babies have more difficulty with this process of maturation, in the majority of cases they are able to overcome these difficulties.

Since in the last years low birth weight is not longer considered identical with prematurity, it is time to compare the premature and the dysmature low birth weight babies with respect to hyperbilirubinaemia. For the clinician the difference is clear enough: many of his dysmature infants do not become jaundiced at all, but naturally the clinical impression gives no sufficient information.

In the Obstetric Clinic in Amsterdam we made a survey during the years 1965 and 1966 of all low birth weight babies, correlating birth

* Department of Physiology and Pathology of the Newborn, Wilhelmina Gasthuis, University of Amsterdam.

weight and length of gestation. The gestation was calculated by Miss
HUIDEKOPER from the Obstetric Department from the first day of the
last menstruation, and in cases of doubt also from the data obtained
during the prenatal examinations.

As you will see tomorrow, Prof. KLOOSTERMAN and Miss HUIDE-
KOPER made curves of intra-uterine growth based on many thousands
of infants, born at Amsterdam. These figures are comparable, though
not identical with those of Dr. LUBCHENCO and co-workers from Denver,
Colorado. The mean weights in the Amsterdam study are somewhat
higher than the Denver studies, which among other factors may be
caused by a difference in altitude.

To compare premature and dysmature babies I have chosen the
group of singleton infants with a birth weight of 1501 to 2500 grams
(table 1). The advantages of studying this group are in the first place
that in this group so few children died within the first week of life,
before having developed hyperbilirubinaemia or not: on a total
amount of 305 infants only 12 died in the first week, which means that
the ultimate conclusions to be derived will not be influenced to a
great extent by the loss of these babies from the survey.

Table 1. *Analysis of* 305 *singleton babies within the range of* 1501-2500
*grams, born* 1965 *and* 1966, *in the obstetric clinic university of
Amsterdam*

| | |
|---|---|
| Total | 305 |
| Died within 1st week | 12 |
| | 293 |
| Discarded because of insufficient data concerning duration of pregnancy | 26 |
| | 267 |

A secundary advantage is that in this group the premature babies,
defined as born before the end of the 37th week = before 259 days,
are present in about the same amount as the dysmature babies. As
a definition of dysmaturity I chose the infants with a birth weight of
less than the 10th percentile. When using the 25th percentile too many

mild cases would have been included. Now the two groups cover each about 50 % of the total amount of infants born in this weight group. It was to be expected that some babies had to be excluded, because of the fact that the length of gestation was too uncertain. We excluded 26 infants. Of course this does not mean that in all the other infants the duration of pregnancy was absolutely certain; I preferred to call the remaining group of infants (267) the group with *reasonably* accurate data concerning the duration of pregnancy.

As a matter of fact I had to discard all babies with diseases which could lead in itself to hyperbilirubinaemia: Rh or ABO haemolytic disease of the newborn (table 2). As you will see in table 5I included one infant in which haemolysis played probably a dominant role. As the cause of the haemolysis remained unknown I preferred to include that baby, (girl, 2090 grams, 34 weeks, had to be exchanged twice). Only one infant of a mother with diabetes mellitus was in this group; most infants from diabetic mothers have a birth weight of more than 2500 grams. A few infants of non-Caucasian parents were excluded. When one of the parents was non-Caucasian, the baby was included. One intra-uterine infection which could lead to low birth weight as well as to hyperbilirubinaemia was discarded. The baby, suffered from cytomegalic inclusion body disease, was not very small for date, 2370 grams at 37 weeks, which is just under the 10th percentile; the maximum bilirubin was only 5.4 mg/100 ml on the 3rd day of life. Hypoglycaemia developed in this baby.

I would prefer to speak about the group of 10 infants with congenital

Table 2. *Babies with reasonably accurate data length of pregnancy*

| | | |
|---|---|---|
| Total | | 267 |
| Discarded because of RH- or ABO-hemolytic disease | 9 | |
| Mother diabetes | 1 | |
| Indonesian, Hindostani, Chinese, Negro-parents | 8 | |
| Congenital malformations | 10 | |
| Intrauterine infections (cytomegalic inclusion disease) | 1 | |
| | | 29 |
| To be analyzed for hyperbilirubinaemia | | 238 |

malformations at the end of my paper, as they comprise a special group
which has to be distinguished from low birth weight caused by intrauterine malnutrition.

There remain then 238 babies, 101 boys and 137 girls. This is not
the excess of boys we would expect, but in this group it is maybe not
completely surprising. In the patient material of these two years
there was a big excess of boys only in the smallest group of infants of
501 till 1000 grams, of which only one survived. Prof. KLOOSTERMAN
suggested, when I showed him our figures, that the excess of the girls
might be caused by the fact that more boys had a birth weight of
more than 2500 grams and were for that reason not included in this
group.

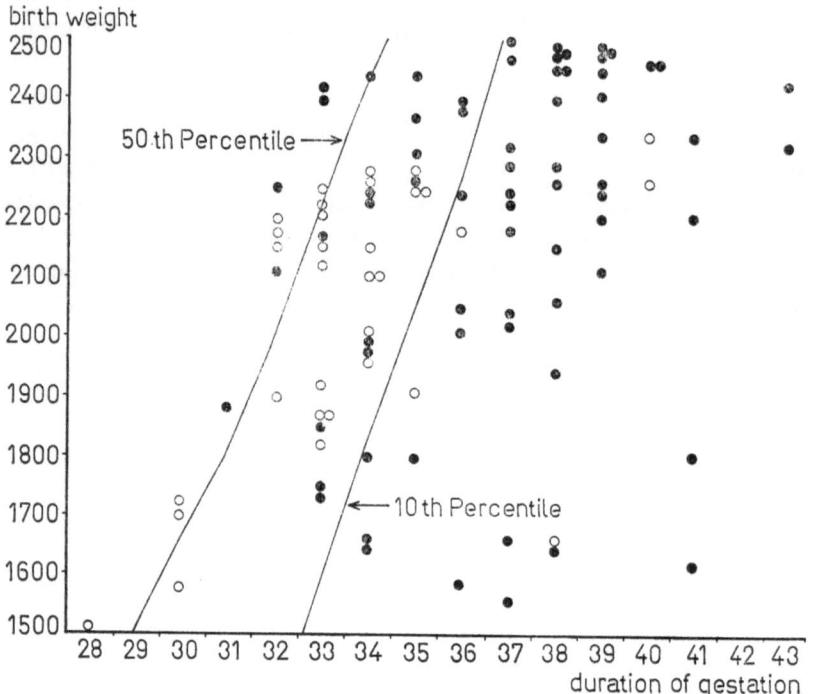

*Fig.* 1.  Maximal blood bilirubin level related to birth weight and duration of
gestation. Scattergram of 101 newborn boys. 50th and 10th percentiles according
to intra-uterine growth curves of KLOOSTERMAN and HUIDEKOPER.
O  maximal bilirubin level ⩾ 15 mg/100 ml
●  maximal bilirubin level < 15 mg/100 ml

As the boys and girls are separately analyzed and compared with the 50th and 10th percentiles for their respective birth weight according to length of gestation, the excess of girls is, for the study-object of today, the hyperbilirubinaemia, not relevant. In all babies who became visibly jaundiced the bilirubin content of the blood was daily and sometimes, when the bilirubin content was high, three of four times daily checked. The method used was the method of Malloy and Evelyn in a micromodification: 0.1 ml capillary bloodserum was obtained by heelprick. The total bilirubin was estimated. The one-minute bilirubin was not estimated in all cases, but even in the cases with high bilirubin values in the blood, the direct reacting bilirubin was not higher than 0.4 to 0.7 mg per cent. As all the babies were born in the hospital, they were weighed immediately after birth.

As many, and especially the dysmature infants, did not become visibly jaundiced at all, and were for that reason not daily checked, it seemed to me of little use to make curves of mean bilirubin content of the blood for each day of life. In order to compare the premature and the dysmature infants, I have chosen as a criterium of hyperbilirubinaemia a bilirubin value of 15 mg/100 ml; with that level in the blood all the babies are without any doubt visibly jaundiced. Although I could have taken all the babies with peak bilirubins of 10 mg per cent or more, I thought it would be better to take the babies with a peak of 15 mg/100 ml or more, in order to be completely sure that not one baby should have been overlooked.

First I made a scattergram of the group of boys (fig. 1). The 50th and 10th percentiles are indicated according to the intra-uterine growth curve of KLOOSTERMAN and HUIDEKOPER. It can be seen that in the large majority of dysmature babies the bilirubin content of the blood does not exceed 15 mg/100 ml. Two of the boys are near the 10th percentile, and both are premature as well as dysmature indicated by the triangle on the scattergram. The other three are far below the 10th percentile and about half of the infants who were premature by gestation and had a birth weight in the neighbourhood of the 50th percentile had a peak bilirubin of 15 mg/100 ml or more.

Table 3 shows in figures what is also visible on the scattergram (fig. 1): only 5 of 52 boys or about 10 per cent with a birth weight of less than the 10th percentile had a bilirubin content of 15 mg/100 ml or more, whereas no less than 27 of the 49 boys, which is about half

of them, who were not only premature but also had a birth weight
above the 10th percentile, had hyperbilirubinaemia of 15 mg/100 ml
or more.

In the girls essentially the same picture is seen (fig. 2): again in
the dysmature girls little hyperbilirubinaemia was present, whereas

Table 3.

---

101 Boys          1501—2500 grams

52 < 10th  Percentile;  bilirubin ⩾ 15 mg/100 ml:  5
49 > 10th  Percentile;  bilirubin ⩾ 15 mg/100 ml: 27

---

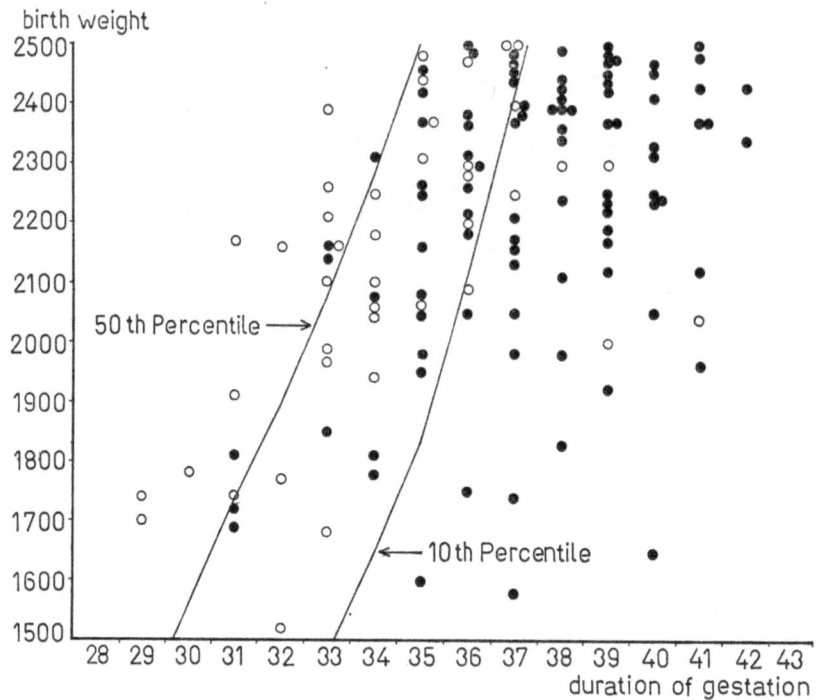

*Fig.* 2.  Maximal blood bilirubin level related to birth weight and duration of
gestation. Scattergram of 137 newborn girls.
O  maximal bilirubin level ⩾ 15 mg/100 ml
●  maximal bilirubin level < 15 mg/100 ml

many premature girls had peak bilirubins of more than 15 mg per cent. Only 7 of 68 girls with a birth weight below the 10th percentile had hyperbilirubinaemia, whereas 35 of 69 premature girls with a birth weight above the 10th percentile had a peak bilirubin of 15 mg/ 100 ml or more (tabel 4). Only 4 infant girls were both premature and dysmature, one of them near the 10th percentile line, a girl of 36 weeks, had hyperbilirubinaemia.

Table 4.

| 137 Girls | 1501—2500 grams |
|---|---|

68 < 10th Percentile; bilirubin ⩾ 15 mg/100 ml:  7
69 > 10th Percentile; bilirubin > 15 mg/100 ml: 35

Table 5.

| Bilirubin 20 mg/100 ml or more |
|---|

13  In premature boys
 0  In dysmature boys

 8  In premature girls
 3  In dysmature girls
    (Of which 1 haemolysis of unknown cause)

Not only that so much less dysmature infants have hyperbilirubinaemia than premature infants have, the hyperbilirubinaemia in dysmature babies seems to follow also a milder course: it does not reach as high peak values as in premature infants. This become clear in table 5: at least in the boys a bilirubin content of the blood of 20 mg/100 ml or more was reached in 13 of the premature boys and not once in dysmature boys; in the dysmature girls this is less convincing as two dysmature infants had a peak bilirubin of 21.1 and 21.6 respectively whereas only 8 of the premature girls had maximum bilirubins of more than 20 mg/100 ml. As exchange transfusion in our hospital is done when the bilirubin content exceeds 23 mg/100ml or is likely to exceed this figure, it has not been necessary to exchange

16

these two girls. Only in special cases which had severe other disturbances like asphyxia, respiratory distress syndrome, accompanied with
severe acidosis, the exchange transfusion is performed before the
bilirubin content has reached 20 mg/100 ml. The one girl with haemolysis is included, but she had a very rapid rise in bilirubin content
indeed and had to be exchanged twice. No cause of any bloodgroup
incompatibility, glucose-6-phosphate-dehydrogenase deficiency, infection or other disease could be found, the child was and remained in a
good condition without other symptoms of disease.

Table 6 shows a similar picture as the number of exchange transfusions corresponds to a large extent with the bilirubin values of
higher than 20 mg/100 ml.

Table 6.

| Exchange transfusions |
| --- |
| 12  In premature boys |
| 0  In dysmature boys |
| |
| 9  In premature girls |
| 1  In dysmature girls |
| (The case with the haemolysis) |

Table 7 shows the group of infants with congenital malformations
which might influence the intra-uterine growth. Five had a birth weight
below the 10th percentile and all five infants were full-term. In the
infant with ectodermal dysplasia the diagnosis was not made in the
neonatal periode, but only after a few months during the follow-up.
The other five infants were premature according to their length of
gestation, though especially the case with trisomy $D_1$ might have been
a small for date baby too. The baby with adrenal hyperplasia and
pseudohermaphroditism had of course no really congenital malformations but as inborn errors of metabolism belong to the group of
the congenital diseases in the broadest sense, I included that baby in
this group because of possible influences of the endocrine disturbances
on intrauterine growth and maturation.

As none of these ten premature or dysmature babies with congenital
malformations had hyperbilirubinaemia of 15 mg/100 ml or more,

the total results of the survey are not influenced by their exclusion.
Nevertheless I think it was necessary to discuss them apart from the
other infants.

Although it is not my task to talk about hypoglycaemia, the combination of hyperbilirubinaemia with hypoglycaemia (blood glucose
below 30 mg/100 ml) occurred in only two of the dysmature babies,
while as we have seen hyperbilirubinaemia above 15 mg/100 ml was
present in 12 dysmature infants and we found hypoglycaemia in 17
infants. It seems therefore that hypoglycaemia does not play a dominant role in the pathogenesis of hyperbilirubinaemia in the dysmature
newborn baby.

Table 7.

| | | | | | 10th percen-tile | max. bil. |
|---|---|---|---|---|---|---|
| V. | Hemihypertrophy | ♂ | 1790 | 41 | < | 14.7 |
| B. | Multiple malf. (Ears, nails, heart, hip, oligophrenia) | ♂ | 2170 | 39 | < | —— |
| G. | Down syndrome + cong. heart | ♀ | 2120 | 39 | < | 5.5 |
| E. | Encephalocele | ♀ | 2400 | 39 | < | —— |
| K. | Ectodermal dysplasia | ♂ | 1890 | 38 | < | —— |
| v.B. | Trisomy 13—15 (D₁) | ♀ | 1860 | 34 | > | 13.8 |
| B. | Oesophageal atresia + hemi-vertebrae | ♀ | 2360 | 35 | > | ? |
| G. | Anal atresia + rectoperineal fistula | ♀ | 2460 | 36 | > | —— |
| R. | Spina bifida with meningo-myelocele | ♂ | 2430 | 36 | > | —— |
| Z. | Adrenal hyperplasia | ♀ | 2310 | 36 | > | 13.4 |

Summarizing I think we might postulate that, when the hyperbilirubinaemia in the newborn is a consequence of insufficient adaptation
to extrauterine life and the full-term infant is better equipped to cope
this problem than the premature baby, the dysmature infant behaves
more like the full-term infant than like the premature infant with the
same birth weight, but born after a shorter gestation, or in other
words, the duration of pregnancy seems to be more important than

the birth weight or, in still other words, the intra-uterine maturation of the liver is in this respect more important than the adaptation to extra-uterine life. This is what we might have expected considering other aspects of dysmaturity e.g. the development and maturation of the central nervous system and of the kidneys.

# DISCUSSION

DISCUSSION PAPER PROF. JONXIS

*Dr. Widdowson* (in the chair): Thank you very much indeed. The paper of Prof. JONXIS is now open for discussion. I wonder if you could make clear to us from the beginning what, if any, food the babies are having on the third day when the R.Q. is so low.

*Prof. Jonxis:* It is humanized milk. Some of the babies received glucose 5 per cent intravenously, but most of them had milk 50 ml/kg. This formula contains 7 per cent of lactose, so the infants got already 3.5 g lactose/kg daily. The infants had a very good supply of carbohydrates. This makes it very difficult for me to understand the low R.Q.

*Prof. R. Schwartz:* I wish to comment on this beautiful study Prof. JONXIS and his associates have prepared for us. These are lovely data to be able to look at and to speculate about a little bit.

It seems to me that we reach the point now of having to think about different organs and their metabolism now we have a fair appreciation of what is happening in the whole body. First of all with reference to whether increased fat mobilisation and free fatty acids are inhibiting glucose uptake. I believe that the Randle data are with reference to muscle mainly. I wonder if you would care to speculate concerning muscle metabolism versus the rest of the body with reference to the maintenance of blood glucose you described.

What is happening to the brain? I wonder if your group, I'm sure you have thought about this, has even considered the adult data on oxygen consumption of the brain as an approximation. When you have so very low R.Q.'s one wonders if the brain is burning glucose at even close to adult levels and probably much less than that. The rest of the body must then have an even lower R.Q. I think we have to look at other metabolic views to put these together with this kind of information. It is very interesting and provocative but I have no explanation.

*Dr. Loeb:* May be I can give you some elements to your question concerning liver catabolism in the dysmature newborn infant. We studied these infants in the first hours after delivery together with some normal infants. We made determinations of non-esterified fatty acids, pyruvic acid and lactic acid. We performed this determination three times: just after delivery, after 24 hours and after 72 hours. Our first results are the following: concerning non esterfied fatty acids we had indeed no difference between our normal children and the dysmature children. Also with lactic acid there was no difference. It seems however that the values for pyruvic acid are higher in the dysmature babies than in the normal babies.

*Dr. Gruenwald:* I wonder whether I understand your data correctly to mean that even the dysmature infants who have been emaciated and are free of fat, still actually have enough fat in their body to perform all these things you have shown. Do I understand this correctly?

*Prof. Jonxis:* Yes, that's correct. But our exposure to cold was a very moderate one and the duration of the experiment was rather short. When you calculate how many mgs of fat are really metabolized during this experiment, you come only to a few mg/kg/minute. There must be a large difference between a long exposure to real cold and a short term exposure to very moderate low temperatures. Dr. HOMMES, do you remember the exact values?

*Dr. Hommes:* It is about 4 mg/kg/min of fat. That amount of fat is surely still there.

*Prof. Minkowski:* Did you determine the ratio of glycerol and free fatty acids? As you remember the group from Prague showed that this ratio is quite different in the normal newborn and in the praemature. I think this ratio is 1 : 5 in normal full-term infants and 1 : 1.5 in praematures.

I wonder if it would not be of interest to know the catecholamine excretion. As you know the dysmature infant is reacting in a very peculiar way as STERN and coworkers have shown. After injection of insulin the dysmature infants did not increase their catecholamine excretion. In an experiment done by LEE from Oregon Medical School they have shown that a higher catecholamine excretion in such a kind of cooling would occur only in 1 out of 3 times.

*Prof. Jonxis:* We have not yet collected these data.

*Dr. Loeb:* I'm not sure that determination of catecholamine excretion in the urine can help us. It has been demonstrated in older children that when you give insulin, catecholamine excretion has not to be higher, even if there is hypoglycaemia. It is not necessary to have adrenals in order to correct severe hypoglycaemia due to injection of insulin. I wonder if the catecholamine excretion can be of any value to understand for instance hypoglycaemia in the newborn.

*Dr. Räihä:* I would like to ask Prof. JONXIS one question about the decrease of R.Q. in praemature and dysmature babies. Was that mainly due to a decrease of $CO_2$ production or to an increase in oxygen consumption?

*Prof. Jonxis:* There is a marked increase in oxygen consumption. The $CO_2$ production is also increasing, but not as fast as the oxygen consumption.

*Dr. Räihä:* I asked this because there are certain experimental conditions in which you produce a very low R.Q. by oxidizing special substrates. When you give an animal alcohol for example, he will oxidize the alcohol and the oxygen consumption is the same, but the $CO_2$ production will go very low. In that condition you have a decrease in R.Q. almost to zero.

DISCUSSION PAPER PROF. R. SCHWARTZ

*Dr. Widdowson* (in the chair): Thank you very much Prof. SCHWARTZ. Dr. MAJAJ has asked me if he could demonstrate to us a few slides. I suggest to begin with those.

*Dr. Majaj:* Prof. SCHWARTZ said, that the mechanisms involved in hypoglycaemia are diffcult to understand. I should like to mention a study which might possibly explain one of the mechanisms of hypoglycaemia (Lib. Med. J. 19, 177, 1966).

It has been shown by MERTZ and coworkers that physiological levels of insulin along with chromium are required for glucose or galactose uptake into the epididymal fat tissue of the chromium deficient rat. It was thought that chromium enhanced the effects of insulin, not only on glucose metabolism but also in other systems, by facilitating the initial reaction of the hormone with its acceptor sites on membranes. This was the basis of this study.

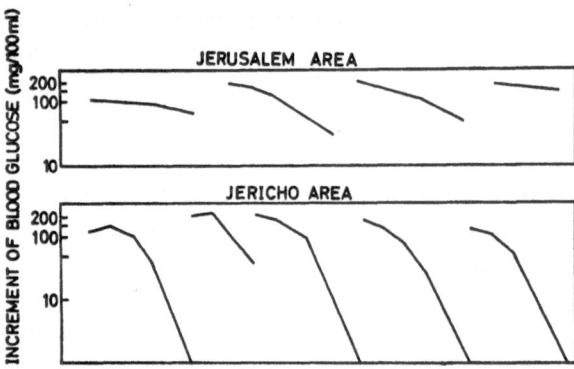

*Fig.* 1.   Initial intravenous glucose tolerance curves of infants from the Jerusalem and Jericho areas.

Hypoglycaemia and impaired glucose utilization are generally associated with kwashiorkor and have been reported in malnourished infants from most areas of the world. Four malnourished Jordanian refugee infants from the Jerusalem area had severely impaired glucose utilization and an average fasting blood glucose level of 59 mg/100 ml. However, five similar infants from the Jericho area had nearly normal glucose utilization and an average fasting blood glucose level of 78 mg/100 ml (fig. 1). Treating the Jerusalem area infants with 250 µg of chromium by mouth resulted in a marked improvement of glucose utilization and an elevation of the average fasting blood glucose level to 80 mg/100 ml in all cases (fig. 2).

Although the exact diet consumed prior to admission to the hospital

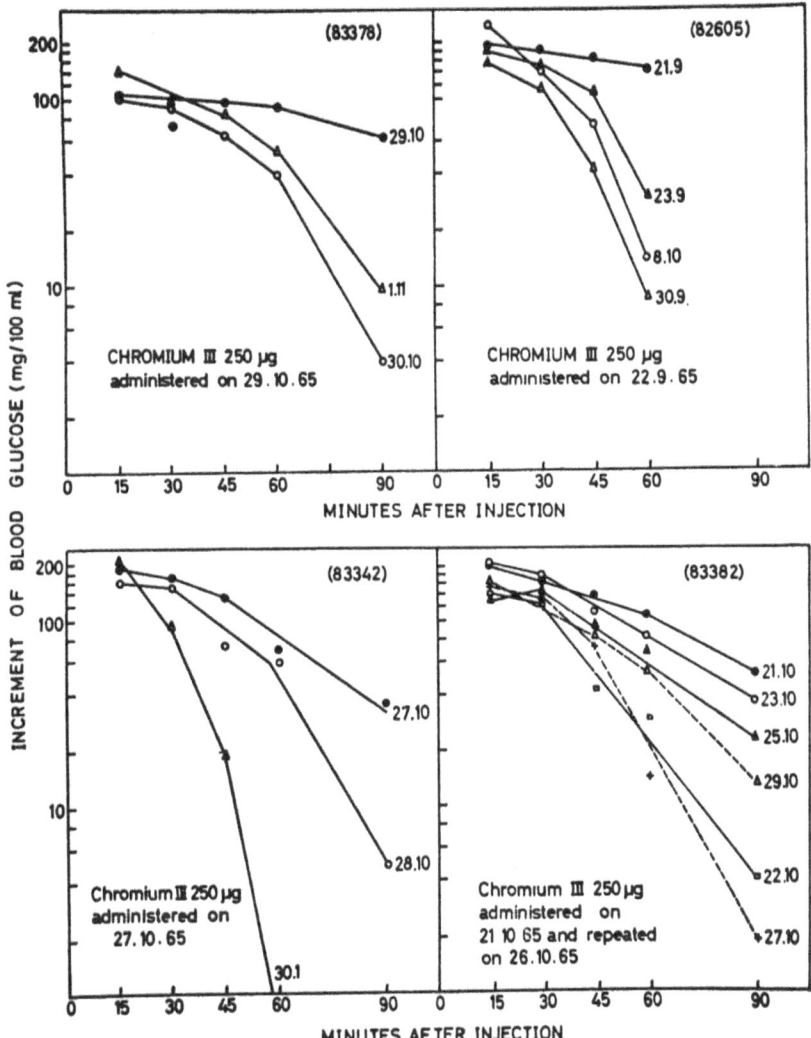

*Fig.* 2.   Intravenous glucose tolerance curves of infants from the Jerusalem area before and after chromium administration. The numbers at each curve designate the date at which the tolerance test was performed.

was unknown, it should be noted that in general the families of infants from both areas received similar food rations from the United Nations. A deficiency of chromium endemic to the hill region around Jerusalem was suspected. This deficiency of chromium does not seem to be endemic in the Jericho area. This is possibly due to differences in the chromium contents of the water supplies in the two regions. An analysis of water from the two regions done by Dr. MERTZ showed chromium contents of the order of 1 part per billion from Jerusalem water supply and 5 parts per billion from the Jericho area. In addition to this 5 times higher content of chromium in the Jericho water it is expected that due to the much hotter and drier climate in Jericho perspiration would require greater intake of water and thus concentration of chromium in the body.

Previous work has shown that in the presence of insulin chromium enhances the transport of glucose across the cell and mitochondrial membranes; its effect on hypoglycaemia, however, has not been reported. A possible chromium deficiency in these infants offers new insight into the high mortality and slow recovery of the severely malnourished infant probably due to intracellular energy depletion.

*Dr. Koldovsky:* What type of chromium was given in your study?

*Dr. Majaj:* It was $CrCl_3$ dissolved in water. You can give it by mouth.

*Dr. Loeb:* There are two points I should like to discuss with Prof. SCHWARTZ. Concerning the results of the glucagon tests I agree completely with you. Our results are in the same way. We have a much lesser response in dysmature infants.

Looking at your glucose infusion studies I think that your results parallel very good the results of the glucose tolerance tests. Indeed the newborn has the same glucose tolerance as the adult. The k-value is around 1.4 in the newborn and 1.7 in the adult. We know that a few days after birth and surely after a few months the k-value is around 3.6. So we can understand the difference you observed after the infusion of glucose.

But there is one point I can't understand. In the newborn you have a lower glucose tolerance. As you showed in the animal experiment you found a higher glucose output and hypoglycaemia. Can you give an explanation of this?

*Prof. R. Schwartz:* This appears to be a conflict. When you give an acute load, the glucose disappears more slowly. Yet we have here a liver in a very young animal putting out glucose at a very high rate.

Since we are studying a steady state it is apparent that the glucose is metabolized.

Your question is which tissues are metabolizing the glucose. Under a steady state the glucose must be going somewhere. I don't know where it is going. People speculate about the brain. The brain may be consuming all the glucose and that's where the hypoglycaemia does come from. I don't believe that myself, because I think we don't have enough data actually either in animal nor in man.

In terms of how much glucose is extracted, metabolized, disposed of or what other term you like to use for isolated tissues, these are data we do need. I don't know how much is taken up by fat on the one hand and by the muscles on the other hand.

I don't think there is a discrepancy really between the acute load and the constant infusion data. Because, if the premise on which we made these studies is correct in extrapolating it from the adult, as one raises the blood sugar in a steady state, the liver shuts off. What we are doing is just replacing glucose in the liver from the outside. This is a little different from the acute load in which the disposal of the glucose is probably in large measure what the liver takes up. Under the steady state we are just looking at what the rest of the body is taking up. Probably during the steady state very little of the glucose is being taken up by the liver, the liver is being shut down. There must be some exchange but it is very little and probably not important.

The slow rate of disposal in the newborn is, I think, probably due to a slow perfusion of the liver or to a decreased uptake of glucose. We see the same thing with fructose and galactose. All three sugars are taken up very slowly in the newborn compared to the older individual. I don't think there is a real discrepancy. Likely there are two different physiological phenomena.

*Dr. Nicolopoulos:* Prof. SCHWARTZ, what is the dose of glucagon you are using in your studies? Could you correlate the results of your glucagon tests with the mode of delivery and with the clinical course of these infants?

*Prof. R. Schwartz:* I'm not absolutely certain but I think almost all infants were delivered by vaginal route. Actually we are not using just glucagon tests. We are using the technique of epinephrine preceding glucagon. So what we do is administer a very small dose of epinephrine subcutaneously, wait ten minutes and then give the big dose of 300 µg per kg of glucagon. We believe we are giving pharmacological doses. The response to glucagon cannot be a question of whether we are stimulating adequately. Whether the glucagon gets to the liver is of course another question, but we believe the dose is sufficient. In the puppies we gave the glucagon intravenously and we gave astronomical doses of glucagon.

I was wondering if someone would ask whether glucagon is stimulating gluconeogenesis, because this has been one of the most recent contributions that has been made in this area. The question comes up how rapidly will glucagon stimulate gluconeogenesis. I thought it was a matter of many hours, at least in a in vitro system. Apparently it is not. Dr. PARK and his colleagues at Vanderbilt University have demonstrated that gluconeogenesis is stimulated by glucagon in a matter of minutes, in half an hour or something like this.

*Dr. Reynolds:* I would like to ask Prof. SCHWARTZ if he feels that pituitary growth hormone in the newborn has any role to play in the maintenance of blood sugar level.

*Prof. R Schwartz:* I would guess that all the hormones, pituitary growth hormone, corticosteroids, glucagon, epinephrine and so on, are important. The question is, are they important acutely or are they more important in maintaining a chronic status. I don't think we really know. The effects of growth hormone on free fatty acid release for example are very acute. Perhaps this is an indirect mechanism if the relationship between free fatty acids and glucose, as suggested by RANDLE, is a valid one by which growth hormone might work. Whether it works directly or indirectly I don't know. There are preliminary data. Dr. LOEB tells me he is getting some data on growth hormone levels in young infants. Dr. CORNBLATH, as you know, has reported on this. The growth hormone levels don't change during the first few days of life. One thing is interesting about them: the levels are paradoxical in oral glucose loads. It is an interesting phenomenon in the newborn period. I don't understand it. I think it is important. Whether it is very important is another question I prefer not to answer.

*Dr. Gruenwald:* To what extend and in what form might the response to glucagon be used to diagnose intra-uterine deprivation?

*Prof. R. Schwartz:* Let me urge a word of caution. The glucagon test as we described it in apparently well infants, is very useful as a physiological tool to understand what is going on. I would guess that under circumstances where one has a very sick infant, one might be lead astray. For example there is a fascinating study in rats in which under certain circumstances, I believe they have to do with starved rats, one can give a dose of glucagon and show not a rise but an actual fall in blood glucose. So when you look at the blood glucose alone one would say there is no effect of glucagon on the liver. However if one looks at lactic acid one will find a rise.

In type 1 glycogen storage disease, there is an absence of glucose-6-phosphatase. In a child with this disease the blood glucose level may be low and when you give glucagon it may fall. If you look at the lactic acid it will already be high depending on the period of starvation, but it will rise after glucagon. Now presumably what happens there, is that the glycogen is broken down, the glucose cannot be released from the liver but it can follow the glycolytic pathway and finally appear as lactic acid.

*Dr. Gruenwald:* So the glucagon test is useful in an otherwise normal infant that has not glycogen storage disease but is just deprived?

*Prof. R. Schwartz:* It is probably useful there.


DISCUSSION PAPER DR. STRICH

*Prof. R. Schwartz* (in the chair): The paper of Dr. STRICH is now open for discussion. First of all I should like to ask Dr. DAAMEN to open the discussion.

*Dr. Daamen:* I appreciated very much your lecture and your beautiful slides on cerebral damage in hypoglycaemia. Postmortem alterations are the cause of great difficulties in evaluation of morphological microscopical findings. There is some degeneration after death. How do you avoid this degeneration after death, how do you fix the brains? How soon were the postmortems done?

*Dr. Strich:* This question has been brought up many times. We have compared these brains very carefully with other material where the postmortem has been delayed up to 96 hours. In one of my cases the postmortem was done nine hours after death, which is pretty soon by our standards. We have never seen any of these changes in brains of other babies that have died and where postmortem has been delayed for a long time. I don't think these are just ordinary postmortem changes. We fix the brains by suspension in 10 per cent formaline.

*Dr. Räihä:* Is there any correlation between the pathological changes you find in the human babies with hypoglycaemia and changes in any experimental situation where you induce hypoglycaemia?

*Dr. Strich:* I don't know about any experiments on foetuses or young animals. Hypoglycaemia in older animals gives histological findings very similar to these, including changes in the anterior horns. We were gratified that the changes particular in cats have been very similar indeed.

*Dr. Räihä:* I should like to comment on your statement that the heart is as sensitive to hypoxia as the brain. In this regard we have done some studies in our laboratory. It is mainly Dr. MÄENPÄÄ who has done this. We have subjected foetuses and newborn rats to hypoxia and we have followed the changes in adenosinetriphosphate in the tissues. It is very striking that in foetal and newborn hearts the ATP level does not decrease during anoxia as rapidly as in adults. The ATP level stays high for up to 20 minutes and then it decreases rapidly and at this moment it is impossible to resuscitate the animal. We studied also the brain and the liver. In these organs the ATP level falls more rapidly although there is a difference as compared to adult animals. I think at least biochemically we can say that the newborn heart is more resistent to hypoxia than the brain.

*Dr. Strich:* Yes, I think it depends very much on exactly how long after birth you study this. SHELLEY and other people have gone into this as you know. Certanily at birth, just before or during the period of birth, the glycogen content of the heart is very high. The heart can then survive through anaerobic glycolysis. But a few hours later when this glycogen has been used up, if I understand the experiments of MOTT and others correctly, then the heart is much more sensitive to hypoxia than it is actually at birth (MOTT, J. C. (1961) Brit. Med. Bull. 17: 144).

*Prof. François:* Did you determine in any of your cases insulin activity in the blood and glycogen content of the liver? What are the histological findings of the pancreas?

*Dr. Strich:* Insulin estimations were done in two cases; the results were normal. These results have not been published. The histology of the pancreas has been done (NAEYE, R. L. (1965) Arch. Path. 79: 284). The pancreas was very small as were all the other organs. The pancreas exocrine tissue is more reduced than the islets in dysmature infants. So when you look at sections of the pancreas it seems the islets are very big but in fact the islets are normal and the rest of the pancreas is small. Glycogen content of the liver was only done in one case and was very low indeed.

*Dr. Gruenwald:* I suppose one of the main reasons of studying neuropathology is the assumption that similar changes, perhaps to a lesser extent, occur in survivors. I would think that while you found these changes in dead infants you might find in some survivors more localized lesions.

My other comment is: the degeneration of the white matter which you showed in the posterior horn of the lateral ventricle, is, I believe, frequently found without hypoglycaemia in infants deprived in utero. I don't know why, but I have seen it in a number of cases just in that same paraventricular localization. So I would guess that these particular lesions may have preceded the hypoglycaemia. I cannot prove it of course.

*Prof. De Bruijne:* Do you think there are irreversible functional disturbances without demonstrable histological lesions?

*Dr. Strich:* This is a very vital question of course. I'm afraid I don't know. There has been one study on electrone microscopic changes in hypoglycaemia and anoxia (WEBSTER, H. DE F. and AMES, A. (1965) J. Cell. Biol. 26: 885). They used rabbits retina originally. They could never keep the tissue in good condition long enough to produce any damage due to hypoglycaemia. Even half an hour of complete lack of glucose did not produce any changes. We don't know yet what the submicroscopical changes, which may or may not be reversible, are.

*Prof. R. Schwartz:* This is a very important discussion here. I would like to perpetuate this for a few minutes. You comment that the effects of hypoglycaemia are only seen when one has hypoglycaemia of long duration. What we are talking about are demonstrable pathological lesions, as you have just emphasized.

From the point of view of survivors one wonders what the brain can sustain in terms of ultimate development. I don't think that we have any information and that we really know what asymptomatic hypoglycaemia in the normal newborn means, let alone in the dysmature. I just urge a word of caution here in the interpretation whether a low blood sugar is 'good or bad.'

*Prof. Minkowski:* As you know some of the hypoglycaemic dysmature babies recur with hypoglycaemia later on, one or two years old. Retrospectively some of the so called idiopathic hypoglycaemic children have a story of prenatal wastage. In this case I wonder if you could compare the brains of children who have died of recurrent hypoglycaemia. This would probably give an answer to the question of Prof. SCHWARTZ because in those cases one has repeated attacks of hypoglycaemia before they die finally.

*Dr. Strich:* I haven't got any information. It would be very interesting to have a look at the brains of survivors of neonatal hypoglycaemia.

*Prof. R. Schwartz:* Thank you very much Dr. STRICH.


DISCUSSION PAPER PROF. DE BRUIJNE

*Prof. R. Schwartz* (in the chair): The paper of Prof. DE BRUIJNE is open for discussion.

*Dr. Papadatos:* I was impressed with the statement of Prof. DE BRUIJNE that only one infant had haemolysis of unknown cause. At the University Alexandra Maternity Hospital in Athens we had about 1000 praemature babies above 1500 g during the last five years. In this group 4.5 per cent underwent transfusion, of which 30 per cent had severe hyperbilirubinaemia of unknown cause. When I say unknown I exclude incomptability of blood groups, enzyme deficiency and so on.

Now I should like to ask you: did you take into accounts in your group of infants with hyperbilirubinaemia the feeding history of the baby? Did they get breast milk?

*Prof. De Bruijne:* Well, I can tell you that most of our praemature babies got breast milk during the first few days of life. However, it was not normal breast milk but it was freeze-dried pooled human milk.

*Prof. Minkowski:* I wonder if we should still keep this classification of level of indirect bilirubin: less than 15, between 15 and 20, and more than 20 mg/100 ml. Determination of indirect bilirubin by micro-methods is varying with the standard of each laboratory. When you give such a level four or five determinations should be done within the same day. Because if you don't determine bilirubin four or five times, the day that the bilirubin level is rising, you might miss the peak. What about your praemature infants, were they all normal infants? Didn't you have any cases of respiratory distress syndrome? In those cases when you have elevation of $pCO_2$ and decrease of pH, the hazard of kernicterus exists with a bilirubin value of as low as 10 or 12 mg/100 ml.

*Prof. De Bruijne:* We actually do bilirubin determinations once a day as soon as the baby becomes visibly jaundiced. When the jaundice is more outspoken we do determinations at least two times and if necessary three or four times a day.

As to your other question concerning the respiratory distress syndrome: in our group of patients resporatory distress did occur. We never had a case of kernicterus in our group with a bilirubin value as low as 10 or 12 mg/100 ml.* We had one infant who developed kernicterus with RDS and a bilirubin level of 19 mg/100 ml. I don't know at what bilirubin level you are performing exchange transfusions in otherwise healthy babies. In some clinics this level is 18 mg/100 ml, in other clinics 24 mg/100 ml. We use the level of 23 mg/100 ml with our method of determination. We never had kernicterus except the already mentioned case of RDS with a bilirubin level of 19 mg/100 ml. The infant died shortly afterwards and the postmorten showed histo-logical changes of kernicterus.

---

* Recently we observed a praemature baby (birthweight 1710 g), who had severe adidosis due to RDS and a bilirubin value of 16.9 mg/100 ml on the 6th day. The baby died 8 days old. At postmortem kernicterus was detected.

17

*Dr. Koldovski:* I would just extend Prof. Minkowski's comment to the question of the critical level of bilirubin using some data we have obtained last year in our laboratory. Schmidt and coworkers in the United States have drawn attention to the significance of albumin binding capacity for bilirubin. We have used this approach and have analysed serum bilirubin in children with different bilirubin levels. In our institute children with Rh-incomptability are collected from a great area, so we had enough material. The critical situation of those children was more related to the free not-albumin bound bilirubin level. Most of the bilirubin on the sephadex column is going together with the albumin. In 5 to 10 per cent the bilirubin is going free from albumin in those children who are in poor condition. When the bilirubin level is high and the bilirubin all travels together with the albumin, there is a very good probability that no other exchange transfusion is needed. But we have seen that some children who were in very poor condition and where a new transfusion was needed or kernicterus definitely developed, also 12 hours after transfusion had again this bilirubin unbound to albumin. From my opinion now, and this will be published in Biologia Neonatorum (11: 204, 1967), this study is a very useful approach to define in clinical terms which children are in danger. With a sephadex-G25-separation you can see either that your yellow colour has travelled out in 30 minutes or that the colour remains for six or seven hours. I don't say this is a complete solution of the problem, but I think it can be of some help for the people who are responsible for the treatment of infants with hyper-bilirubinaemia.

*Prof. R. Schwartz:* Dr. Koldovsky, will you comment on free fatty acids and albumin binding?

*Dr. Koldovsky:* In our institute some experiments have been done (Res. Czechoslov. Med. 11: 161, 1965) that have extended the original observation of Odell from the United States about the competition of free fatty acids and bilirubin for the binding capacity of the albumin. In increasing the level of free fatty acids you get a change in the level of bilirubin. But in these experiments the change was only 2 or 3 mg/100 ml. It shows that this competition exists, but what is the significance of these 3 mg/100 ml, how much is this critical or not?

I should like to add a few words to the experiments I just mentioned before. The albumin binding could give a lot of thinking. It could be a low level of albumin, or the albumin binding sites could be occupied by other substances for instance FFA, or, and this is the speculation, the albumin could be a 'sick' albumin and could have not good binding sites.

*Dr. Valaes:* In my opinion the question of susceptibility to bilirubin toxity is quite different from the question of bilirubin levels in the various groups of infants. We have extensive experience with this new standard Dr. GRUENWALD mentioned. We are confident, we have now reproducible, constant bilirubin values, which is a prerequisite for any sort of study in this field.

We have also had some experience with the method suggested by Waters and Porter, to estimate the free binding sites of albumin with use of phenolsulfonphthalein. We are unfortunate enough to receive many babies with kernicterus and some had high PSP values. So at least that method was not good for separating the babies who are in danger of kernicterus. (Pediatrics, 39, 876, 1967).

Now coming to the main question whether babies who are dysmature have really lower bilirubin values, I want to remind that babies of toxaemic mothers have also as a group lower bilirubin values than their controls of similar birthweight and gestation. I think there are implications in this fact which we really can't answer for the moment, but I wonder if the placental-foetal unit and its steroid production has anything to do with it in terms of inhibition of foetal serum to glucuronide formation.

*Prof. De Bruijne:* We have adapted our laboratory methods to American standards and we have regularly control sera from the United States. We think that at this moment the laboratory is working very well.

# OBSTETRICAL AND PREVENTIVE ASPECTS OF DYSMATURITY

# THE OBSTETRICIAN AND DYSMATURITY

G. J. KLOOSTERMAN*

The aim of obstetrics is the birth of a healthy baby, born to a healthy mother. By preventive and curative measures the obstetrician tries to attain this end and in doing so you could look at him as the pediatrician of the unborn baby. That the obstetrician sometimes misses his mark is to nobody better known than to pediatricians to whom the obstetrician sometimes handles babies who require the utmost of pediatric skill to survive.

In the beginning I thought that the organisers of this excellent congress made a mistake by asking the obstetrician as one of the last speakers of this symposium. In daily life the sequence is the other way round: first comes the obstetrician and than the pediatrician or, still worse, the neurologist, worst of all, the pathologist. So I thought in my naïvety, but the organisers of this congress make no mistakes and I was wrong in supposing even a slight one. The sequence is all right and at the end of my paper I hope to explain why.

First some remarks about dysmaturity. We should like to define this as intra-uterine starvation or, like GRUENWALD puts it, as chronic fetal distress. It is something pathological and therefore not identical with 'small for date', although many 'very small for date babies' are dysmature as well. Still it is possible that a very small baby is not dysmature but a real dwarf without any sign of dystrophia, whereas a rather heavy child can show symptoms of distress that can be called dysmaturity. Examples of this last situation are often found in cases of postmaturity or maternal diabetes. Dysmaturity is a conflict between the needs of the unborn child and the trophic capacities of the mother during a period of at least some weeks. If, for example the foetus has gained a weight of 4000 g after 40 weeks of pregnancy

* Department of Obstetrics and Gynaecology, Wilhelmina Gasthuis, University of Amsterdam.

and labour does not start before 46 weeks in spite of successive degeneration of the placenta, than the baby will be born after 46 weeks with
a birthweight of, let us say, 3800 g and, if it is alive, with severe
symptoms of dysmaturity.

Dysmaturity is to some extent synonymous with relatively too late
born whereas prematurity is synonymous with relatively too early born.
This is perfectly clear in the case of dysmature children, born after a
prolonged pregnancy (for example after 44 weeks) and in the case of
normal developed but very unripe children, born before 28 weeks,
but between these extreme and clear and rather rare examples,
frequently situations are found where both conditions go together.
This means, that many children have to choose between a to early
birth, followed by neonatal death by unripeness and a birth, preceded
by an intrauterine death. This means also, that the obstetrician
sometimes tries to save the unborn child by suppressing uteruscontractions and more often by stimulating uterus contractions.

On the whole we have to be very careful with these activities because it is highly probable that Nature is already doing the same thing.
Already the Father of Medicine, HIPPOCRATES, wrote 2500 years ago
the following about this subject: 'When there is no more food for the
young in the egg and it has nothing on which to live it makes violent
movements, searches for food and brakes the membranes. The mother,
perceiving that the embryo is vigorously moving, smashes the shell.
In just the same way, when the child has grown big and the mother
can not continue to provide him with enough nourishment, he
becomes agitated, breaks through the membranes and incontinently
passes out into the external world free from any bounds. In the same
way, among the beasts and savage animals, birth occurs at a time
fixed for each species without overshooting it, for necessarily, in each,
nourishment will become inadequate. Those which have the least
food for the foetus come quicker to birth, and vice versa. And that is
all I have to say upon the subject' ends Hippocrates.

Today, 25 centuries later, I think that we can say something more
upon the subject. We don 't believe any more that the child leaves
the uterus under its own power, but we know that it is expelled by
the uterus. The uterus does not start to contract because the baby
gets hungry, but it is highly probable that the blocking effect exerted
by the placenta on the uterus is coming to a standstill or even declines

whereas the stimulating effect on the uterus, exerted by the growing baby, becomes stronger and stronger. But by assuming that the same organ which provides the unborn child with nourishment is responsible for the duration of pregnancy and that on the whole the trophic capacity of the placenta is linked to its hormone production and

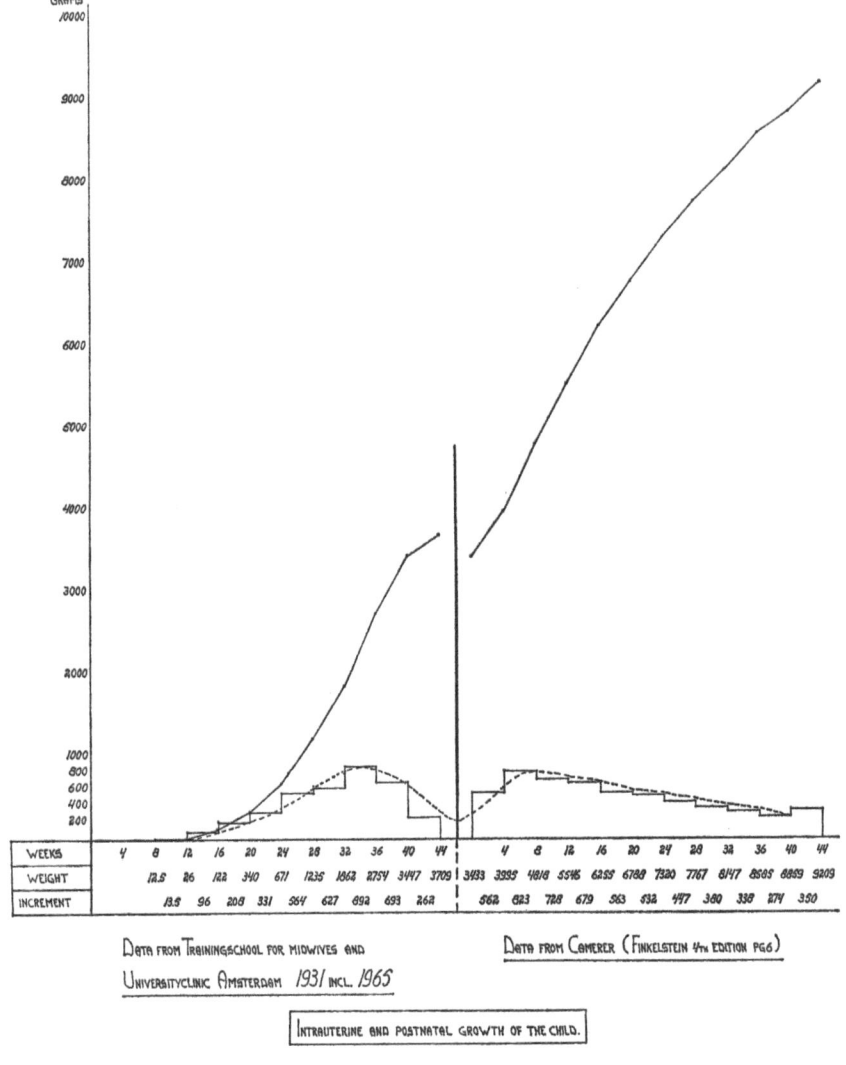

*Fig.* 1.

blocking capacity of uteruscontractions, we follow the same line of reasoning as Hippocrates.

An argument for the correctness of this line of reasoning can be found in figure 1. This graph represents a study of nearly 80.000

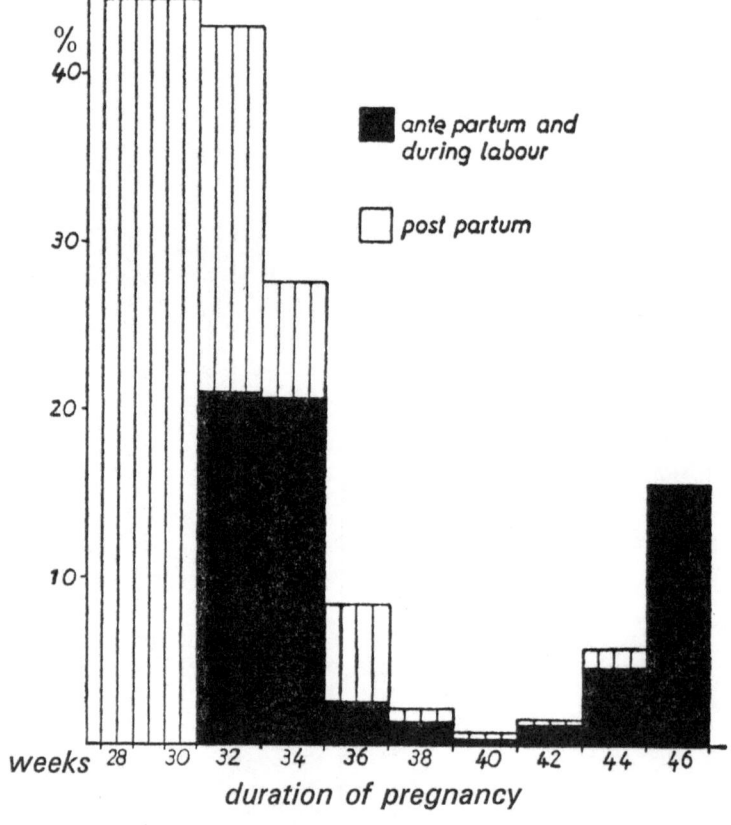

*Fig.* 2. Stillbirth rate and postnatal mortality. In this figure the percentage of intra-uterine deaths is represented by black columns and that of postnatal deaths by hatched columns.

birthweights, collected by Miss HUIDEKOPER in our clinic and combined with data about the infant growth-rate collected by CAMERER. It is plainly apparent that the growth shows a fairly sharp decline during the last few weeks before birth, to rise again shortly after birth. The decline in growth-rate prior to birth cannot be accounted for by a diminished tendency to grow, originating in the child itself, but must be due to a temporary obstruction which is no longer present after birth. This obstruction can be explained by the fact that under normal conditions the capacity of the placenta for providing

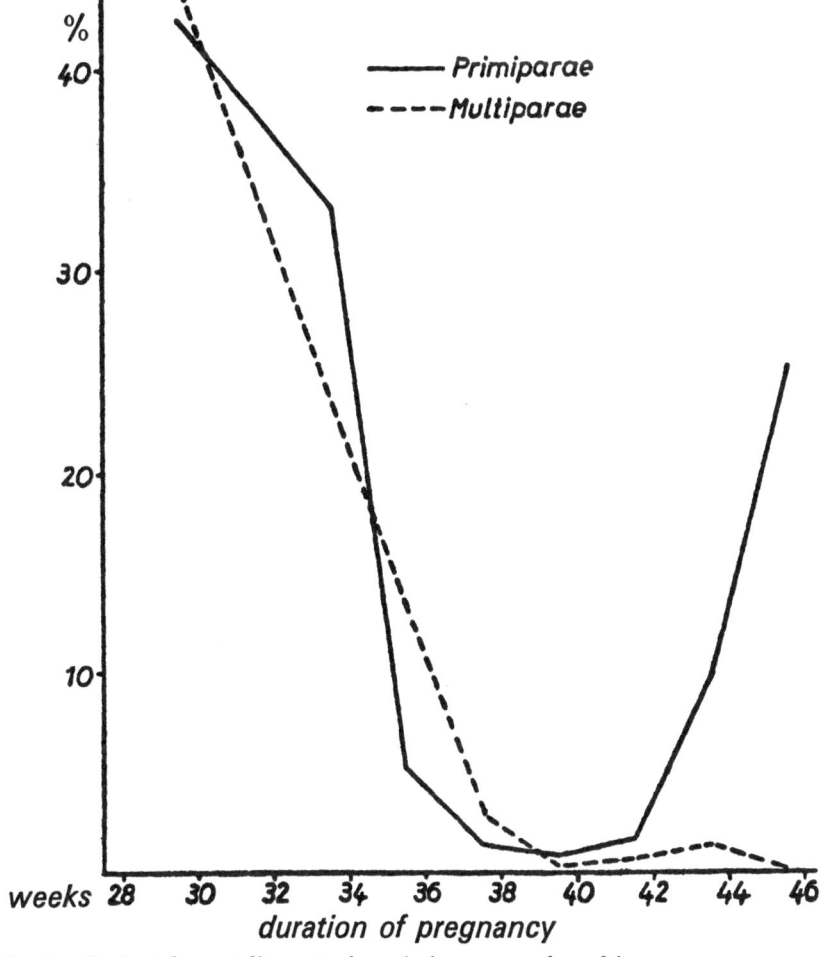

*Fig.* 3.  Perinatal mortality rate in primiparous and multiparous women.

nourishment has reached its peak some time before birth. Is the uterus very slow to react than the child will be born long after this moment, showing symptoms of dysmaturity or even being stillborn; is the uterus very eager to react, than the child can be born long before the placenta has reached the peak of its trophic capacity and the child will be born very premature and unripe, dying shortly after birth by immaturity. But very often a child will be born too early (that is: before 38 weeks) with symptoms of dysmaturity. In that case we have to admire the

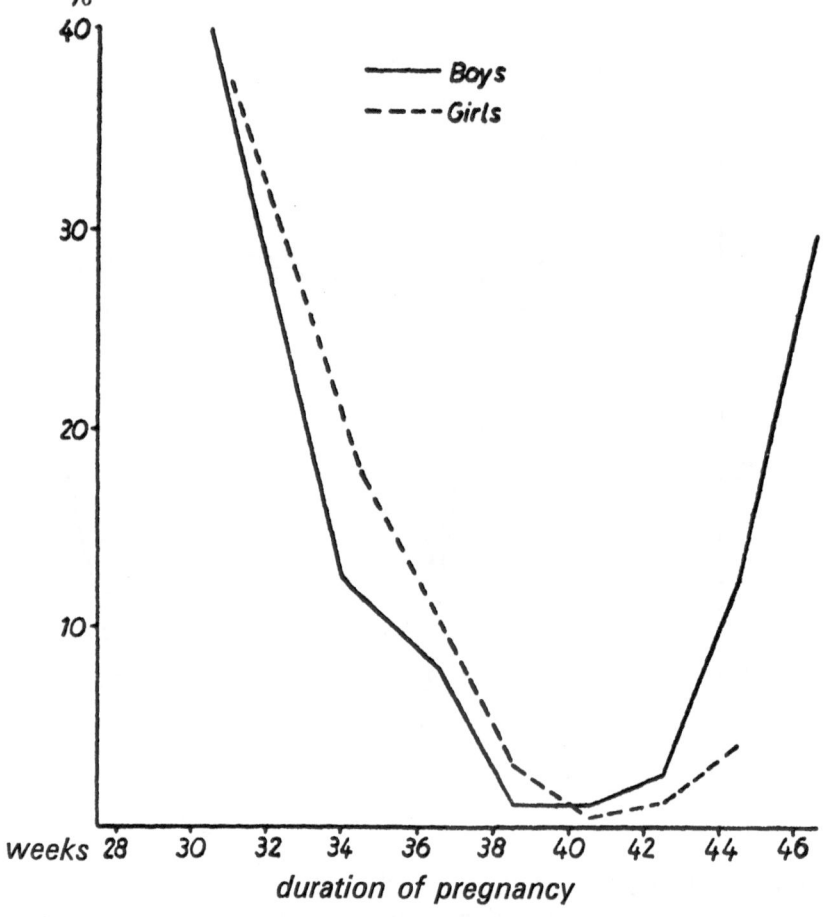

*Fig.* 4. Perinatal mortality rate after different weeks of pregnancy for boys and girls.

wisdom of nature to send a baby earlier into the outer world because the intra-uterine conditions were too bad for a longer stay. Were the child born at an earlier date, it would have been more unripe. Were it born at a later moment it would have been more dysmature or even dead.

The struggle of the obstetrician against dysmaturity seems most easy and grateful in cases of postmaturity, that is pregnancy prolonged till more than 42 weeks, and the most obvious way seems to be shortening of pregnancy by induction of labour or performing a Caesarean. Since 1948 we have studied this problem. In the first five years we have been completely conservative in accordance with our education, but in 1952 it became evident that postmaturity was not harmless as can be seen in figure 2. A striking fact was, that of the 14 children who died after 297* days of pregnancy not less than 13 children were children of primiparous women. As can be seen from figure 3, postmaturity is dangerous in primiparous women and hardly so in multiparous women. Another striking fact was, that of the 14 children who died after 297 days of pregnancy, 11 were boys and 3 were girls (fig. 4). This marked preponderance of boys dying in cases of prolonged pregnancy cannot be explained by the fact that pregnancy is protracted considerably more often when the foetus is a boy than when it is a girl. In a material of 25.910 pregnancies we found a sex ratio of 1 girl to 1.05 boys. After 42 weeks the ratio was 1 girl to 1,03 boys (Table 1).

Table 1. *Sex ratio of neonati according to duration of pregnancy.*

| Duration of pregnancy in weeks | Number of boys | Number of girls | Sex ratio |
|---|---|---|---|
| 21–29 | 354 | 299 | 118 |
| 30–35 | 754 | 653 | 117 |
| 36–38 | 2139 | 1912 | 115 |
| 39–41 | 8377 | 8196 | 102 |
| 42–46 | 1645 | 1590 | 103 |
| Total | 13269 | 12650 | 105 |

* In this study we defined 40 weeks as the period of 277—283 days after the first day of the last menstrual period, and more than 42 weeks as more than 297 days. In the literature more than 42 weeks means: after the 300th day of pregnancy.

Pregnancy continuing beyond the normal duration is obviously more dangerous to boys than to girls. This points to placental insufficiency as a probable cause since we know that boys are heavier than girls of the same fetal age (fig. 5) but their placental weight is the same (fig. 6); in other words, boys ask more from their placenta than girls do and probably this is extra dangerous when the placenta is at the end of its career.

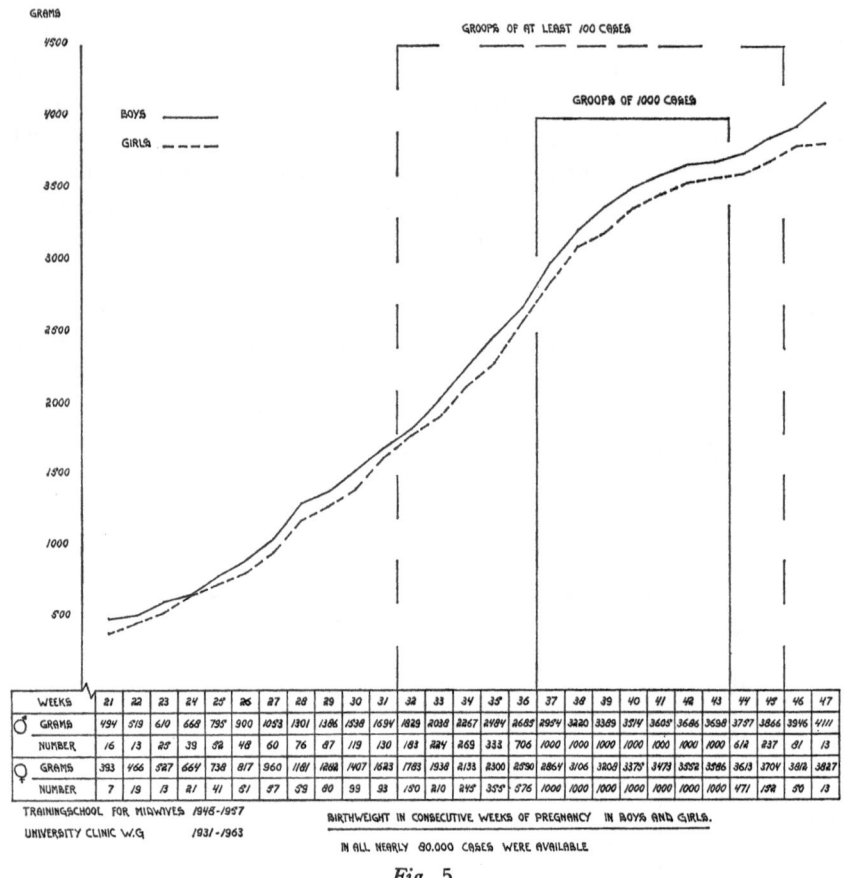

| WEEKS | 21 | 22 | 23 | 24 | 25 | 26 | 27 | 28 | 29 | 30 | 31 | 32 | 33 | 34 | 35 | 36 | 37 | 38 | 39 | 40 | 41 | 42 | 43 | 44 | 45 | 46 | 47 |
|---|---|---|---|---|---|---|---|---|---|---|---|---|---|---|---|---|---|---|---|---|---|---|---|---|---|---|---|
| ♂ GRAMS | 494 | 519 | 610 | 668 | 795 | 900 | 1053 | 1301 | 1386 | 1538 | 1694 | 1829 | 2038 | 2267 | 2484 | 2685 | 2954 | 3220 | 3389 | 3514 | 3605 | 3686 | 3698 | 3787 | 3866 | 3946 | 4111 |
| NUMBER | 16 | 13 | 25 | 39 | 52 | 48 | 60 | 76 | 87 | 119 | 130 | 163 | 224 | 269 | 333 | 706 | 1000 | 1000 | 1000 | 1000 | 1000 | 1000 | 1000 | 612 | 237 | 61 | 13 |
| ♀ GRAMS | 393 | 466 | 527 | 664 | 738 | 817 | 960 | 1161 | 1262 | 1407 | 1623 | 1783 | 1938 | 2133 | 2300 | 2590 | 2864 | 3106 | 3208 | 3375 | 3473 | 3552 | 3596 | 3613 | 3704 | 3812 | 3827 |
| NUMBER | 7 | 19 | 13 | 21 | 41 | 51 | 97 | 59 | 60 | 99 | 93 | 150 | 210 | 245 | 355 | 576 | 1000 | 1000 | 1000 | 1000 | 1000 | 1000 | 1000 | 471 | 192 | 50 | 13 |

TRAININGSCHOOL FOR MIDWIVES 1948–1957
UNIVERSITY CLINIC W.G 1931–1963

BIRTHWEIGHT IN CONSECUTIVE WEEKS OF PREGNANCY IN BOYS AND GIRLS.

IN ALL NEARLY 80.000 CASES WERE AVAILABLE

*Fig.* 5.

Another argument, pointing to placental insufficiency was the following: if we arranged all postmature children according to the weight of the placenta (weighed without cord and membranes and thoroughly wiped clean of bloodclots) the result was striking. Perinatal mortality ranked highest in the group of placentae less than 400 g and went regularly down to zero in the group of placentae of 700 g and more (fig. 7). The mean weight of the placenta of the living postmature children was 580 g against 452 g of the children who died.

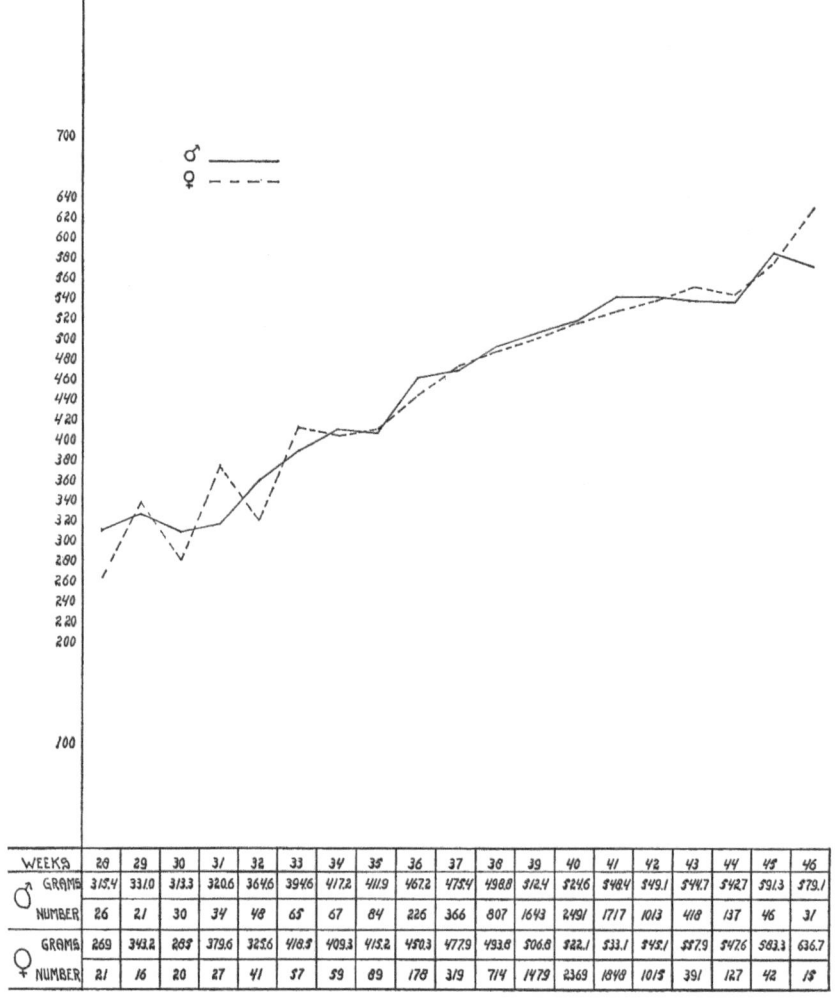

| WEEKS | 28 | 29 | 30 | 31 | 32 | 33 | 34 | 35 | 36 | 37 | 38 | 39 | 40 | 41 | 42 | 43 | 44 | 45 | 46 |
|---|---|---|---|---|---|---|---|---|---|---|---|---|---|---|---|---|---|---|---|
| ♂ GRAMS | 315.4 | 331.0 | 313.3 | 320.6 | 364.6 | 394.6 | 417.2 | 411.9 | 467.2 | 475.4 | 498.8 | 512.4 | 524.6 | 548.4 | 549.1 | 544.7 | 542.7 | 593.3 | 579.1 |
| NUMBER | 26 | 21 | 30 | 34 | 48 | 65 | 67 | 84 | 226 | 366 | 807 | 1643 | 2491 | 1717 | 1013 | 418 | 137 | 46 | 31 |
| ♀ GRAMS | 269 | 343.2 | 288 | 379.6 | 325.6 | 418.3 | 409.3 | 415.2 | 450.3 | 477.9 | 493.8 | 506.8 | 522.1 | 533.1 | 545.1 | 557.9 | 547.6 | 583.3 | 636.7 |
| NUMBER | 21 | 16 | 20 | 27 | 41 | 57 | 59 | 89 | 178 | 319 | 714 | 1479 | 2369 | 1848 | 1013 | 391 | 127 | 42 | 15 |

WEIGHT OF PLACENTA IN CONSECUTIVE WEEKS OF PREGNANCY (IN BOYS AND GIRLS)

TRAININGSCHOOL FOR MIDWIVES 1948-1957
UNIVERSITY CLINIC W.G.          1957-1962

*Fig. 6.*

The widespread view that the infant grows to an abnormal size in prolonged pregnancy, so that it will be increasingly liable to die from a disproportion between its size and that of the birthcanal is untenable.

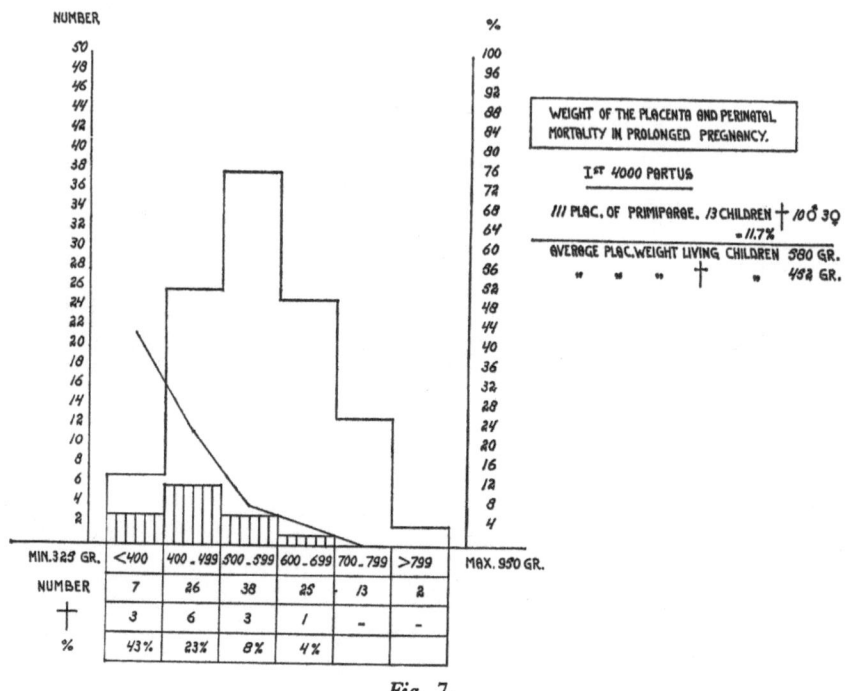

*Fig. 7.*

Overdevelopment and prolonged pregnancy are two entirely different things, which are scarcely correlated. Many authors have already drawn attention to that fact (ZANGEMEISTER, WIJSENBEEK, HOSEMANN, KORTENOEVER). Our own investigation showed that the mean weight of the children born after the 297 day of pregnancy was 3.595 g as against 3.462 g in the infants born at term. The mean weight of the postmature children who died was 3.630 g. This shows that postmature children are only slightly heavier than children born at term and that postmature children, who die, are virtually as heavy as the live-born infants of this group, while there was only one case that could be considered as overdeveloped (5.200 g).

So we found several arguments in favour of placental insufficiency as a cause for the higher risk of the postmature foetus:

1. Children with a low placental weight are much endangered than children of the same size with a higher placental weight.
2. Boys are much more endangered than girls.
3. Children of primiparous woman are much more endangered than children of multiparous woman.
4. 86 % of the postmature children who died perinatally did so before birth against 59 % of the children who were born before the 279th day.

These results are in perfect accordance with the well known publication of CLIFFORD that appeared in 1954, after our investigation. CLIFFORD found 85 percent of the postmature deaths to be fetal deaths, we 86 %. CLIFFORD found postmaturity to be a problem of the primiparous woman and no problem to the multiparous woman, we found the same.

After this investigation we decided to continue with our expectant attitude in cases of postmaturity in multiparous women, but to abandon this attitude in primiparous women. After the first of January 1953 we tried to induce labour by chemical induction in all primiparous women who went beyond the 297th day of pregnancy. We were well aware of the fact that this decision also could have its drawbacks. Shortening the duration of pregnancy would be an advantage, but doing so by chemical induction could probably result in hypertonia of the uterus and, by that, endanger the oxygenation of the foetus, a danger especially to be feared in cases of placental insufficiency. Still, it seemed worth trying. The patients were hospitalized for this purpose. Initially 30 ml of caster oil was administered, followed by 200 mg of quinine given every hour for 4 hours, after which one Voegtlin unit of pituitrin was administered every hour. When 2–3 injections failed to induce any response, the dose was gradually increased to 2 U per injection. Treatment was discontinued after 6–8 injections or even earlier when labour seemed to have started or the tonus of the uterus had increased. When labour did not start, then the same treatment was applied again 2 days later.

We followed this way of conduct till June 1957. During these 4 years another group of 4 000 women (with single pregnancies only) was delivered. Among them were 112 primiparae who went beyond 297 days of pregnancy (to 111 postmature primiparae in the first

18

group of 4.000 women). These 112 women received in total 220 chemical inductions. The result was, that no primipara had a pregnancy of more than 44 weeks; in comparison with the first group we had shortened pregnancy with an average of slightly more than 3 days, but the perinatal mortality was virtually the same as in the first group, namely 12 in 112 = 10.7 % in the second group against 13 in 111 = 11.7 % in the first group. Among the 12 children who

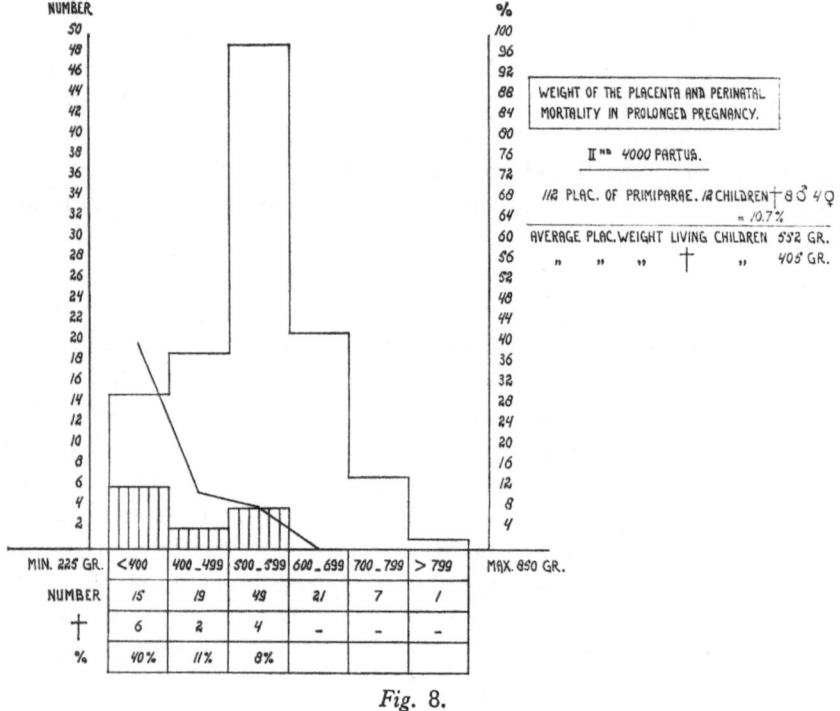

*Fig. 8.*

died perinatally were 8 boys to 4 girls. The mean placental weight of the living postmature children was 552 g; of the children who died the placental weight was 405 g. Again there was no mortality among children who had a placenta of more than 700 g and again ranked the mortality highest in the group of children with a placental weight of less than 400 g (fig. 8). Chemical induction, at least in the way we had applied it, had given no significant improvement, very probably due to the fact that the rather rough way of chemical induction had neutralized the advantage of the shortening of pregnancy.

We decided to continue our efforts, but now in another way. The dangers of placental insufficiency can be reduced by prescribing complete bedrest in the hospital and perhaps also to some extent by low salt diet. The importance of complete bedrest is, apart from clinical experience, also demonstrated by the experiments of McClure Brown, who could show that the uterine bloodflow improves with a thirty percent if the pregnant women changes from the standing position to the horizontal position. The importance of low salt diet is less generally known, but we found strong clinical evidence for it in cases of habitual intra-uterine death without toxemia or hypertension and we could show that it prevents to some extent oedema of the placenta. Perhaps it acts favourable on the permeability of the placenta. Therefore we choosed for the combination of bedrest and low salt diet. To make out whether a very carefully given chemical induction could have some advantages we also decided to give every second postmature nullipara a chemical induction, but this time only by the intravenous method, using synthetic oxytocine (piton S) to a maximum of 8 mU/minute. In the meantime our sphere of action had shifted from the trainingschool of midwives to the Obstetrical Department of the University of Amsterdam. (This explains the much higher numbers of pregnancies controlled per annum after 1957).

From January 1958 till January 1965, 15.906 women (twinpregnancies not included) were controlled in our out-patient department and delivered in our clinic. Among them 536 primiparae went beyond 297 days of pregnancy. The perinatal mortality was 19 children = 3.5 %. For the first time we had made a significant progress from 11.2 % perinatal mortality in the first 223 to 3.5 % in the last 536 postmature primiparae. The difference in perinatal mortality 7.7 ± 2.1 is highly significant. That the treatment (and we think in the first place the complete bedrest in hospital) had given a real improvement is also shown by the fact that especially the high mortality rate in the group with small placentae had gone down sharply (from 9 in 22 till 5 in 45 = from 41 % to 11 %, see figure 9).

A comparison between the 260 patients who belonged to the active group (careful chemical induction on top of the treatment with bedrest and low salt diet) and the 276 patients who belonged to the conservative group (only bedrest and low salt diet) showed that the results were slightly better in the first group (7 of 260 = 2.7 % and 12

of 276 = 4.3 % perinatal mortality). Although the differences are
not big enough to call them significant and although the difference
in duration of pregnancy in the two groups amounted to only 1.04
days in favour of the active group we decided to treat since January
1966 all postmature nulliparae in the same way i.c.: hospitalisation,
complete bedrest, low salt diet and chemical induction twice a week

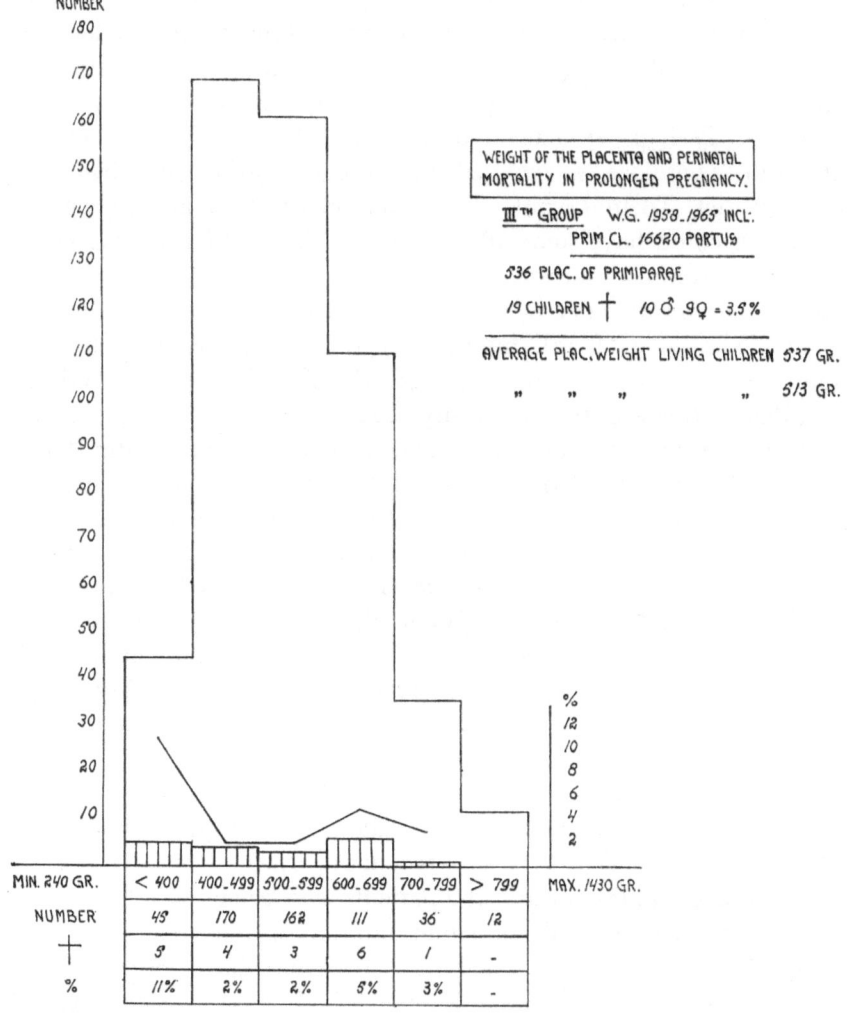

*Fig.* 9.

with intravenous oxytocin, starting from 5 mU/minute to 8 mU/minute.

We are well aware of the fact that the last word of the problem of postmaturity has not been spoken. The fact remains that more than 80 % of all postmature nulliparae are complete healthy women who are treated by us without a real indication. As soon as methods are developed to distinguish between physiological and pathological postmaturity we can stop with this undiscriminate way of treatment. Up till now these methods are not sufficiently available. Cytological methods are unreliable according to our experience. Amnioscopy (SALING) seems promising, but is, done every second day, also a burden for the expectant mother. Clinical signs (high resttonus of the uterus, decrease of the amount of amniotic fluid, going down of body weight, hypertension or high age of the mother, history of infertility) are important, but not always present as a warning. The hormone excretion in the urine, especially pregnandiol and oestriol can be of some help, but this is only possible in women who are already hospitalized. Moreover, this method is very expensive and not suited for big numbers of patients.

In concluding we propose to treat nulliparous women who go beyond the 42th week of pregnancy in the above mentioned way. This means that we will try in the first place to improve the foetal condition by improving placental circulation and only in the second place will take refuge in interruption of pregnancy. Nevertheless, to prevent dysmaturity and intra-uterine death (both conditions are very much akin, for dysmature children are children that got through by the skin of their teeth) in prolonged pregnancy we can theoretically also choose liberally the second solution, that is interruption of pregnancy by induction of labour or performing a caesarean section and in that way reduce the abnormal duration of pregnancy to a normal one. But when we now look at dysmaturity in a much earlier period of pregnancy, for example 8 weeks before term, then it is clear that every possibility to improve the foetal condition is much more attractive than taking the foetus out of the uterus and handling it to the paediatrician, for in doing so we replace the supposed danger of dysmaturity by the sure danger of unripeness. In these cases it is much more attractive to improve the foetal condition as much as possible and to gain time till the foetus has reached a gestational age of at least 35 weeks, than to interrupt pregnancy.

Which possibilities do we have to improve foetal condition by improving placental bloodflow? The most important is complete bedrest, by preference in the hospital. Then a low salt diet, also in normotensive women. In exceptional cases with high diastolic blood-pressure (above 125 mm Hg) a careful use of antihypertensive drugs (aldomet) can be of some use but overshooting is very dangerous for the unborn child.

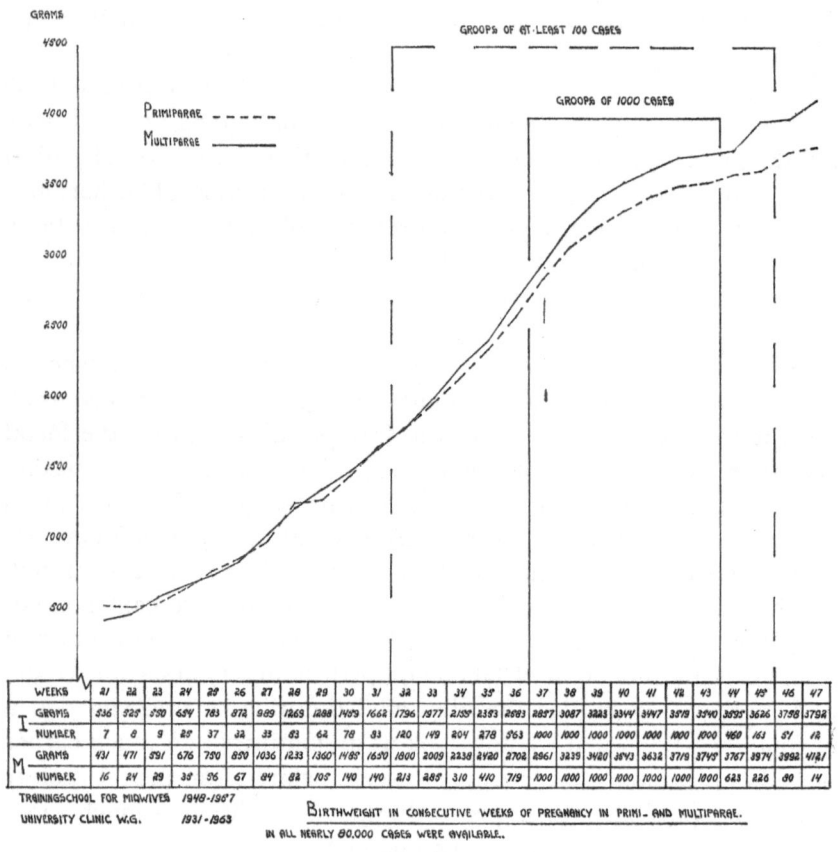

| WEEKS | 21 | 22 | 23 | 24 | 25 | 26 | 27 | 28 | 29 | 30 | 31 | 32 | 33 | 34 | 35 | 36 | 37 | 38 | 39 | 40 | 41 | 42 | 43 | 44 | 45 | 46 | 47 |
|---|---|---|---|---|---|---|---|---|---|---|---|---|---|---|---|---|---|---|---|---|---|---|---|---|---|---|---|
| I GRAMS | 536 | 525 | 580 | 654 | 783 | 872 | 989 | 1263 | 1488 | 1449 | 1662 | 1796 | 1977 | 2155 | 2383 | 2683 | 2827 | 3087 | 3223 | 3344 | 3447 | 3578 | 3540 | 3635 | 3626 | 3758 | 3752 |
| I NUMBER | 7 | 6 | 9 | 25 | 37 | 22 | 33 | 63 | 62 | 78 | 93 | 120 | 149 | 204 | 278 | 563 | 1000 | 1000 | 1000 | 1000 | 1000 | 1000 | 460 | 163 | 51 | 12 | |
| M GRAMS | 431 | 471 | 591 | 676 | 750 | 820 | 1036 | 1233 | 1360 | 1485 | 1650 | 1800 | 2009 | 2238 | 2420 | 2702 | 2861 | 3239 | 3420 | 3643 | 3632 | 3718 | 3745 | 3767 | 3974 | 3952 | 4181 |
| M NUMBER | 16 | 24 | 29 | 38 | 56 | 67 | 84 | 82 | 105 | 140 | 140 | 213 | 285 | 310 | 440 | 719 | 1000 | 1000 | 1000 | 1000 | 1000 | 1000 | 1800 | 623 | 226 | 80 | 14 |

TRAININGSCHOOL FOR MIDWIVES 1948-1967  
UNIVERSITY CLINIC W.G. 1931-1963    BIRTHWEIGHT IN CONSECUTIVE WEEKS OF PREGNANCY IN PRIMI- AND MULTIPARAE.  
IN ALL NEARLY 80.000 CASES WERE AVAILABLE.

*Fig.* 10.

If the placental dysfunction is caused by an intramural myoma or septum uteri then in rare cases an operation can improve the situation for a next pregnancy. A spontaneous improvement of the trophic capacity of the mother can be expected in the next pregnancy especially after the first pregnancy, perhaps because the uterus stays better vascularised after the first pregnancy. That after the 32th week of pregnancy the weight of the firstborn child lies behind of the weight of children of multiparous women is shown in figure 10. This difference is $\pm$ 200 g when pregnancy reaches 40 weeks. Avoiding noxious influences like heavy smoking of cigarettes, protecting the mother against malnutrition, especially during the last trimester of pregnancy are also means to prevent dysmaturity. But the most important of all is to raise healthy young girls who will be healthy, tall and happy brides and will have their first babies at a rather young age, at least before the age of 30 and preferably so before the age of 25.

Of all known factors that affect foetal growth:
1. ovular factors, genetically determined or caused by lesions during the embryonic period,
2  maternal factors that is to say, physical habitus, constitution and state of health of the mother before and during pregnancy,
3. the way mother and ovum get into touch with each other, in other words the place and manner of nidation of the ovum, here ovular, maternal and also peristatic factors may have their effect,
4. peristatic factors, i.e. the maternal milieu during the period of pregnancy in the most comprehensive sense,
the maternal factors (point 2) are the most important. An argument in support of this thesis is to be seen in the fact that we found an average weight of 3201 g as birthweight of children, born in the 40th week of pregnancy out of mothers who were smaller than 155 cm and a birthweight of 3659 g (a difference of 458 g) in children who were of the same gestational age but with mothers who were taller than 174 cm.

And so the circle is closed. In the prevention of dysmaturity the obstetrician comes after the paediatrician. A young woman, who is at the moment of conception in a perfect state of health and has been so since her own birth will not give the problems that have been the subject of this congress. The good results of obstetrics in a country to a high degree are due to the general state of health in that country. During pregnancy the obstetrician has to work in the same line, by protecting the expectant mothers against harmful influences and on the whole his aim, to handle a healthy baby to a healthy mother, will more often be achieved by careful watching and protecting the processes of nature than by interfering with them.

## REFERENCES

1. CAMERER, quoted by H. FINKELSTEIN (1938) *Säuglingskrankheiten*, 4e Auflage, Elsevier, Amsterdam: p. 6.
2. CLIFFORD, S. H. (1954) *J. Pediatrics* 44: 1.
3. McCLURE BROWNE, J. C. (1962) *Brit. Med. J.* II: 1080.
4. McCLURE BROWNE, J. C. (1953) *J. Obst. and Gyn. Brit. Emp.* 60: 141.
5. GRUENWALD, P. (1963) *Biol. Neonat.* 5: 215–265.
6. HOSEMANN, H. (1952) *Biologie und Pathologie des Weibes* 7: 828–899.
7. McKEOWN, T. and R. C. RECORD (1952) *J. Endocrin.* 8: 387.
8. McKEOWN, T. and R. G. RECORD (1953) *J. Endocrin.* 9: 418–426.
9. KLOOSTERMAN, G. J. (1956) *Gynaecologia* 142: 373–388.
10. KLOOSTERMAN, G. J. (1966) *Ned. T. Verlosk. en Gyn.* 66: 361.
11. KORTENOEVER, M. E. (1948) Thesis, Leiden.
12. RUNGE, H. (1942) *Zentrallbl. f. Gynak.* 1202.
13. SALING, E. (1966) *Das Kind im Bereich der Geburtshilfe*, Georg Thieme Verlag, Berlin.
14. WIJSENBEEK, L. A. (1926) *Geneesk. Gids* 4: 109.
15. ZANGEMEISTER, W. (1929) *Zbl. Gynak.* 53: 2723.

# DISCUSSION

DISCUSSION PAPER PROF. KLOOSTERMAN

*Prof. R. Schwartz* (in the chair): Prof. KLOOSTERMAN's paper is open for discussion.

*Dr. Wigglesworth:* I really must congratulate Prof. KLOOSTERMAN on what I think is quite the most scientific presentation I have ever heard from any obstetrician on this problem. I'm very interested in many of your results, particularly in the finding that boys have the same placental weight as girls. This perhaps suggests that the difference in birthweight between boys and girls is more likely to be genetic than due to variations in trophoblastic invasion. You have also shown very clearly the difference in mortality rate related to placental weight which I don't think has been shown in this way as clearly before.

I would like to ask particularly whether you have information about the influence on mortality of pathological changes in the placenta other than reduced weight.

*Prof. Kloosterman:* Yes, indeed we did histological examinations of all these placentas. They are studied macroscopically for infarcts. If the baby dies, and in case of a control series, we have done also microscopic examinations. We could show that the incidence of infarction of the placenta goes up after 40 weeks. On the average we have divided the placentas into 4 groups: (1) with no visible infarcts, (2) with slight infarcts, (3) with rather many infarcts and (4) with more infarcts than 25 per cent of the total placenta. Only group (3) and (4) are of pathological significance in our opinion: then we find 10 per cent on the average belonging to that group. In cases of post-maturity it is 20 per cent.

In our opinion the size of the placenta is of more importance than local and focal damages in the placenta. This is in contradiction with many studies on this object; all try to find some particular damage in the placenta and have not looked for the size of the placenta. It seems a rather silly business in our present time to do determinations of the weight of the placenta with a balance you can buy for 5 or 10 guilders. This study could as easily have been done in the 17th century. But I think there is a an explanation for this. This investigation is only possible in a clinic where you have women who came already in the 3rd month of pregnancy for control. 50 years ago everybody said: if you have a woman with 46 weeks of pregnancy, that woman has made an error. But if I have seen that woman in the 2nd month of pregnancy already and have done pregnancy tests then, I know absolutely for certain that she is not mistaken when she has carried on for 45 or 46 weeks. I think that this is the most important background for this investigation. In the past obstetricians have wiped away the problem and have said: every woman comes in labour when her time is due. On the whole that's true, but there are exceptions and we have studied them.

*Dr. Reynolds:* I wonder whether Prof. KLOOSTERMAN has taken advantage of this very large and well followed series of postmature pregnancies to look into the hormonal contents of the maternal urine during this period. Particularly I'm interested to know if he has done any oestriol determinations during the weeks following term. They are useful for predicting foetal viability, foetal condition and perhaps placental weight.

*Prof. Kloosterman:* I'm glad you mentioned this, I forgot to speak about it. Of course it's true that our attitude towards postmaturity is still not what it has to be, because we are treating every primiparous woman who goes beyond 42 weeks in the same way. We are well aware that at least 70 per cent of those women don't need any treatment at all. But we can't pick out the right ones beforehand. We are looking for methods to see which patients have to be treated and which can walk around even after 42 weeks.

In the first place we have seen that this is a primiparous problem with some rare exceptions. Secondly there are some clinical signs. When the uterus does not grow anymore, when the rest-tonus of the uterus rises, when the amount of amniotic fluid is going down, when the weight of the patient is going down, when her age is above 35 years, when she has a history of long infertility, in these cases dangers are much bigger and such women have to be treated even sooner for post-maturity than others.

Thirdly we have tried to do cytological examinations of the vagina. LIECHTFUSS and PUENDEL have mentioned that you could see by a cytological smear whether women would be at term or postterm. We have tried at our utmost but we can't see this. And then we went to real hormonal examinations. So we tried to estimate pregnandiol, oestriol, oestradiol and oestron. We have a series of 400 patients. Only a small number of this series went beyond term. This is the dificulty of this study. You don't know beforehand which woman will go beyond term. We only have some patients who did what we expected. I can show you the results in one patient together with a control. In a normal case the hormone content stays at the same level till the moment of birth, but in postmaturity it goes down before birth.

In the normal situation the stretch of the uterus by the growing foetus causes the initiation of labour. But if this moment has been missed, the baby doesn't grow anymore and is even resorbing amniotic fluid, there is no augmentation of stretch of the uterus. Then the initiation of labour has to wait for aging of the placenta. The amount of progesteron is then going down and this initiates the labour. But this labour is much more dangerous for the baby than a normal labour, because the uterus has now a lack of the normal amount of progesteron and other hormones as well. The uterus has a higher rest-tonus already. If you give these women oxytocin then the dangers are bigger I think than in normal women. Perhaps the same holds true for dysmature babies with duration of pregnancy for 34 or 36 weeks. For that reason we prefer a caesarean section in those patients. Of course it is impossible and utterly against the heart of an obstetrician to do a caesarean in every case of a primiparous women who goes beyond term.

*Dr. Papadatos:* Is there anything special in the amniotic fluid that would help us in determining gestational age?

*Prof. Kloosterman:* I don't know if there is anything in the amniotic fluid that could help us in determining gestational age. But perhaps it is possible to determine the situation of the foetus. We are taking

samples of amniotic fluid transabdominally. In the first place we look
for meconium stains. If there are meconium stains in the amniotic
fluid we will consider caesarean section in cases where induction of
labour was not successful. Secondly we try to determine the content of
albumin. We have the impression that dysmature babies have perhaps
a lower albumin content in their amniotic fluid. You could also
detect the amount of amniotic fluid by giving evans blue for example.
Perhaps there are some other parameters for examination of amniotic
fluid. If you have a suggestion I would be very grateful.

*Dr. Eggermont:* I should like to know the time of cord clamping in
Amsterdam for the interpretation of the weight of the placenta in
your study.

*Prof. Kloosterman:* By the moment of cord clamping you can influence
the weight of the placenta very much. That can make a difference of
80 tot 120 grams. For that reason all placenta's are weighed after
bleeding. We are used to clamp late, after 2 minutes at least and very
often after 5 minutes. Also in cases of caesarean section we clamp late,
because we remove the placenta and give the baby together with the
placenta to the paediatrician without clamping. We think it could
be of some advantage in prevention of hyaline membrane disaese. After
cutting the cord we don't tie the cord at the placental side, so we let
the placenta bleed completely.

# DEVELOPMENTAL ASPECTS

# CAUSES OF HANDICAP IN THE LOW
# WEIGHT INFANT

C. M. DRILLIEN

## Introduction

That infants of low birth weight have a higher than average incidence of all sorts of handicaps is no longer in dispute, equally there is general agreement that whereas the later progress of most infants of 2000–2500 g is not much different from that of larger born children from similar homes, below this birth weight the incidence of handicap increases steadily as birth weight further decreases (1).

Figure 1 illustrates the condition at 7 years of 175 children of birth weight 2000 g or less born in Edinburgh hospitals between 1953 and 1960. About 90 per cent of surviving children from the original sample were followed up to this age. Those classified as having moderate or severe handicap are ineducable or require special educational provision on account of physical defect or mental retardation or attend ordinary school but suffer from cerebral palsy and/or epilepsy. All those classified as having some handicap are educable in normal school but have educational difficulties in the majority associated with dull or low average intelligence and/or marked behaviour problems, and a few have moderate physical defects such as high myopia which do not necessitate special schooling.

I do not propose to dwell on the problems illustrated here but spend my allotted time considering why it is that some babies of low birth weight present later with a variety of physical, neurological and intellectual handicaps, whilst others of like birth weight escape relatively unscathed.

## Survival rates

The incidence of later handicap illustrated in figure 1 is rather higher than that reported from most other centres and much higher

* Department of Child Life and Health, University of Edinburgh.

than that reported from some. For instance, in the continuing study by DANN and LEVINE (2, 3) of infants with birth weights or minimal post-natal weights of 1000 g or less, the incidence of significant physical defects (apart from frequently observed eye defects) in the two-thirds of the original sample who were later re-examined, was only 16 per cent and only 13 per cent had I.Q. levels below 80. Of the one-third who did not return for re-examination, over one-half were known to be mentally retarded, thus the total incidence of handicap is higher than is at first apparent, but nevertheless is much lower than that found in Edinburgh born children of like birth weight.

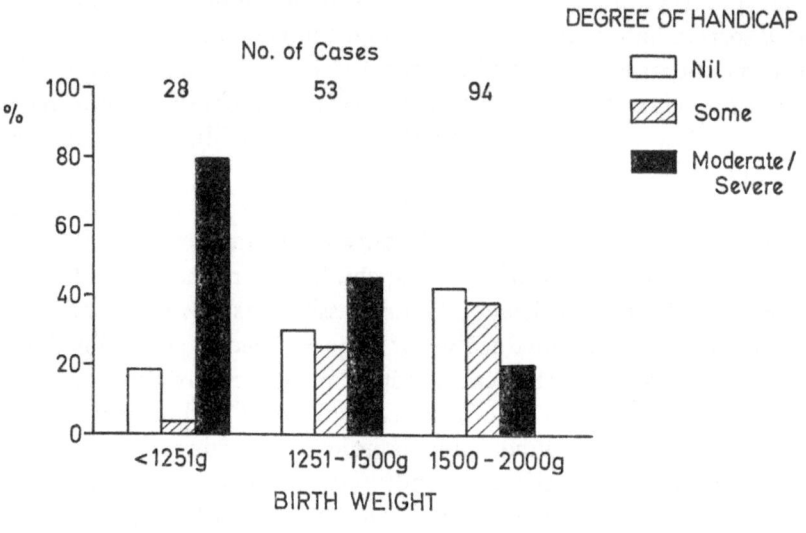

*Fig.* 1.

It may be that there are deficiencies in ante-natal care of mothers and post-natal care of low weight infants in Edinburgh; conversely, it could be that care is too good and that infants already damaged are more likely to survive.

A second look at the study of DANN and LEVINE suggests that when intensive care facilities are immediately available after birth the survival of damaged infants is more likely. Whereas in the Edinburgh group all but a handful of the infants studied were born in maternity hospital and transferred immediately to a premature unit, over two-thirds of the New York babies were transported usually from small private hospitals elsewhere and most had survived for 12—48 hours before transport. DANN and LEVINE reported that a significantly higher proportion of children with later I.Qs. of 100 or over was found among those coming from families having private medical care and concluded from this that social class was the most important variable associated with later mental development. However, nearly all transported babies had private doctors compared with one-third of those actually born in the City Hospital.

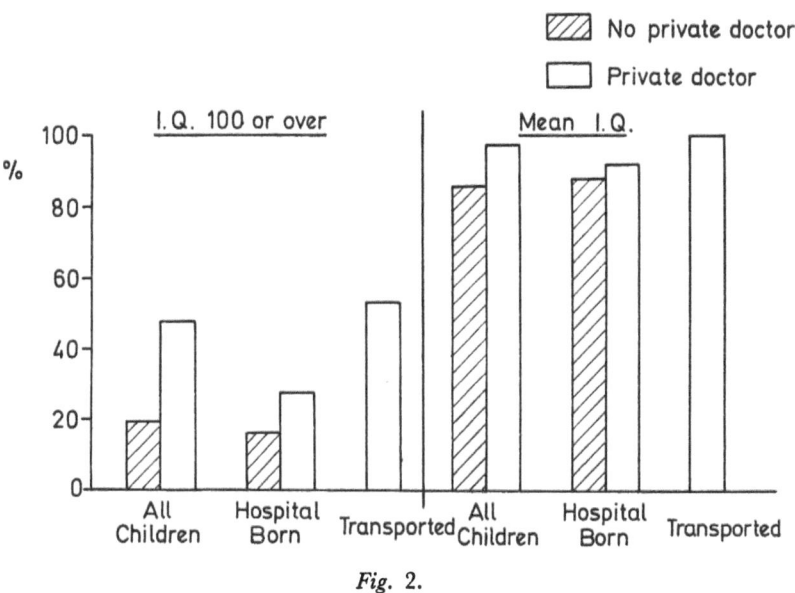

*Fig.* 2.

Figure 2 shows that although among the total sample over twice as many of those with private doctors had later I.Qs. of 100 or over as compared with those having no private doctor, the difference by type of medical care was much less among hospital born infants, and also that among all infants having private care twice as many scored 100 or over in the transported group as did those in the hospital born group. These findings suggest that a more important factor associated with later mental development than social class was whether the low weight infant could survive without special care long enough to be transported to the New York City Hospital.

19

*Sex of infant. Single or multiple birth*

We will now consider certain types of infants who appear to have an added risk of subsequent damage.

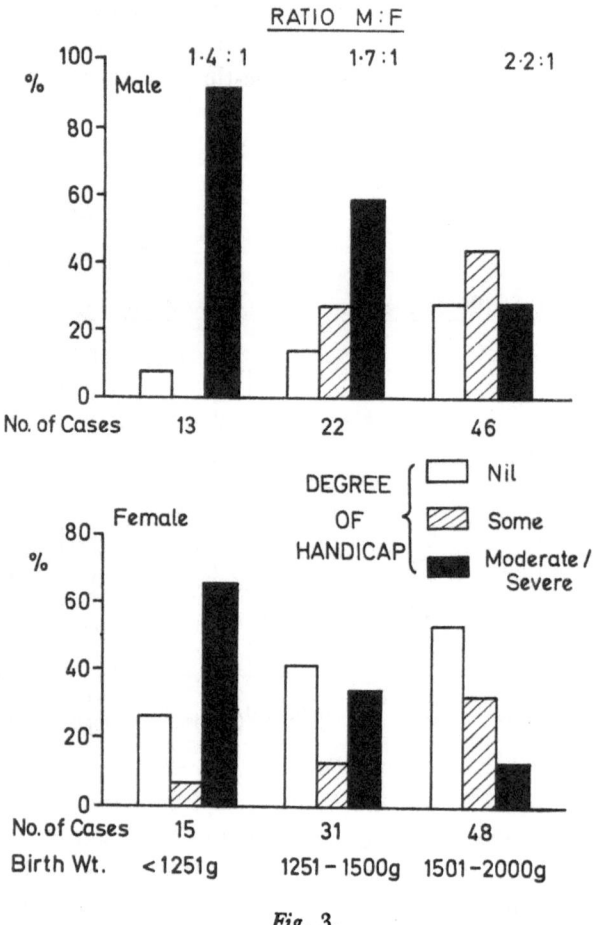

Fig. 3.

Figure 3 shows degrees of handicap by birth weight and sex. There is a significant excess of boys with moderate or severe handicap. The ratio of severely handicapped boys to girls is lowest (1.4:1) at birth weights of 1250 g or less and highest (2.2:1) at weights of 1500—2000 g. This appears to be due to the greater vulnerability of male infants to the adverse effects of severe maternal complications such as toxaemia and chronic disease. The proportion of births associated with these pregnancy complications increased with increasing birth weight within this birth weight range.

Figure 4 illustrates degrees of handicap according to whether the infant was the product of a single or multiple pregnancy. At birth weights of 1500 g or less (but not above this weight) infants resulting from multiple pregnancies had a lower incidence of severe handicap.

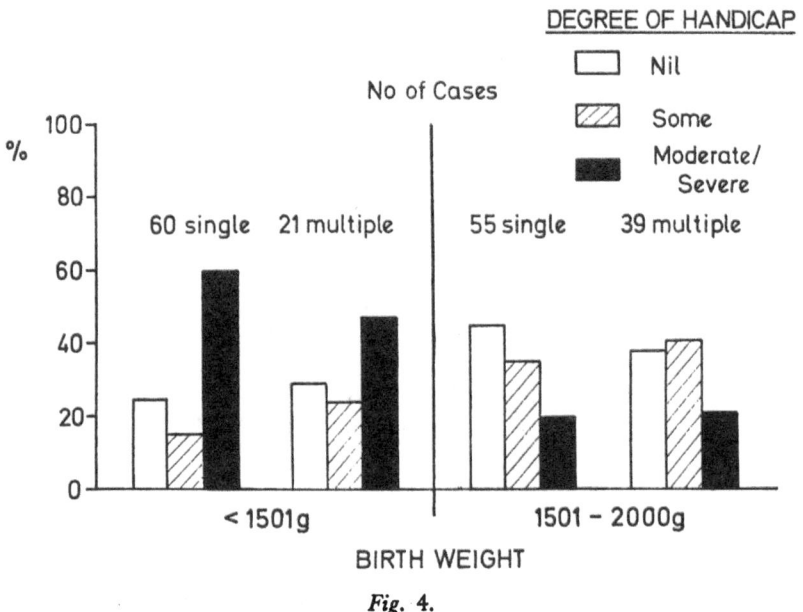

Fig. 4.

*Social class*

Like other workers I have found that women from poor working class homes are more likely to give birth to premature babies and to small for dates babies, and also that at later ages the low weight infant reared in a poor home is more likely to be classified as handicapped. In my total sample of mothers, one-quarter were graded as poor working class, which is three times what would be expected in a total population of births in the same area.

Figure 5 shows that 20 per cent of children *without* and 35 per cent of children *with* severe handicap come from poor working class homes. However, a further breakdown of the severely handicapped into those with mental defect only, and those with neurological and physical defects, with or without mental defect, reveals that the excess of handicapped children from poor homes is accounted for almost entirely by children who are mentally defective only.

It should be remembered that intellectual ability rated as low average or dull in a child whose parents and siblings are of above average ability may indicate as marked a degree of relative retardation and present similar domestic problems as a child who is classified as handicapped because he has an I.Q. of less than 70 and attends special school but whose parents and siblings are themselves of low intelligence.

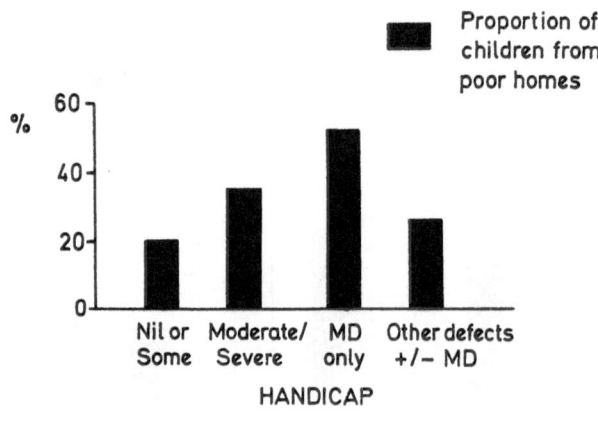

*Fig.* 5.

The next two figures which compare teachers' assesments of educational attainment in English and Arithmetic at age 11 years and I.Q. scores at 12 years, of low weight infants and mature controls by type of home, indicate that relative retardation appears to be most marked in children coming from the best homes.

Compared with mature children the proportion of low weight infants whose ability in both English and Arithmetic is considered poor is most marked in those coming from the best homes and least marked in those coming from the worst (figure 6).

Similarly, on the results of the routine group I.Q. tests at transfer to secondary school the differences in scores between low birth weight and mature children were most marked in those coming from middle class and superior working class homes (figure 7).

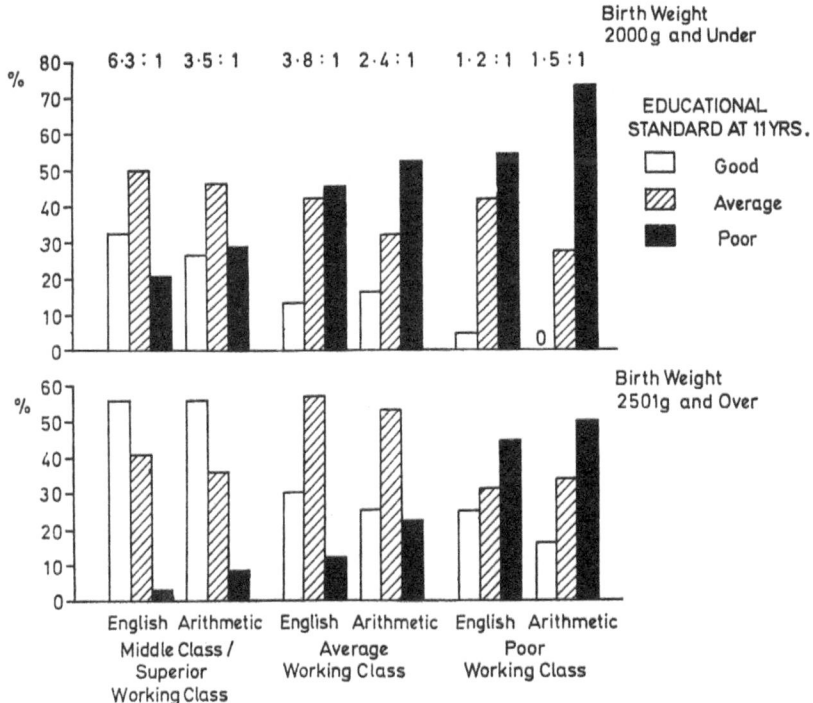

*Fig.* 6.

*Intrauterine growth retardation*

Unlike some other workers I have not been able to confirm that the infant who is markedly underweight for his gestation period is likely to show more handicaps at later ages than the true premature of like birth weight, though it may be that the real effect of intrauterine growth retardation has been masked by inaccuracy of reporting of gestational age in the mid-50's.

Figure 8 shows that though there are rather fewer poorly grown infants among those with no handicap, and rather more among those with some handicap, the differences observed are small, and are in fact more than accounted for by an excess of poor working class mothers giving birth to underweight infants and a few undergrown

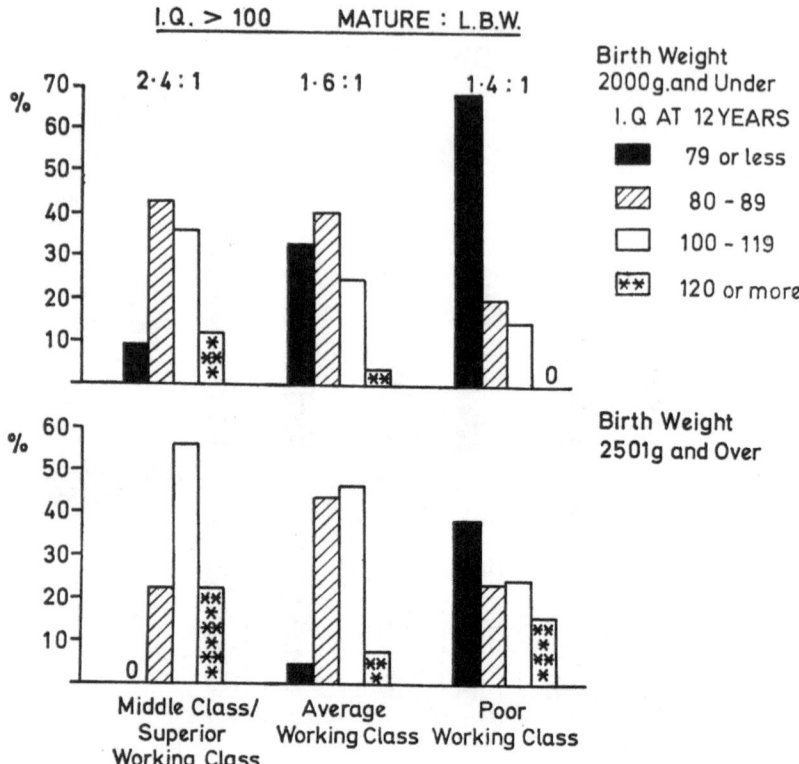

*Fig.* 7.

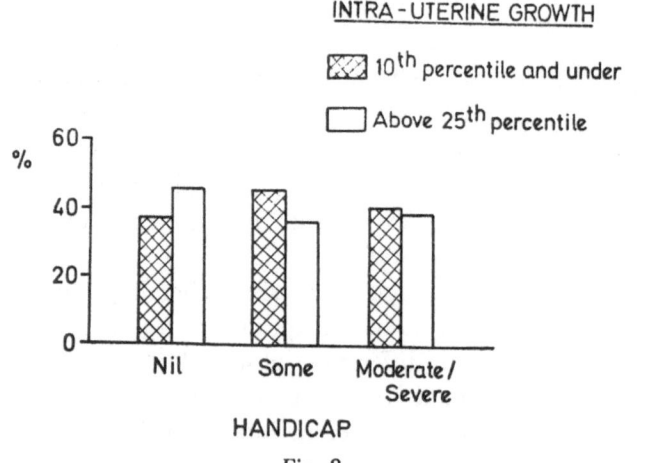

HANDICAP

*Fig.* 8.

children with major congenital anomalies. When these were excluded the small for dates infants showed significantly less handicap at later ages than true prematures of like birth weight.

It seems certain that some cases of mental and neurological defect reported in children who were small for dates were due to hypogly-caemia as has been described by Dr. STRICH (4). These essentially preventable handicaps should be seen far less frequently in the future.

Low weight for gestation period in my group was associated with severe maternal complications but these complications had an adverse effect (particularly on male infants) whether or not intra-uterine growth retardation was present.

In another group of low weight infants which I am studying at present, the most striking difference by intrauterine growth observed in the first 6 months is the much higher incidence of congenital ano-malies (both minor and major) in those who were markedly under-weight for gestational age. Thrity-six per cent of those below the 10th percentile show anomalies likely to have been developmental in origin, 25 per cent of those between the 10th and 25th percentiles and 12 per cent of those whose intrauterine growth was above this level.

This current study is still in the very early stages but my observation on the original group that minor congenital anomalies are increased in those presenting later with more serious mental and neurological defects, leads me to suspect that the excess of handicaps reported in small for dates babies may be due more to growth retardation asso-ciated with developmental malformation than to the adverse effect of foetal malnutrition on a potentially normal central nervous system. However, further long term studies are required here.

*Complications of later pregnancy and delivery*

In no case of severe handicap in my original group did it seem likely that complications of labour or traumatic delivery were prima-rily responsible for later defect. In 3 of the 175 cases handicap most likely originated post-natally.

Of the rest their mothers had or had not suffered from compli-cations during late pregnancy or chronic disease continuing throughout pregnancy in approximately equal numbers of cases, Of those mothers with complications over one-half suffered from toxaemia and/or chronic disease and over one-third from unexplained antepartum haemorrhage, by which I mean haemorrhage unassociated with toxaemia, chronic disease, attempted abortion, or placenta praevia. In all, uncomplicated pregnancy, toxaemia and antepartum haemorrhage accounted for 90 per cent of the total pregnancies.

The incidence of later severe handicap was about the same for those born to mothers who did or did not have pregnancy complications.

*Developmental malformations*

In 13 per cent of the children classified as moderately or severely handicapped the handicap is due to major or multiple congenital anomalies which must have arisen at an early stage of intrauterine existence. However, the commonest and most serious handicaps observed were neurological and mental defects which could also have arisen in early intrauterine life or alternatively could have arisen from damage to a potentially normal central nervous system at a later stage of gestation or post-natally. Some children with mental and neurological defects also show developmental anomalies and in these cases it seems reasonable to hypothesise that the total picture of handicap is likely to be due to developmental malformation rather than to later damage. In addition, of children without severe handicap there are more who have minor physical defects likely to have been developmental in origin, than was found in my mature control group.

*Maternal infertility*

Maternal infertility has been demonstrated as a significant association with a number of congenital anomalies. Infertility was reported by MURPHY (5) in his study of the reproductive histories of all mothers of infants with fatal congenital malformations, born in a 5 year period in Philadelphia; by RECORD and EDWARDS (6) studying congenital dislocation of the hip in Birmingham and in studies of cerebral diplegia (7, 8) and nonfamilial cleft lip and palate (9), in Edinburgh.

It is well known that mothers of mongols are characteristically older than mothers of like parity in the general population. However, in a group which I have been studying it appears that their average age at marriage and at the births of their preceding children is not much different from that of mothers of like social class in the general population. Their older age at the births of their mongol offspring is often accounted for by a long preceding period of involuntary infertility.

Figure 9 illustrates the reproductive capacity of mothers of low weight infants who do and do not have severe handicaps and that of a group of 112 control mothers of 90 normal singletons of birth weight over 2500 g and 22 pairs of twins, both of whom weighed over 2500 g.

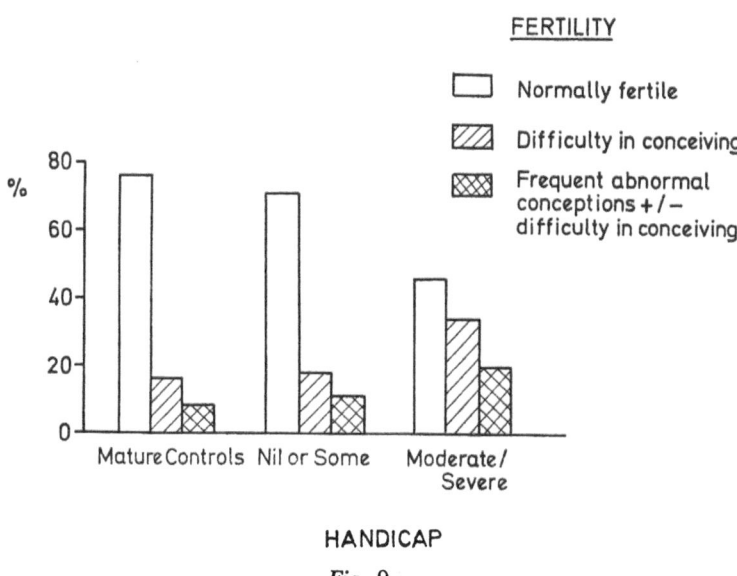

*Fig.* 9.

The incidence of relative infertility was not much different for mothers of control children and low weight children without severe handicap but there was a marked increase both in women having difficulty in conceiving and in those having frequent abnormal conceptions among mothers of handicapped children, which further suggests that some handicaps are likely to be due to developmental malformation.

When incidence of relative infertility was related to birth weight, the highest incidence occurred at weights of 1500 g or less, but among the smallest infants there was not much difference in outcome by fertility of mother. The incidence of maternal infertility was lower in the birth weight range 1500—2000 g but here there was a much higher incidence of handicap noted in the offspring of infertile mothers.

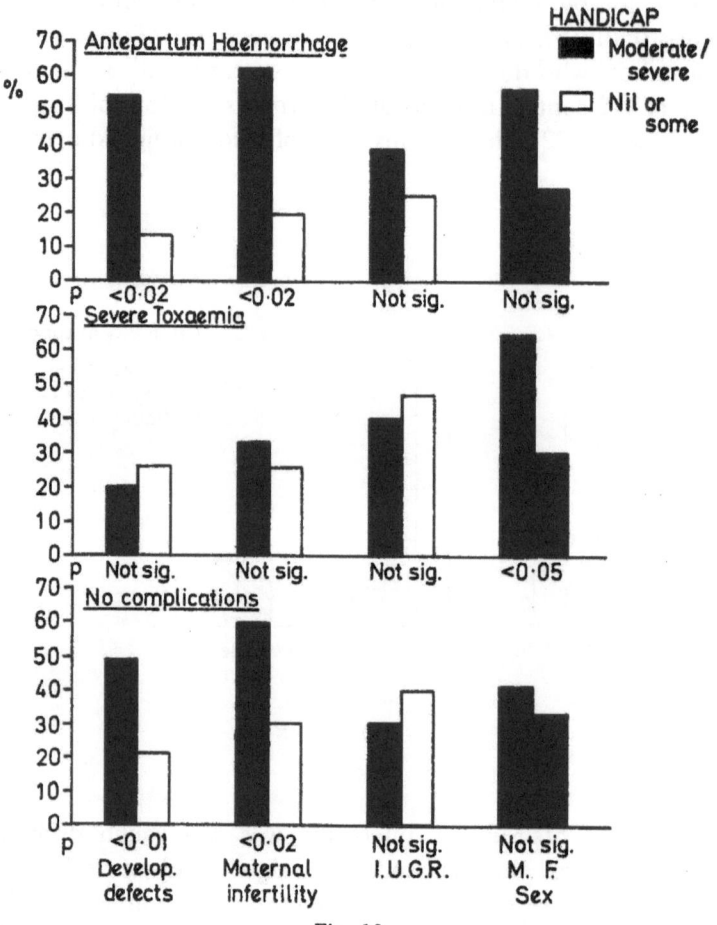

*Fig.* 10.

*Factors associated with later handicap*

I have tried to bring together some of the factors already discussed which may be associated with later handicap, in figure 10, which deals with children who have or do not have severe handicap, divided into the three main pregnancy groups: uncomplicated pregnancy, pregnancy complicated by toxaemia and/or chronic disease, and pregnancy complicated only by unexplained antepartum haemorrhage.

The first colum shows the proportion of children with and without handicap who have developmental defects. The overall incidence of major or minor anomalies is lowest in children born following severe toxaemia and in this group there are rather more defects among children who are not seriously handicapped. The incidence is much higher in the other two groups and in both there is a strikingly significant excess of developmental defects among the handicapped.

The second column shows the incidence of maternal infertility. Again the lowest incidence is seen in those mothers suffering from toxaemia and here there is little difference in infertility between mothers of children with and without severe handicap. In the other two groups there is a statistically significant excess of infertility among mothers of handicapped children.

The incidence of marked intrauterine growth retardation is highest in the toxaemia group but in no group is there a significant difference in incidence of growth retardation between those with and without handicap.

The last column shows the proportion of males and females with severe handicap. In all three groups there is an excess of males but this is particularly marked and only statistically significant in the case of infants born to toxaemic mothers.

To summarise this figure, one could say that in the one-quarter of total low weight infants who were born to mothers with toxaemia and/or chronic disease and whose premature delivery was nearly always due to deliberate termination of the pregnancy, pointers to developmental malformation are minimal. Here later handicap seems most likely to be due directly to the adverse effect (particularly on males) of maternal complications.

In the two-thirds of total infants born after uncomplicated pregnancies or ones complicated only by unexplained antepartum haemorrhage, the much higher incidence of congenital anomalies and maternal infertility in those presenting later with severe handicaps suggests that the primary cause of later disability (and also of the unexplained haemorrhage) is developmental malformation, and that the low birth weight and/or premature labour are secondary to this and not primarily the cause of later handicap.

*Handicap and survival*

Finally, to return to what I said at the beginning about the higher incidence of handicap in Edinburgh born children, perhaps one can only make fair comparisons if total groups of live born low weight infants are considered and the proportions dying, surviving with handicap and surviving undamaged are compared.

I have not found any published figures of this sort, but figure 11 illustrates these findings in a group of Edinburgh infants of birth weight 3 lb (1360 g) or less delivered alive in Edinburgh maternity hospitals between 1948 and 1959.

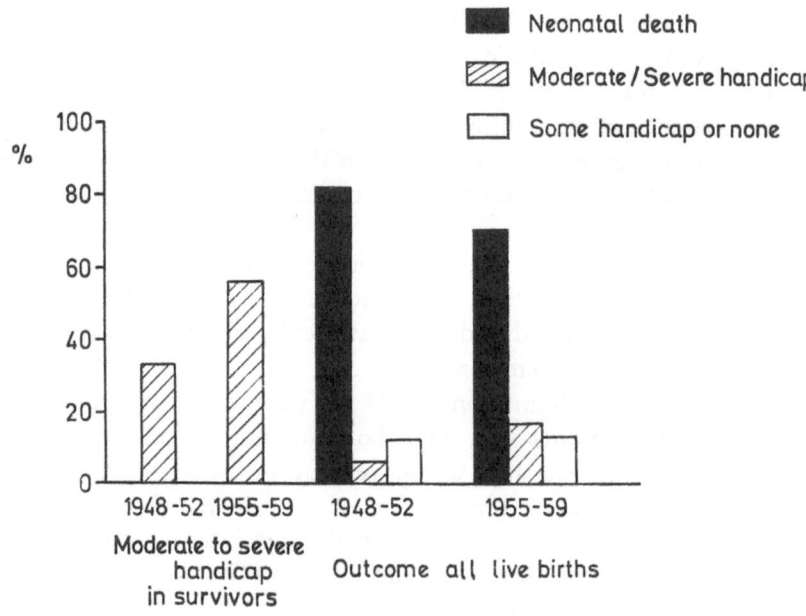

*Fig.* 11.

Less than one-third of children born in the five year period 1948—52 have moderate or severe handicap compared with over one-half of those born 1955—59. However, the survival rate improved from 18 per cent in the earlier to 30 per cent in the later period.

If one looks at the survival of children without severe handicap there is not much difference, 11.5 per cent of those born 1948—52 and 13.2 per cent of those born 1955—59.

These rather depressing figures are hardly surprising if, as my findings seem to suggest, developmental malformation is a major cause of later handicap, and one might expect that as survival rates of very small infants improve, so the proportion of surviving children with subsequent handicaps due to developmental malformation might also increase.

SUMMARY

A study of 175 Edinburgh born children of birth weight 2000 g or less, all of whom have reached the age of 7 years, indicates that the incidence of moderate or severe handicap is influenced by the following factors:
1. Birth weight. Incidence of handicap increases steadily with decreasing birth weight.
2. Sex, single or multiple birth. Incidence is higher in males than females, particularly following birth weights of 1501—2000 g. Incidence is lower in infants of 1500 g or less resulting from multiple pregnancies.
3. Social Class. Among the total sample of mothers three times as many came from poor working class homes as would be expected in the general population.
Children with physical and neurological defects (with or without additional mental handicap) were no more likely than children without severe handicap to be reared in poor working class homes.
Children classified as handicapped on account of mental defect only were nearly three times as likely to come from poor homes. However, the results of I.Q. tests at 12 years and teachers' assessments of educational attainment at 11 years, indicate that as compared with mature control children from similar homes *relative* retardation is no less marked in low birth weight children coming form the best homes.
4. Intrauterine growth. There was little indication that children who had been markedly underweight for their gestation period were any more likely to show later handicap than children of like birth weight whose weight was more appropriate for gestational age.
5. Complications of pregnancy. The incidence of later handicap was approximately the same for those born to mothers who did or did not have complications in the third trimester. Boys appeared to be more vulnerable than girls to the adverse effects of severe toxaemia and/or chronic disease of mother.
6. Maternal infertility. At birth weights of 1501 g or over there

was a significant excess of later handicap in the offspring of mothers who had a history of difficulty in conceiving or frequent abnormal outcome in their other conceptions.

7. Developmental malformations. There was a significant excess of minor and major congenital malformations in those with later neurological and mental handicap, suggesting that in many cases the total handicaps were developmental in origin.

8. Survival rate. The proportion of surviving children with handicap has increased as the survival rate has improved.

CONCLUSIONS

Over one-third of children who had been 2000 g or less at birth, presented with moderate or severe handicap at 7 years.

In one-quarter of cases of handicap this was thought to be due primarily to the adverse effects of severe maternal complications, necessitating premature termination of pregnancy. Males are particularly susceptible to these complications.

In two-thirds of cases of handicap this was thought to result primarily from developmental malformation in the foetus. Pregnancies were uncomplicated or complicated only by unexplained antepartum haemorrhage. One-half of mothers showed impaired reproductive capacity. Two-thirds of handicapped children had minor or major congenital anomalies.

## REFERENCES

1. HARPER, P. A. and G. WIENER (1965) *Ann. Rev. Med.* 16: 405.
2. DANN, M., S. Z. LEVINE and E. V. NEW (1958) *Pediatrics* 22: 1037.
3. DANN, M., S. Z. LEVINE and E. V. NEW (1964) *Pediatrics* 33: 945.
4. ANDERSON, J. M., R. D. G. MILNER and S. J. STRICH (1966) *Lancet* 2: 372.
5. MURPHY, D. P. (1947) *Congenital Malformations. A study of parental characteristics with special reference to the reproductive process.* ed. 2. Lippincott, Philadelphia.
6. RECORD, R. G. and J. H. EDWARDS (1958) *Brit. J. prev. soc. Med.* 12: 8.
7. DRILLIEN, C. M., T. T. S. INGRAM and E. M. RUSSELL (1962) *Arch. Dis. Childh.* 37: 282.
8. DRILLIEN, C. M., T. T. S. INGRAM and E. M. RUSSELL (1964) *Develop. Med. Child Neurol.* 6: 241.
9. DRILLIEN, C. M., T. T. S. INGRAM and E. M. WILKINSON (1966). *The Causes and Natural History of Cleft Lip and Palate.* Livingstone, Edinburgh.

# NEUROLOGICAL FINDINGS IN NEWBORN INFANTS AFTER PRE- AND PARANATAL COMPLICATIONS*

H. F. R. PRECHTL**

In recent years, several attempts have been made to assess the hazards of pre- and perinatal obstetric complications. There is little doubt that obstetric complications carry an increased risk of mortality (1, 2). Moreover, where several obstetric complications are present in combination, it would be expected, a priori, that the risks will be additive. Whilst the exact causes of mortality in any case may be diverse, one major factor is fatal damage to the central nervous system. Post-mortem examination of the brains of babies who would have died after obstetric complications or unfavourable events during the neonatal period have clearly shown the possibility of these factors producing lesions in the nervous system (3, 4, 5, 6, 7). Studies in monkeys (8, 9, 10) have provided evidence of the harmful consequences of experimentally induced perinatal complications.

Whilst mortality-rate studies have a strict criterion available — death of the foetus within a given period of time — the assessment of damage to the surviving infant is much more difficult. Signs have to be found which indicate the baby's condition and these signs must have both high inter-observer reliability and long-term prognostic value. Apgar's technique has merits but is restricted to the first few minutes after birth and deliberately covers only general aspects of physiological status (11, 12). A quite different approach has been used by GRAHAM (13) and GRAHAM et al. (14) who measured behaviour patterns of babies a few days old.

In our own department a detailed neurological examination has been developed for the assessment of babies (15). This examination has good inter-observer reliability and high prognostic value (16, 17).

* This paper is an enlarged version of the Mental Health Research Fund Lecture 1967, held in London.
** Department of Developmental Neurology, State University, Groningen.

In a sample of 102 neonates without neurological signs 86 % were found to be neurologically normal at follow-up between 2 and 4 years later. From 150 neonates with abnormal neurological signs, 73 % still showed abnormal signs at follow-up during a similar period.* Certain constellations of neonatal abnormal signs, which we designated hyperexcitable-, apathetic- and hemi-syndromes respectively, were prognostic of continuing neurological abnormality in 67 %, 59 % and 73 % of cases respectively, when the latter were examined at 2—4 years (17). Preliminary findings from our follow-up studies at 8 years show a similar picture to that found at 2—4 years. This method of examination may thus be regarded as a highly sensitive indicator of long-term neurological functioning. The identification of factors which contribute to neurological abnormality in the newborn is therefore a problem of crucial importance.

The aim of the present paper is to examine some inter-relationships between obstetric complications and the results of this examination. Our hypothesis is that obstetric complications carry a high risk of neurological damage to the surviving infant. The data upon which the present study is based, have been collected over a period of twelve years. The paper will be restricted to presentation of a number of global findings. Full data will be published elsewhere.

METHOD

*The sample*

A neurological examination was carried out on 1515 infants born in the Department of Obstetrics of the University Hospital. In the Netherlands about 70 % of all infants are born at home. The 30 % hospital-delivered babies are therefore primarily cases with a risk of obstetric complications, although a minority goes to hospital for social reasons, such as poor housing.

From this total, the following were eliminated:
1. Babies of women who did not regularly attend the out-patient unit of the obstetric department during pregnancy;
2. Babies whose birthweight was less than 2500 g;
3. Babies with gross malformations;

* The correlation between neonatal findings and the presence or absence of abnormal neurological signs on follow-up gave a value of $\varphi = 0.583$ (p < 0.0001).

4. Babies whose mother was in a poor nutritional state, suffered from psychiatric disease, epilepsy, diabetes or heart disease, or whose basal metabolism was low;
5. Babies whose mothers had suffered prolonged sterility.

Both categories 4 and 5 occurred rarely in our material. Babies whose condition was poor or dangerous in the first week were not subjected to full neurological examination. The sample remaining, after exclusion of the above cases, consisted of 1378 babies.

*The neurological examination*
The standard neurological examination technique has been previously described (15). All infants were examined once, two or three hours after a feed. All examinations were carried out between the second and fourteenth day, 91 % of them being between the third and tenth day. The babies were picked at random from the obstetric department and were examined without knowledge of the obstetric history.

*Data processing*
The obstetric and neurological data were entered on precoded forms and later transferred to IBM punched cards. 76 items were related to the mother, the course of pregnancy and delivery and the general aspects of the infant, and 142 items to the neurological examination. All computations were carried out on a general purpose computer (TR 4) at the Computer Centre of the University.

RESULTS

1. *Incidence of obstetric complications*
An obstetric complication may be defined as any factor or group of factors in the pre- or perinatal environment which increases the risk of foetal mortality. These will be symptoms of maternal disease during pregnancy, signs of foetal distress and mechanical intervention in the delivery. Few of these factors are independent of each other and many are causally related. For example, maternal toxaemia may lead to foetal distress which in turn will lead to instrumental extraction.

In order therefore to give a more precise meaning to the rather loosely-used term 'complication', the following procedure was adopted.

20

For every case, forty-two variables of the obstetric history were analysed and a count was made of the number of variables which did not deviate from optimal conditions (the 'Obstetric Score'), according to generally accepted criteria. Table 1 gives the criteria. In 6.2 % of our sample, all forty-two variables were in the optimal condition, the largest number of *non*-optimal conditions was 15 (figure 1).

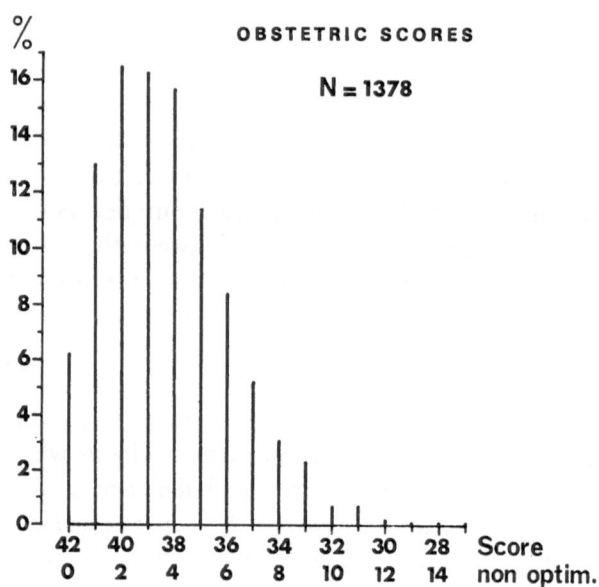

*Fig.* 1.  Percentage distribution of the obstetric scores. Below each score is given the corresponding number of non-optimal conditions.

Table 1.  *Criteria of optimal obstetric conditions*

| *Maternal factors* | |
| --- | --- |
| 1. maternal age primipara | 18–30 years |
|     maternal age multipara | 20–30 years |
| 2. marital state | married |
| 3. parity | 1–6 |
| 4. abortions in history | 0–2 |
| 5. pelvis | no disproportion |
| 6. luetic infection | absent |
| 7. Rh antagonism | absent |
| 8. blood group incompatibility | absent |
| 9. nutritional state | well nourished |

10. haemoglobin level — 70 or more
11. bleedings during pregnancy — absent
12. infections during pregnancy — absent
13. X-ray abdomen during pregnancy — no
14. toxaemia — absent or mild
15. blood pressure — not exceeding 90/135
16. albuminuria and oedema — absent
17. hyperemesis — absent
18. psychological stress — absent
19. prolonged unwanted sterility (2 years) — absent
20. maternal chronic diseases — absent

*Parturition*

21. twins or multiple birth — no
22. delivery — spontaneous
23. duration 1st stage — 6–24 hours
24. duration 2nd stage — 10 min–2 hours
25. contractions — moderate or strong
26. drugs given to mother — $O_2$, local anaesthetic
27. amniotic fluid — clear
28. membranes broken — not longer than 6 hours

*Foetal factors*

29. intrauterine position — vertex
30. gestational age — 38–41 weeks
31. foetal presentation — vertex
32. cardiac regularity — regular
33. foetal heart rate (2nd stage) — 100–160
34. cord around the neck — no or loose
35. cord prolapse — no
36. knot in the cord — no
37. placental infarction — no or small
38. onset respiration — within first min.
39. treatment, resuscitation — no
40. drugs given — nil
41. body temperature — normal
42. birth weight — 2500—4990 g

Table 2 shows some of the most frequently occurring non-optimal conditions.

The data were next divided into six subgroups: those with 0; 1—2; 3—4; 5—6; 7—9; 10 or more non-optimal conditions. The percentage of cases in each sub-group is given for boys and girls seperately, in figure 2.

There were no statistically significant sex differences with respect

to occurrence of non-optimal obstetric conditions. In the subsequent
analysis the data for boys and girls are combined.

Table 2

| Condition | N | % |
|---|---|---|
| Maternal age above 30 years | 342 | 25.0 |
| Moderate toxaemia | 250 | 18.1 |
| Severe toxaemia | 108 | 8.5 |
| Other than vertex presentations | 235 | 17.2 |
| Non spontaneous delivery | 427 | 31.0 |
|    Caesarean sections | 81 | 6 |
|    Middle forceps | 75 | 5.4 |
|    Low forceps | 133 | 9.7 |
| Prolonged labour $\geqslant$ 24 h. | 170 | 12.3 |
| Second stage longer than two hours | 96 | 7.0 |
| Tight cord around the neck | 101 | 7.3 |
| Foetal brady-cardia < 100/min | 188 | 13.6 |
| Postpartum apnea > 1 min | 224 | 16.3 |

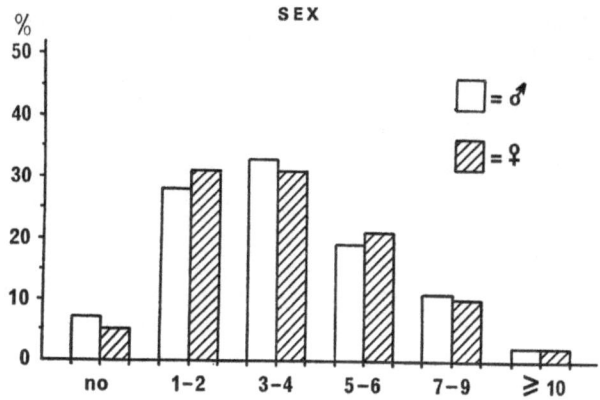

Fig. 2.   Incidence of non-optimal conditions in boys and girls.

2. *Inter-relationships between non-optimal obstetric conditions*
It is of interest to examine which conditions occur in combination
with others and which do not. This summary will be confined to three
examples only, illustrating respectively: complications of pregnancy,
delivery and foetal state.

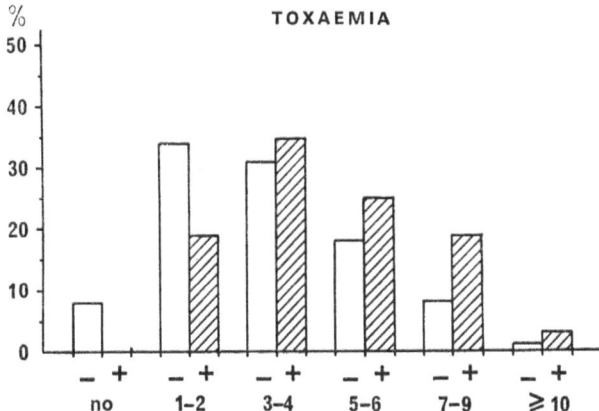

*Fig.* 3.   Percentage of the non toxaemic (—), and moderate and severe toxaemic cases (+) (N = 370) in each subgroup of non-optimal conditions. The difference is significant.

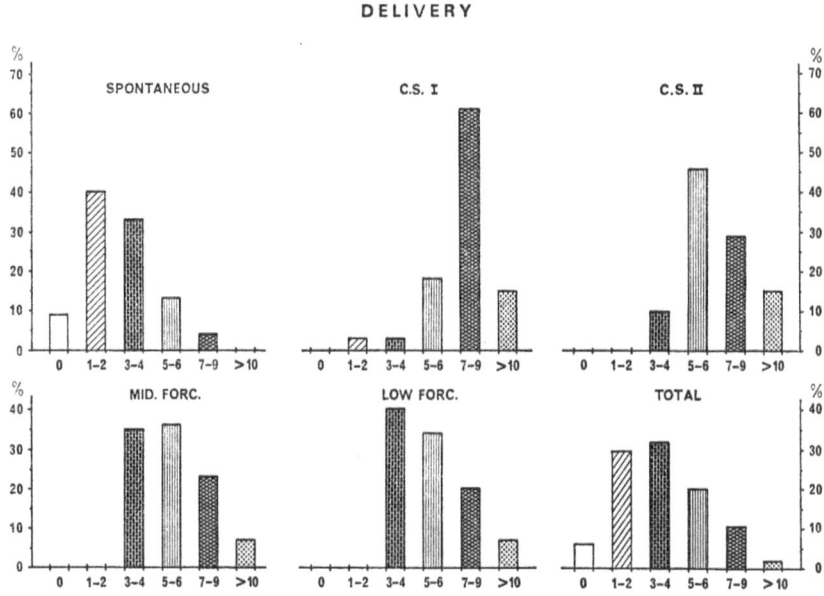

*Fig.* 4.   Type of delivery and obstetric subgroup. Spontaneous delivery, elective caesarean sections C.S.I (N = 33), non-elective C.S.II (N = 48), middle forceps (N = 85), and low forceps (N = 133) are presented seperately.

## a) Toxaemia

If all cases with moderate or severe toxaemia (characterized by blood pressure ⩾ 140/95, and albuminuria and oedema respectively) are compared against the rest, with respect to the distribution of complications, it will be seen that there is a marked tendency for the toxaemia cases to occur in association with a large number of other non-optimal conditions (figure 3).

## b) Delivery

A similar picture emerges, as might be expected, for instrumental, as compared with spontaneous, deliveries (figure 4).

## c) Foetal heart-rate and apnea

Signs of foetal distress, such as tachy- or brady-cardia during the second stage (figure 5) and postpartum apnea longer than 1 minute (figure 6) behave similarly to the complications above.

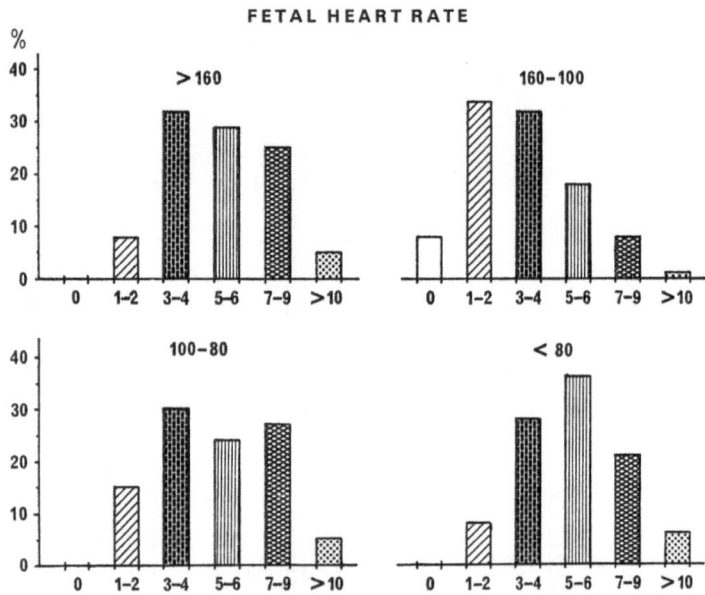

*Fig.* 5.  Foetal heart rate and non-optimal conditions. The tachycardia group with a heart rate > 160/min (N = 59) and the two groups of bradycardia 100—80/min (N = 101) and < 80/min (N = 89) are all significant different from the group with normal heart rate (100— 160).

3. *Non-optimal obstetric conditions and neurological symptoms*

Most of the items of the neurological examination are assessed on an ordinal scale with three or four points. For instance, the palmar grasp reflex is recorded as being absent (—), being weak or just discernable (+), giving a good sustained response for 10 seconds (++), or giving an exaggerated forceful grasp (+++). The rooting response is recorded as being absent (—), showing only a weak turn toward the stimulated side (+), giving a full turn and a grasp with the lips (++), and consisting of a very vigorous turn with grasping (+++). The intensity of the Moro reflex is recorded as low, middle or high. In the case of the palmar grasp reflex and rooting response, the (++) category may be regarded as the optimal response, whereas for the Moro reflex, the optimal response would be that of intermediate intensity and threshold.

If we assume that for each item of the neurological examination there is an optimal response, we may examine the frequency with which cases with varying numbers of obstetric complications, fall into the optimal and non-optimal categories.

For the purpose of this analysis the data were divided on the basis of the obstetric complications into three sub-groups:

1. A 'low risk' group (N = 264; 19.2 %) with 0 or only 1 non-optimal condition;
2. A 'middle risk' group (N = 943; 68.4 %) with 2 to 6 non-optimal conditions;
3. A 'high risk' group (N = 171, 12.4 %) with 7 or more non-optimal conditions.

The word 'risk' is used to denote a raised probability of mortality during delivery and the first two weeks of life. It involves no assumptions about the possible outcome of the neurological examination.

For illustration the distributions of response intensities of the palmar grasp reflex (figure 7) the rooting response (figure 8) the Moro-response (figure 9) and the head control in sitting posture (figure 10) are shown for the low and high risk group.

58 neurological items were selected which, as above, could be assigned a position on a 4-point ordinal scale. Contingency tables were constructed showing the frequency with which patients from the

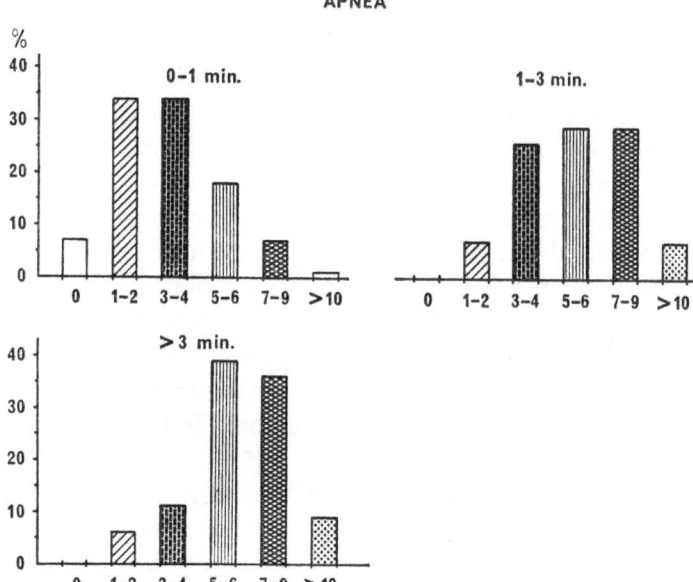

*Fig.* 6.   Onset of respiration and incidence of non-optimal conditions. The longer
the apnea the more other non-optimal conditions are present. The difference is
highly significant 1—3 min N = 187, > 3 min N = 37.

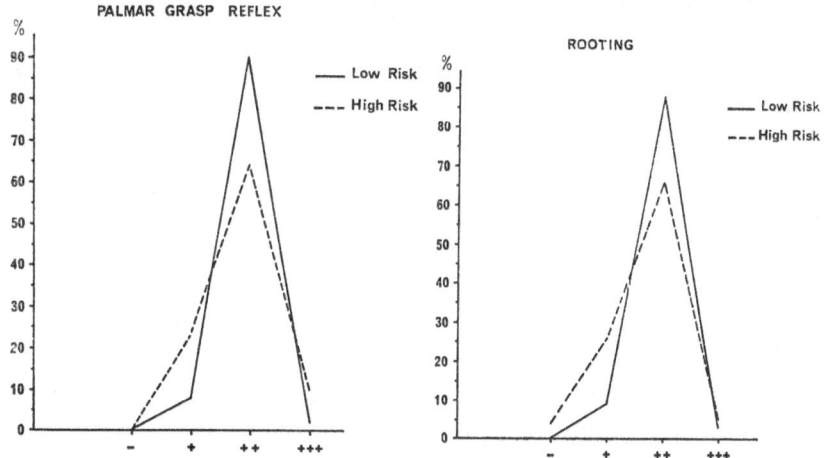

*Fig.* 7.   Distributions of response intensities of the palmar grasp reflex in the low
and high risk groups. The difference is significant. ($\chi^2 = 22.2$; p = 0.001).

*Fig.* 8.   Distributions of response intensities of the rooting response in the low and
high risk group. The difference is significant ($\chi^2 = 22,2$; p = 0.001).

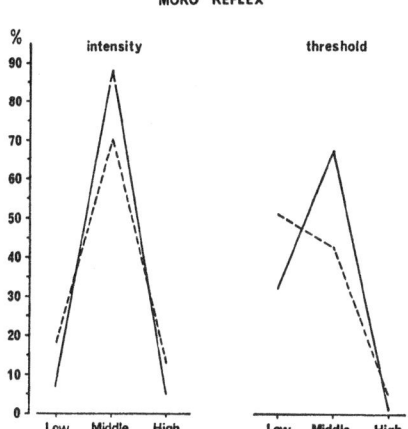

*Fig.* 9. Distributions of the response intensities and threshold of the Moro-response in the low (solid line) and the high risk (broken line) group ($\chi^2 = 19.8$; p < 0.01 and $\chi^2 = 19.9$; p < 0.01 respectively).

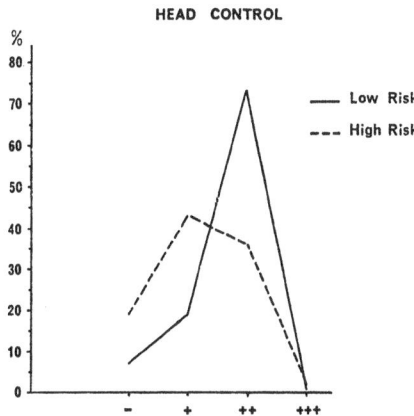

*Fig.* 10. Distributions of the scores of head control in sitting posture in the low and the high risk group ($\chi^2 = 20.1$; p < M 0.01).

three 'risk' groups fell into different positions on each scale. In 42 of the tests, the differences between expected and observed frequencies as measured by $\chi^2$ tests, were significant at least at the 1 % level of confidence. The 'low-risk' group predominantly showed those responses described as 'optimal', whereas the 'high-risk' group showed *relatively few optimal responses*. In all 42 of these items, the 'middle-risk' group was intermediate between the other two with respect to the number of optimal responses. In other words, there is a highly significant association between the number of non-optimal obstetric conditions and neurological abnormalities in the newborn.

The relationship between non-optimal obstetric conditions and neurological abnormality is seen even more clearly, if we carry out the following transformation. For each ordinal item of the neurological examination, a score of '1' was given if the baby's response was in the 'optimal' category. It was thus possible to obtain a 'neurological score', the number of items of the neurological examination upon which the baby gave an optimal response. For all babies on whom the full neurological examination had been carried out (N = 1000) the neurological scores were plotted against the corresponding number of non-optimal conditions.

It was found that the mean neurological score decreased as the number of obstetric complications increased (figure 11).

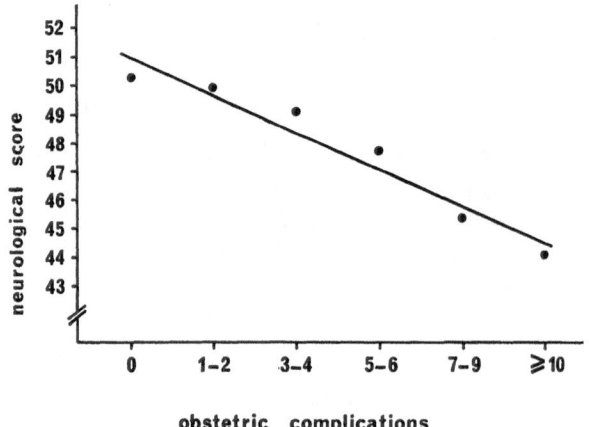

*Fig.* 11. Mean neurological scores plotted against the corresponding number o non-optimal conditions.

The neurological scores were next separated into three main groups, taking the following cut-off points: scores equal to or less than 47 (abnormal); scores between 48 and 52 (suspected abnormal) and scores between 53 and 58 (normal). The babies in each of these 3 groups were then allocated, on the basis of their mother's obstetric score to the high, middle and low risk groups. The relationship between the neurological and obstetric findings is shown in table 3.

Table 3.

| Neurological Scores | Risk Group | | | Totals |
|---|---|---|---|---|
| | Low | Middle | High | |
| ⩽ 47 | 73 (101.7) | 375 (363.4) | 83 (65.9) | 531 |
| 48—52 | 84 (87.9) | 316 (314.1) | 59 (57) | 459 |
| 53—58 | 107 (74.3) | 252 (265.5) | 29 (48.1) | 388 |
| Totals | 264 | 943 | 171 | 1378 |

Figures in parentheses are expected frequencies.

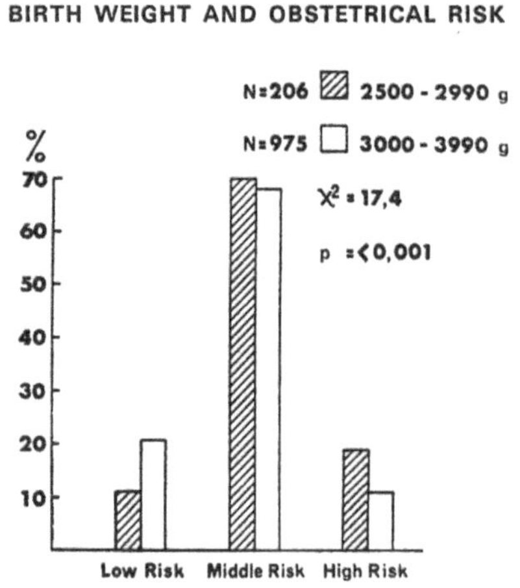

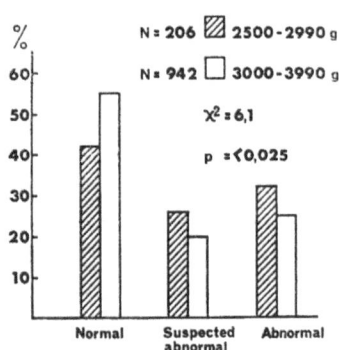

BIRTH WEIGHT AND OBSTETRICAL RISK
N=206 2500 - 2990 g
N=975 3000 - 3990 g
$\chi^2$ = 17,4
p =<0,001
%
70
60
50
40
30
20
10
Low Risk
Middle Risk
High Risk

BIRTH WEIGHT AND NEUROLOGICAL FINDINGS
%
N = 206 2500-2990 g
N = 942 3000-3990 g
$\chi^2$ = 6,1
p =<0,025
60
50
40
30
20
10
Normal
Suspected abnormal
Abnormal

*Fig.* 12. Comparison of percentages of lower and higher birth weight babies in low, middle and high risk groups.

*Fig.* 13. Comparison of percentages of lower and higher birth weight babies in neurological normal, suspected abnormal and abnormal groups.

There was a very highly significant difference between the observed and expected frequencies with which the three neurological subgroups were represented in the three risk groups ($\chi^2 = 38.5$, d.f. $= 4$, $p < .001$). It is clear therefore that there is a high association between obstetric complications as measured by the obstetric scores and the occurrence of neonatal neurological abnormalities. It is of interest to examine the relationship between the obstetric and neurological findings and birth-weight. Babies with a relatively low birth-weight of 2500—3000 g were compared with those whose birth-weight was 3000—4000 g. The percentages of babies in each range who fell into the three obstetric groups, low, middle and high risk, are shown in figure 12. Babies with the lower birth-weight are significantly over-represented in the high risk and under-represented in the low risk groups respectively. Similarly, the lower birth-weight babies are significantly under-represented in the neurologically normal and over-represented in the suspected abnormal groups respectively (figure 13).

### 4. Obstetric risks and neurological syndromes

If a group of symptoms occur repeatedly in combination they may be said to constitute a syndrome. We have previously described a combination of low intensity of general motor activity and of sucking, rooting, hand- and foot-grasping, head-lifting in prone position, recoil of forearms and the labyrinthine reflex, the *apathy syndrome* (16). Similarly, babies showing lowered resistance to passive movements of the neck, trunk, shoulder, elbow, hand, hip, knee and ankle joints, have been described as hypotonic. Significantly more babies showing both the apathy syndrome and hypotonia were found in the high risk group than in either the middle or low risk groups (figures 14 and 15). The apathy syndrome was also found significantly more often among the babies whose birthweight was relatively lower (2500—3000 g) (figure 16). Babies with asymmetries of posture, tendon reflexes and skin reflexes (which we have previously described as the *hemisyndrome*) were equally distributed among the three risk groups. Interestingly, however, babies with the hemisyndrome and those with facial palsies, had a significantly raised incidence of occurrence after forceps delivery and version-extraction. Babies who are what we have called *hyperexcitable* (16) were significantly over-represented in the middle risk group. Hyperexcitability occurred significantly more frequently amongst the boys.

### 5. Neurological scores and classical neurological signs

We have so far argued that there is a high positive correlation between non-optimal conditions and neurological abnormality as measured by our standardised procedure. Because neonatal abnormalities using

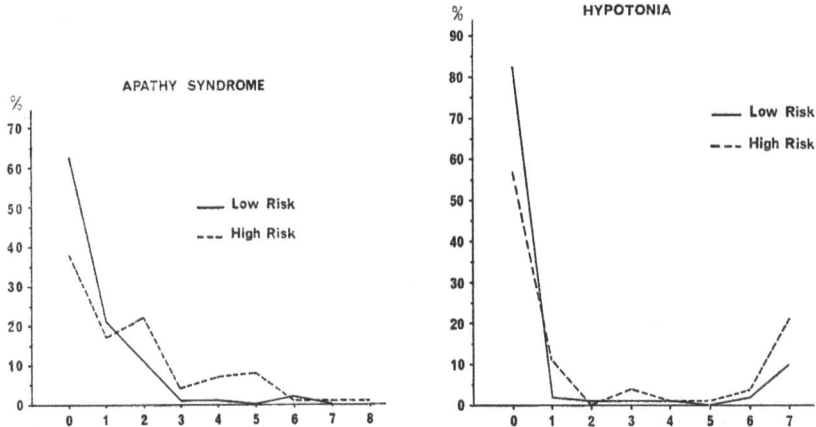

*Fig.* 14. Distributions of apathy scores in low and high risk groups.

*Fig.* 15. Distributions of the hypotonia score in the low and high risk groups. The rise at the right end of the curves is due to the generalized hypotonic babies who obtained the highest scores.

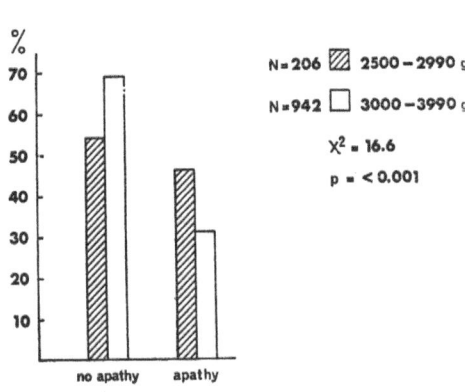

*Fig.* 16. Comparison of percentages of lower and higher birth weight babies with respect to the presence or absence of the apathy syndrome.

this technique are predictive of continuing abnormality and future behavioural disturbance (17) we believe it is essential that full neuro-logical examination is carried out on all babies who are obstetrically at higher risk. It might be argued however, that since the full exami-

nation is a time-consuming and expensive procedure, it is sufficient
to record the presence of obvious neurological signs which any well
trained obstetrician or paediatrician could not fail to see. In fact, 25
of our babies showed one or more obvious-neurological signs: facial
palsies; bulging fontanelles; deviation of eye position; absence of
sucking; Moro or palmar grasp reflexes; severe floppiness or marked
asymmetry. It is of interest to examine the distribution of the neurological scores of these babies relative to that of the remainder. No
baby with an obvious neurologically abnormal condition, ever obtains
fewer than 4 non-optimal sub-test items, i.e. it is never misclassified as
normal by our examination. On the other hand, a very large number
of babies with no classical neurological signs, obtain the same neurological scores as those *with* such classical signs. It is clear therefore
that examination merely for gross signs of pathology will result in the
omission of a considerable amount of neurological abnormality which
is prognostically ominous. Thus, the presence of 'classical neurological
signs' is not exclusive evidence of neurological abnormality. Moreover,
we have shown that neurological abnormality, as measured by the
full standardised procedure, increases in relation to the number of
non-optimal obstetric conditions. It therefore follows that the urgency
for *full* neurological examination of the newborn increases also as a
function of the number of non-optimal conditions present.

DISCUSSION

The identification of what constitute obstetric hazards remains still an
urgent clinical problem. An approach to this question through mortality rate studies has great merits, but the answers must remain incomplete, since the majority of infants survive obstetric complications.
Among these babies however may be many who suffer major or minor
impairment of brain function. The early recognition of nervous dysfunction is of great importance both with respect to the possibility
of early treatment, and in relation to handling difficulties arising
during the development of the mother-infant relationship. Many
studies seem to indicate that besides handicaps such as cerebral palsy,
due to pre- and peri-natal brain damage, minor brain dysfunctions,
undramatic from the clinical neurological point of view, may lead
to severe problems in the life of children and their parents. Although
well controlled studies are still scarce, the available data are alarming.

In the context of these aspects the need for early indicators of risks is evident. The attempt to design risk registers which would select those babies from the population who are at special risk of brain damage is a major task. If only for the purpose of practical management, criteria are needed which do not select for special attention half or even more of all newborn babies. In the light of our study, one possible approach is through the obstetric score. It will be remembered that obstetric scores were highly correlated with neurological findings which were themselves predictive of continuing abnormality. In practice, this would mean filling in a checklist of non-optimal conditions which results in a risk score. This is obviously a more reliable strategy than to look only for the presence of particular dangerous obstetric conditions in the baby's history.

As a further result of our study new criteria are suggested for the interpretation of the quantative results of our neurological test items. Although it was possible previously to indicate the optimal intensity of responses, it was still questionable for many responses, at which points of the scale one should speak of an abnormal response, a fact we have indicated in our Manual for the neurological examination of the full-term newborn infant (15). Differences found between the neurological item scores of the obstetrically high risk group and those of the low risk group are very suggestive of a more valid demarcation of neurological abnormality. For example, with respect to the rooting response, the differences between the two risk groups are apparent in the scores (—) and (+), but the incidence of (+++) is no higher in the high risk group than in the low risk group. This offers a possible operational definition of 'abnormal' as being the (—) and (+) responses only, in contrast to the normal responses (++) and (+++) In the case of the palmar grasp response, on the other hand, the (+++) response would still be considered as abnormal.

This new information is valid for many test items of the neurological examination. There remain certain neurological signs which are undoubtedly abnormal, such as the absence of sucking or of the Moro response, persistent deviation of the eyes. Our study has shown however, that application of these generally accepted criteria of abnormality alone would leave many neurologically abnormal babies unrecognized. The French technique as advocated by St.-Anne Dargassies (18) uses only such qualitative signs. The quantitative assessment of neurological signs is not however a mere academic refinement of neurological examinations but a clinical necessity.

## SUMMARY

A group of 1378 full-term newborn infants, born in the Obstetric Department of the University Groningen were subjected to a standardized quantitative neurological examination in their first 10 days of life. Data on pregnancy, delivery and condition of the infant at birth were available.

Since previous correlation analysis of neurological results with obstetric complications failed to give instructive results a new approach was carried out. 42 variables of the pre- and paranatal history were analysed and counted if they deviated from optimal condition, giving an obstetric risk score for each baby. The distributions of response intensities of many neurological items were shown to be different in the low, middle and high risk groups. This held true also for some syndromes. Number of optimal neurological responses was negatively correlated with the number of non-optimal obstetric conditions.

It was shown that non-optimal conditions tended to occur in association with each other. The more a condition deviated from the norm, the greater the number of other non-optimal conditions associated with it. A simple count of the number of such non-optimal conditions present, offers promise as a means of identifying those babies at risk of neurological damage.

It is suggested that the criteria for assessing what is an abnormal neurological response may be refined by reference to the responses of our low and high risk groups.

ACKNOWLEDGEMENTS

My thanks are due to Prof. L. A. JOOSSE and Prof. B. S. TEN BERGE of the Dept. of Obstetrics, University Groningen for their interest and co-operation over the many years of this study. I am also indebted to my coworkers Drs. D. J. BEINTEMA, J. DIJKSTRA, A. V. D. GAAG, W. LAVANT, B. C. L. TOUWEN for their part in collecting the data. Without the great assistance of Dr. D. SMITS, director of the Computer Center of the University and Dr. R. WIPPLER and Mrs. J. H. VAN DIJK-V. D. HORST the data processing would have been impossible. I want to express my warm appreciation for the help of Dr. S. J. HUTT in the preparation of the manuscript. This study was supported by a grant from the Association for the Aid of Crippled Children New York.

## REFERENCES

1. DE HAAS-POSTHUMA, J. H. (1962) *Perinatale sterfte in Nederland. Onderzoek naar factoren, die de perinatale sterfte beïnvloeden.* T.N.O. Van Gorcum en Comp., Assen.
2. BUTLER, N. R. and D. G. BONHAM (1963) *Perinatal mortality.* E. & S. Livingstone Ltd., Edinburgh and London.
3. DEBRÉ, R. and E. BARGETON (1955) *Arch. Franc. Pediatr.* 12: 673–684.
4. NORMAN, A. P. (1956) *Brit. Med. J.* 37–40.
5. MALAMUD, N. (1959) *J. of Neuropathol. and Exp. Neurol.* 18: 141–155.
6. CLARK, D. B. and G. W. ANDERSON (1961) *J. Neuropathol. Exp. Neurol.* 20: 275–278.
7. MORF, E. und J. BRETSCHER (1966) *Gynaecol.* 161: 211–215.
8. RANCK Jr., B. and W. F. WINDLE (1959) *Exp. Neurol.* 1: 130–154.
9. WINDLE, W. F. (1960) *Pediatrics* 25: 565–569.
10. WINDLE, W. F., M. I. R. DE RAMIREZ DE ARELLANO, M. RAMIREZ DE ARELLANO and E. HIBBARD (1961) *Rev. Neurol.* 105: 142–152.
11. APGAR, V. (1966) *Pediatr. Clin. N. Amer.* 13: 645–650.
12. DRAGE, J. S. and H. BERENDES (1966) *Pediat. Clin. N. Amer.* 13,: 635–644.
13. GRAHAM, F. K. (1956) *Psychol. Monogr.* 70: 20 and 21.
14. GRAHAM, F. K., M. PENNOYER, B. CALDWELL, M. GREENMAN and A. F. HARTMANN (1957) *J. Pediat.* 50: 177–189.
15. PRECHTL, H. F. R. and D. J. BEINTEMA (1964) The neurological examination of the full term newborn infant. *Little Club Clinics in developmental Medicine* no. 12. Publ.: The Spastics Society Medical Education and Information Unit in Association with William Heinemann Medical Books Ltd. London.
16. PRECHTL, H. F. R. and J. DIJKSTRA (1960) Neurological diagnosis of cerebral injury in the newborn. In: *Prenatal Care,* ed. Noordhoff, Groningen, 222–231.
17. PRECHTL, H. F. R. (1965) *Proc. Roy. Soc. Med. London* 58: 1991–1994.
18. DARGASSIES, S. SAINT-ANNE (1962) *Biol. Neonat.* 4: 174–200.

# DISCUSSION

DISCUSSION PAPER DR. DRILLIEN

*Prof. Jonxis* (in the chair): Thank you very much for your clear exposition about this for all of us so important subject. Your lecture is very important for giving us information on the cause of the handicap. We should like to know if a special treatment is a good or a bad one. Only after five years or more we may learn what the value of a special treatment is. In order to reach a conclusion we shall have to study special groups very carefully and I have the feeling that up till now few paediatricians are doing these follow-up studies. Dr. DRILLIEN's paper is now open for discussion.

*Dr. Wigglesworth:* I have two questions for Dr. DRILLIEN. First of all I should like to ask if she has any idea why the poor male sex is so feeble and more prone to handicap than the female sex. Secondly whether she can tell us anything on possible relationships between feeding of these babies in the immediate newborn period and later handicap.

*Dr. Drillien:* Well, as to the first question it is obvious that the female is the superior sex from conception to the grave. From the teleological point of view this is because the female is carrying on the race and the part of the male takes only a fraction of time.

About feeding, you may have noticed that I left out in the last slide the years 1953 and 1954. During that time the incidence of handicap in those two year groups was very high. It happened to be that in those two years I first started collecting data about prae-matures. This very high incidence of handicap aroused my interest. It was so obvious even at that very young age. Those two years were when we were practising delayed feeding. I don't mean we were

21*

feeding at 48 hours instead of 12 hours, I mean that the babies were not fed often before the 5th or 6th day. Our mortality figures improved dramatically in that period. So I think this had some effect on survival. Our nursing techniques were not so good then. But I'm sure that the high incidence of handicap in this group of babies was caused by extremely delayed feeding. Whether you should feed at 12 hours or before or whether you should feed at 36 hours I'm rather in favour of early feeding as long as you have got skilled nurses. When you have not enough confidence in your nursing staff probably you do better to delay feeding until 24 hours.

*Dr. Gruenwald:* The group of babies below the 10th percentile you have analysed presumably includes both mature growth-retarded and pre-term growth-retarded infants. In other words in this group are infants who are pre-term *and* growth-retarded. I wonder whether you have ever separated the pure groups, the pure pre-term and the pure growth-retarded infants. This might perhaps pin-point the kind of damage a little better than when you include the transitional forms and the combination forms.

*Dr. Drillien:* The majority of them were undergrown and pre-term. I haven't done anymore on this group from the point of view of birth-weight and gestational age because I have not enough confidence in the accuracy of the data. But this is a thing I'm doing with the current group.

*Dr. Lubchenco:* I can give a little bit of information. We used birth weight for our follow-up study of children who were approximately ten years of age. We looked at only those under 1500 g at birth. Eighty per cent were below the median of our curves for birth weight. We found that the combination of birth weight and gestational age was extremely important. The handicap-rate fell directly as the gestational age progressed. Under 1500 g the handicap-rate of moderate to severe disease was nearly 85 per cent for the infants with a very short gestation and very low birth weight, i.e. smaller than 950 grams and younger than 28 weeks, to about 20 per cent for infants of 1350— 1500 grams and gestational ages over 33 weeks. We also looked at caloric intake in relation to birth weight, gestational age, and later outcome. There seemed to be a positive independent effect of calories over and above gestational age and birth weight. The more calories during the first week after birth, the better was the outlook. The effects of caloric intake on later outcome by follow-up studies, however, are very difficult to evaluate.

*Dr. Drillien:* I'm greatly encouraged by the fact that Dr. LUBCHENCO apart from myself finds a high incidence of handicap in her low birthweight babies, as I have heard from many people that the postnatal care of praematures in Denver is excellent.

*Dr. Dreyfus-Brisac:* We tried in Paris to differentiate exactly between true praemature children and children with low birthweight for gestational age. I would like to show you the results of the study we have done with the EEG. We have studied 96 small for date infants (see table 1), 91 were born between 37 and 43 weeks, 5 were born before 37 weeks (mean 39.1 weeks). The birthweight ranged between 890 g and 2570 g (mean 1895.4 g), the length was between 33 cm and 45 cm (mean 43.4 cm) and the occipito-frontal circumference was between 25 cm and 36 cm (mean 30.7 cm).

Table 1

| Gestational age at birth | Electroencephalographic age | | | |
|---|---|---|---|---|
| | Correct | Correct but imprecise | Incorrect | Unknown |
| 30—36 weeks 5 cases | 4 | | | 1 |
| 37—39 weeks 54 cases | 41 | 6 | 2 | 5 |
| 40—43 weeks 37 cases | 28 | 5 | 2 | 2 |
| Total 96 cases | 73 | 11 | 4 | 8 |
| | | 84 | | |

The results of the electroencephalographic study have been classified in 4 groups: correct, imprecise, uncorrect and unclassifiable (see table).

84 EEG gave a correct appreciation of the gestational age with the criteria already described (C. DREYFUS-BRISAC, World Neurology). Among them, 11 were imprecise, mainly by absence of the sleep patterns, which allow the differentiation between infants of 37—39 weeks of gestational age, and those of 40 weeks or more.

8 EEG were unclassified, being either incomplete, without waking or sleeping patterns, either too pathological.

The 4 errors of classification will be studied in more detail.

Of this series of 96 babies we have seen 31 children again after 3 years. Among them there were 3 with severe encephalopathy and 15 with mild retardation at school. 13 were quite normal.

*Prof. De Bruijne:* Do you think it is possible that the increase in handicap can be counterbalanced by our better treatment of hypoglycaemia, of hyperbilirubinaemia and disturbances of acid-base metabolism?

*Dr. Drillien:* I have the impression from this new group I'm collecting in the last 18 months, that there are rather fewer handicaps. But in this group they are still very young. In my other group quite a lot of children, who were, I thought, not doing too badly in the first two years, have turned out in school to have handicaps. I'm quite sure the factors mentioned by Prof. DE BRUIJNE may have an additional effect. Hypoglycaemia of course we should not see anymore because this is preventable. I can't answer your question, but maybe in five years time.

*Prof. Minkowski:* I first like to confirm the number of handicapped children that Dr. DRILLIEN found in her series. In our follow-up study during 15 years of 315 low birthweight infants, both praemature and dysmature, we have only 200 children who are prefectly normal. The other 115 are more or less severely handicapped.

I would like to ask you what do you exactly mean by developmental malformation? Do you mean developmental malformations of the brain? This is difficult to prove.

*Dr. Drillien:* By developmental malformation I meant something going wrong early in pregnancy during the period of organogenesis. In the new group we are studying we may be able to get a clue. My dental colleagues tell me that by examination of the deciduous teeth, when they fall out, they may be able to tell us something was going wrong — but not what — and roughly at what stage in gestation. I'm very hopeful that this will give us some indication at what stage in gestation something went wrong if anything went wrong.

*Prof. Kloosterman:* I should like to say some words in defence of the poor males. If you take the birthweights as points of origin, then you have males who are more early born than the girls among your sample. Then you are composing the girls in a more favourable situation than the boys. I think you have to correct for gestational age. This will be possible if you get more reliable data from your obstetrician.

*Dr. Drillien:* I don't think this is such an important factor, because most of the difference in birthweight between males and females arises in the last 6 weeks of normal gestation. Before that period there is nearly no difference in weight. Most of my infants were praematurely born and there was not much difference by gestational period in the weights of males and females.

*Prof. Kloosterman:* We found a difference from 20 weeks already. Another thing of course is that both sexes have the same size of placenta. So at least before birth the mother is handicapping a little bit her poor boys.


DISCUSSION PAPER DR. PRECHTL

*Dr. Dreyfus-Brisac:* In your follow-up studies you have lost many children, have you seen all the children again between 2 and 4 years?

*Dr. Prechtl:* There was certainly a drop-out, but it was a small one. I have not mentioned the 8 years follow-up study which we have carried out on a smaller group. Over the 8 years we had a drop-out from all causes, including death, of only 18 per cent.

*Prof. Stahlie:* This syndrome of hyperexcitability in the young baby, have you been able to correlate this with calcium values in the blood?

*Dr. Prechtl:* Yes, this was one of the first things we examined. When we saw those babies who are so hyperexcitable that they produce a startle or a Moro reflex at the slightest disturbance, calcium and glucose levels were checked. Of course there are babies who are very hyperexcitable with low calcium or low glucose. But the majority of the babies whom we called hyperexcitable had normal values.

CLOSING SESSION

# SUMMING-UP AND GENERAL DISCUSSION

It is my task to present to you a summary of this meeting and to stimulate a general summarizing discussion. If I might say, this is not an easy task.

The theme of this meeting was 'aspects of prematurity and dysmaturity'; I think we could have used the term 'aspects of perinatal development' as well. Indeed, I have been fascinated by the fact, that we have discussed these days some fundamental problems of development and differentiation. We all here, as paediatricians, obstetricians, biologists, are deeply involved in problems of growth and development. One of the most fundamental mysteries of biology which we are going to unravel in future research on growth and development is the biochemistry and genetics of differentiation.

*Development* can be described as a series of synchronous events, characterized by adaptive functional change: such changes may be a decrease or abolition in function, an increase or commencement in function, or an alteration of function.

*Differentiation* can be most simply defined as an increase in the complexity of structure and function. As differentiation continues, the increase in the complexity of function and structure necessitates the development of specific regulatory processes, and a number of very precise, mostly feedback regulating systems have been discovered, in which hormones act as 'messengers'.

There is every reason to state that differentiation of cells and tissues does not occur by a 'sorting-out' process of genes into different cells, but that each cell in a multi-cellular organism has the same genetic information as every other cell. All phenomena during development can be related to information from the genetic material being transcribed to its final form, a protein, which is mostly an enzyme. We still do not know the genetic mechanism of differentation and development, but the recent advances in our understanding of the genetic process and of the biosynthesis of specific proteins, together with advances in the techniques of cell culture and chemical analyses are so promising that it will be possible to solve this fundamental problem of differentiation in the future, not in the near future, but in a future which we can foresee.

It seems evident that differentiation means a differential activation of genes in different cells and tissues at a specific time. This concept of 'critical periods' during differentiation seems to me a very important one.

A beautiful example of the phenomenon of appearance of a protein at a specific time, the disappearance of this protein and its replacement by a protein with a similar function, is the replacement of fetal hemoglobin by adult hemoglobin. The great problem of course is what sets the clock.

Dr. HERBERT SCHWARTZ has reviewed this subject and he has shown that careful and detailed study of this 'switch-over mechanism' may clarify some of the problems I just mentioned. Other examples of this phenomenon were discussed by Dr. SERENI in regard to glycogen and lipid metabolism. Before birth there is enzyme-maturation of those enzymes which synthesize glycogen, right after birth enzymes as glucose-6-fosfatase which release glucose become very active. Lipogenesis occurs before birth, lipolysis with release of FFA occurs after birth. Dr. SERENI also discussed the interesting observation of a sharp increase in the rate of nucleic acid and protein synthesis after birth which occurs at least in the rat. Cortisol and perhaps thyroxine seem to play a permissive role in this process. What is the meaning of this rapid change in enzyme synthesis after birth and how can it be explained in the light of our current ideas about protein biosynthesis?

Dr. KOLDOVSKY presented new data on the development of enzymes and absorption processes in the small intestine of the fetus. He also discussed the effects of adrenocortical steroids as cortisol (and aldosterone as well) on the appearance and disappearance of invertase and the beta-glucosidase lactase at a specific period of development in the rat. Adrenalectomy counteracts both changes, but subsequent administration of a steroid induces again both changes. This is a beautiful example of molecular differentiation: lactase disappears when the rat is weaned and invertase activity increases; cortisol apparently is involved in both events. Such phenomena could be explained by the Jacob and Monod theory: a structural gene is 'repressed' or 'derepressed' as the operator gene turns it on and off. Hormones, at least some hormones, may well act this way. Molecular differentiation has enlightened the old words of the philosopher: *life is a series of little deaths, out of which life always returns.*

Now let us turn to growth of the organism as a whole. Why does an organism grow? What controls growth? These are fundamental questions which we cannot answer as yet. However, the subject has been studied extensively during recent years and we have been very fortunate to have a number of experts in this field at this Symposium.

Many factors influence foetal growth. Drs. GRUENWALD, LUBCHENCO and OUNSTED discussed this subject. These are exogenous factors (socio-economic, congenital anomalies, toxaemia, altitude, smoking a.o.), and endogenous factors. It is apparent that maternal factors play a most distinctive role, as Dr. OUNSTED beautifully analysed. Correlation of birth-weight in maternal half-sibs is much higher than in paternal half-sibs. Dr. OUNSTED also discussed the most interesting correlation of length of the mother, her own birth-weight and birth-weight of her child. If a low birth-weight, as a result of intra-uterine conditions, has a long-term effect on adult size twenty years later, and this again determines birth-weight in the next generation, then indeed we might conclude that the preparation for pregnancy begins already during foetal life.

Dr. OUNSTED's speculation about the role of the placental 'pro-lactin-like growth hormone' in the trophoblastic invasion of the maternal decidual tissue is a tempting one. Placental size depends primarily on the extent of this trophoblastic invasion, and placental size correlates with birth-weight.

I think all of us were particularly pleased to listen to Dr. LUB-CHENCO's presentation. She really has provided us reliable standards for antenatal growth and almost all speakers at this meeting showed slides based on her curves.

If there is retardation of growth in utero, not all organs are retarded to the same extent. As Dr. GRUENWALD showed in the human, and Dr. WIGGLESWORTH and Dr. WIDDOWSON in the animal, the liver is markedly underweight, but the brain weight is much less abnormal. What then regulates the growth of each individual organ?

The experimental approach to problems of dysmaturity seems most promising. Drs. WIGGLESWORTH and WIDDOWSON presented fascinating papers with many interesting data for the clinician who can relate these studies with the experiments of nature in the human. Again such experimental studies support the idea of 'critical periods' during development. Retardation of growth during some periods of development is followed by 'incomplete catch-up': although there is the same rate of growth compared with animals who have been normal throughout, the experimental animals end up as small adults. This again has great implications for human pathology.

Some effects of undernutrition in the young animal are most interesting. The skeletal development in a runt is retarded but more advanced than in a normal fetus of the same weight. Total water content is almost the same as in a normal fullterm animal, and different from that in the foetus of the same weight and normal duration of pregnancy. Obviously further studies of *body composition* are indicated in the dysmature animal and dysmature human as well. Other aspects of dysmaturity in the human as decreased glycogen content of the liver can be beautifully produced in the experimental dysmature animal.

To me it also seems very important to analyse in these studies not only cell mass, but also the number of cells. It makes a great difference if growth-inhibitory factors affect the organism at a time when cells are dividing rapidly or at a time when cells are just growing, increase in size. Irreversible effects can be expected to occur when cells are dividing, when they increase in number. Of course, organs are different in this way: for instance the brain stops quite early with cell-division, and this may explain why the brain has a relatively normal weight in the dysmature human baby or animal as compared with other organs.

What is the role of the placenta? We knew already that the placenta is an organ with multiple functions. The recent concept of the feto-placental unit as an integrated endocrine organ has added another most important function. Dr. REYNOLDS reviewed this subject and he has added the results of a whole series of most ingeneous experiments. What is the meaning of this? Teleologically speaking the protection of the fetus against the androgens of the mother would be most important. We know that administration of androgens to the young animal fetus, as for instance the rat, is followed by sterility in the female and abnormalities in behaviour at older age. The syndrome is called the 'early androgen syndrome'. You might well recall that ALDOUS HUXLEY in his 'Brave New World' in 1932 already sterilised the 'in vitro cultured' embryos by adding androgenic hormones.

The placenta detoxifies maternal androgens; the fetus itself does not produce much androgens because the enzyme 3-beta-ol dehy-drogenase is lacking. But this implies that he neither can transform progesterone from pregnenolone, as an immediate precursor for cortisol and aldosterone. However, the placenta supplies the fetus with great amounts of progesterone.

Morphological studies of the placenta, in normal and pathological conditions, are very difficult indeed as Dr. GRUENWALD pointed out. However, it is clear that further work in this field will provide another approach to study the role of the placenta in dysmaturity. Dr. WIGGLES-WORTH presented his new technique of studying the arterial blood supply, as a good example of such a new approach.

Many questions remain here unanswered. What determines the end of gestation and the moment of birth? Ageing of the placenta has been suggested as an important factor, but the underlying mechanism has to be elucidated. It will be necessary to develop reliable diagnostic methods to analyse this ageing process for clinical purposes.

What then is dysmaturity? Professor KLOOSTERMAN has defined it as intra-uterine starvation, and I like his remark that 'such a child in some way is born too late'. It is important to realize that, although we often speak of dysmature infants when they are born after a preg-nancy of 42 weeks and more, an infant can be dysmature and born between 28 and 38 weeks of pregnancy. Such an infant is dysmature and premature as well.

Estimation of foetal age by careful physical and neurological examination is not as easy as some people suggest, at least in my own experience. Of course we were delighted to watch the beautiful film of Professor MINKOWSKI and his collaborators on the neurological assessment of foetal age.

I have no objections against the term dysmaturity. Although I can appreciate Dr. GRUENWALD's point of view, I think that the dysmature infant is retarded not only in length and total weight, but also in weight of individual organs, functions of organs and even in the development of regulatory functions. Of course we must realize the fact that the degree of retardation is not the same for all of these parameters.

The dysmature infant faces the paediatrician with a whole series of clinical problems in the immediate postnatal period and during infancy. Professor JONXIS discussed the specific changes in RQ and $O_2$

consumption during cold exposure in the dysmature infant as compared with the full-term born and premature infant.

Professor ROBERT SCHWARTZ analysed the factors involved with
glucose control in the neonate: maternal nutrition, placental transport, maturity of the infant, and early versus late feeding after birth.
There is very good evidence now, I think, that early feeding will
decrease the number of complications involved with hypoglycaemia
and hyperbilirubinaemia. It is my opinion that if inadequate nursing
care prevents early oral feeding in these infants, intravenous administration of fluids should bridge the intermittent period between
birth and the day when sufficient fluid and calories can be given
orally. Professor DE BRUYNE demonstrated that dysmature infants
have a higher frequency of hyperbilirubinaemia. Further work in
this field has to be done in regard to standardisation of bilirubin
measurements and treatment of the syndrome.

Dr. STRICH showed us the severe pathological changes in the
nervous system as a result of neonatal hypoglycaemia. Many important problems are here open for further investigation: how to study
cerebral blood flow in relation with anoxia; is there an energy supply
of the brain other than glucose, and many more.

The obstetrical aspects of dysmaturity were discussed by Professor
KLOOSTERMAN. His results of careful prenatal control and treatment
after the 42nd week of pregnancy are most impressive and represent
the best traditional Dutch obstetrics. Dr. WIGGLESWORTH expressed
the admiration of the audience.

The results of the combined efforts of obstetricians and paediatricians in the prenatal and postnatal care of the low birth-weight infant
were discussed by Drs. DRILLIEN and PRECHTL. These results are rather
depressing, but we are looking forward to see the further follow-up
studies of new samples of infants which were treated during recent
years with more intensive care during the neonatal period. Qualitative and perhaps quantitative methods are now available to follow-
up the neurological development in infants and children, and no one
could better illustrate these methods than Dr. PRECHTL.

There is a great need for expanded basic research relating to the
developing nervous system, particularly to determine the incidence
of brain damage in infants with low birth-weight.

It has been a good meeting, I think. Progress has been defined as the activity of today and the assurance of tomorrow. The art of progress is to preserve order amid change and to preserve change amid order. If this is true, this meeting has illustrated the progress in the field of perinatal development.


## SUMMING-UP BY PROF. KLOOSTERMAN

Before I fullfill my task to put together what has been said during this conference on the role and function of the placenta in dysmaturity, I should like to express my thanks to the organizers of this symposium. They have brought together a group of workers of different disciplines all interested in the same object, but looking at it from different angles. In doing so everybody stimulates the interest of members of other disciplines to new ideas or reconsideration of their old ones. This has been a very useful and interesting experience. This sort of symposium is in my opinion the ideal of what a symposium should be. One interest, one place, one language — I hope that Shakespeare will forgive us — but different disciplines, different personalities and different nations. One aim and different ways to reach it.

Now what has been said during this symposium about the placenta in general and its significance for dysmaturity in peculiar. Dr. REYNOLDS started and showed us that the placenta is able to synthesize progesteron de novo from acetate without interference of the foetus, but that for the production of the oestrogens, especially oestriol, the foetal-placental unit is necessary. This means that for some important functions like synthesis of oestrogens the foetus is dependent on certain enzymes that are only present in the placenta. This means also that a hormone that is very important for the maintenance of pregnancy, namely progesterone, is formed in the placenta without interference of the foetus. This means that the placenta from a biochemical point of view is very important and as far as steroid synthesis is concerned in some aspects even more important than the foetus itself.

Then we heard interesting data from Dr. GRUENWALD who emphasized the fact that microscopic studies of the human placenta reveal many differences with the placenta of even such close relatives like Rhesus monkeys. He made probable that the arterial blood flow of maternal origin in the placenta is between the different cotyledones

or tambours and not direced towards the center of these cotyledones
as far as morphological studies can show.

Interesting thereafter were the investigations of Dr. WIGGLESWORTH
who could show by method of injection-preparations that the flow is
directed towards the center of the lobules and that morphological
studies and physiological studies have to be combined.

Dr. WIGGLESWORTH and Dr. WIDDOWSON showed us that, if the
bloodflow in the arteries in the beginning of pregnancy is interfered
with, not only the foetus but also the placenta stays small. Very interesting is what Dr. WIGGLESWORTH mentioned about the fact that in
rats the placenta is not growing anymore after 19 days of pregnancy.
If the placenta at that moment is of a small size, then even improvement in blood flow in the mother after that date will not be able
to let grow the placenta. To some extent you could compare pregnancy with a three-step-rocket. In the first part of pregnancy the uterus
is growing, then the uterus stops growing, but the placenta is lanced
and will grow still for several weeks or months depending on the species. Then the placenta stops growing and the foetus continues growing
as the last step of the whole rocket and then after some time even the
foetus stops growing and it is lanced into the outer world. It was most
stimulating to hear this idea. At least so is my interpretation of what
I got from him.

Dr. OUNSTED has given very interesting remarks, and most stimulating, about the fact that the size of the placenta is influenced by
genetic differences between mother and child. In cases of Rhesus-
sensitization we know the placenta is on the whole rather big and
there is of course a difference between mother and child. On the other
hand we could show that the placenta in the case of boys and girls is
not different in size. This has been a very interesting thing that stimulates to further work to make out which maternal factors or factors
in antagonism between mother and child can influence the size of
the placenta.

In conclusion I should say that it is very important to look at the
placenta not only as an organ of the foetus, but also as an organ that
is more influenced than any other organ by maternal conditions. I
should like to conclude with stressing the fact that Dr. GRUENWALD
has put here, that the definition of placental insufficiency is handled

in different ways. Perhaps it could be very important, if we could come to accordance about this question. You could look at the definition of placental insufficiency as the whole supply of the mother given to the foetus, because it goes through the placenta. If the bloodstream in the placenta is insufficient by maternal causes, then you can speak of course of placental insufficiency. But it gives an extension to this idea. You also could speak of placental insufficiency only in cases where the placenta itself is the factor that narrows the blood supply because the size and the condition of the placenta are below normal level.

I should propose to speak of placental insufficiency in a broad sense. Then everything is included, also maternal conditions, shock of the mother and insufficient blood supply of the uterus. Speaking of placental insufficiency in a narrower sense, we have to find a very small placenta or a placenta that is damaged by infarctions and so on. If everybody could follow this advice of Dr. GRUENWALD, I think this should be a very important conclusion of this congress.

*Dr. Ounsted:* I should like to comment on the statement of Prof. KLOOSTERMAN about the size of male and female placenta. At variance with the findings of Prof. KLOOSTERMAN other workers (HENDRICK, C. H. (1964) Obst. and Gynaec. 24, 3, 357, and Mc. KEOWN, T. and RECORD, R. G. (1953) J. Endocrinol. 10, 73) reported that male placentae were larger than female.

*Dr. Matsaniotis:* Although I am an outsider in this field, I would like to make a general remark concerning the placenta: this organ reminds me of another remarkable organ with which we are much more familiar: the thymus. Just a few years ago nobody knew anything about the thymus, which proved to be a master-organ of all defensive mechanisms.

It would be a very good idea to preserve frozen samples of every peculiar-looking placenta or of every placenta associated with a peculiar-looking baby, which could be examined in the future when we know much more about the function of this most important organ.

*Dr. Gruenwald:* I don't know if this belongs to this point, but I would only suggest that we should make distinction between two forms of insufficiency of the supply-line. I personally should like to reserve the term placental insufficiency for a real defect of the placenta itself. We should separate insufficiency of the supply-line to the foetus which is chronic in duration, has lasted for a long time and has lead to growth retardation, from shorter lasting insufficiency which has lead to wasting in a foetus that grew normally untill not very long before birth. I have a suspicion that the late sequelae in both groups will be different. I suspect that the foetus that has just wasted for some days will probably grow up normally on the average. The growth-retarded group, that has stopped growth long before birth, might be expected to show more severe and perhaps different sequelae. If we keep these two groups together we may make the interpretation difficult. This will of course necessitate the definition of groups and criteria that have not yet been developed but should be developed in the near future.

*Dr. Lubchenco:* I hesitate but feel that I should raise a voice of objection to using the terms 'placental insufficiency' and 'dysmaturity'. It seems to me that we are still at the stage of describing these different groups of babies. Maturity is such a difficult term to define at this particular time because there is maturation of the skeleton, maturation of the enzyme systems, and so on. For these reasons it was decided not to use the word 'maturity' in the classification of newborns recommended by the American Academy of Pediatrics. I wonder again if one should not use something like 'intrauterine growth retardation' or 'small for gestational age' rather than 'dysmaturity'.

*Dr. Wigglesworth:* In defining placental insufficiency, I would agree with Prof. KLOOSTERMAN, I don't think that you can restrict the term placental insufficiency to any group with abnormal placentas. You never know to what extent any abnormality of the placenta is secondary to an abnormality of its supply-line. It is quite impossible to seperate the two, although it is obviously reasonable as Dr. GRUENWALD suggested to separate classes of babies.

So I think one will have to include under the term placental insufficiency, the very wide group that Prof. KLOOSTERMAN suggests and subdivide them later when better criteria are available.

*Prof. Kloosterman:* I like to comment on the objections of Dr. LUB-CHENCO. Dysmaturity has something to do with intra-uterine starvation. It is a conflict between the needs of the baby and we don't know these needs. There are children who like to become nine pounds at the end of pregnancy and there are others who are completely satisfied with six pounds. They show this tendency also in later life. Therefore dysmaturity is very difficult to detect at the period of birth, because we can't ask the baby what his intention has been. I should like to warn against changing now the definition because also in other ways we can make it more clearly and easily to detect it. We have made the same mistake in the past.

Praematurity has been defined in the past as a birthweight of less than 2501 g, because this definition was easy and everybody could handle it. This definition has made studies in this field more difficult for 20 years, because we had an easy definition but it was not the truth. Therefore I should like to warn against dysmaturity as a definition of a child below a certain weight, because there are seemingly well developed children who are dysmature, and there are very small children who are not dysmature. It is better to use a term without an easy definition than changing for a term with a very sharp definition, very easy to handle, but not in accordance with difficult biological facts.


SUMMING-UP BY DR. RÄIHÄ

Dr. VISSER asked me kindly yesterday if I would say a few words concerning chemical differentiation during the perinatal period in relation to praematurity and dysmaturity. During this symposium we have heard some very interesting papers which have been devoted to biochemical changes around birth. The basic processes for protein synthesis appear to be similar for all species, but it is not clear whether all species or even organs possess similar control mechanisms. We know today that many biochemical and functional processes continue to develop long after organogenesis and reach full maturity at various stages before and after birth. We have a great deal of knowledge about the specific developmental pattern of certain enzymes around birth such as tryptophane pyrrolase, tyrosine trans-aminase, many intestinal enzymes, enzymes concerned with urea synthesis etc., but this is still very descriptive information, and we know very little about factors which control this development in the mammalian cells. Dr. SERENI pointed out the possible role of corticosteroids and thyroid hormone in regulating liver nucleic acid and protein synthesis, but aside from this all reports here have been purely descriptive. When we know more about mechanisms which regulate normal biochemical development around birth we can turn to the problem of the effects of dysmaturity. Here, we could use as a tool the nice methods described by Drs. WIDDOWSON and WIGGLESWORTH, to produce experimental dysmaturity. I think it is safe to say that any defect in biochemical development which might be due to prae- or dysmaturity has to do with the regulatory processes and not with the basic genetic information for protein synthesis. Thus, we want to know whether there are some 'critical periods' during development when a change in the environment can affect irreversibly the pattern of biochemical development in a similar way as we have seen physical growth to be affected in Dr. WIDDOWSONS rats nursed in small or large litters. These environmental factors could be changes in humoral balance, changes in concentration of intracellular intermediates and substrated or changes in $O_2$ and $CO_2$ tension etc. We know e.g. from the work by Kaplan and coworkers (J. Mol. Biol. 15, 18, 1966) that $O_2$ tension as such controls the synthesis of the muscle type LDH (M-LDH).

It is evident that the knowledge of control phenomena at the level of RNA and protein synthesis in the mammalian cell will shed light on many so far unexplained pathologic processes and many open paths to their treatment.

SUMMING-UP BY PROF. R. SCHWARTZ

I was pleased to hear that Prof. VISSER used the term perinatal development in his new definition of the symposium. As human biologists I suppose our ultimate goals are the survival and the reproduction of the species. We just might ask why we ave concerned about such a small group as the dysmature or even the praemature infants who have such ill-defined problems, and who have such a poorly defined future. Again as a biologist we might just comment that this is one brief aspect of the continuum from fertilization of the ovum to senescence. We might think that understanding of the biochemical and physiological adjustments at this time may well provide answers to the more stable processes of later development.

What are the problems of the clinician? We just heard one conflict already expressed and that is the problem of definition. We have the problem of the awareness and recognition between the immature, the abnormal immature, the mature and the abnormal mature infant. We have the problems of anticipation that Prof. KLOOSTERMAN commented on. It is fine to talk about the postmature infant, you have a time sequence to focus on, but when you talk about the abnormalities of the pre-term infant we are less able to anticipate problems.

We are still at the stage, as Dr. LUBCHENCO pointed out, of description of growth-differentiation. We just may go back and be very simple and consider viability and pre-term, term and post-term infants. We are talking about 'normals' and 'abnormals'. I would prefer to be very simple-minded and not use the term dysmaturity or any of the related other terms, but rather to think of what is normal and what is abnormal. Actually it has been pointed out already this morning, that the definition of the normal is a very incomplete and inadequate one. I think we will have to wait until people like Drs. DRILLIEN, LUBCHENCO and PRECHTL eliminate in longterm follow-up studies those children that end up with handicaps that we can define psychological or orthwerise in order to go back and re-examine the infants we have called normal. Even the growth curves that Drs. GRUENWALD and LUBCHENCO have shown us contain at the lower end infants who are abnormal. This is one of the things that concerns Dr. LUBCHENCO considerably.

Our developmental norms have been expressed mainly in anthropometric terms and we should be equally concerned about physiological, biochemical and psychoneurological development.

Once we learn to classify, understand and to recognize abnormalities in immature praemature and dysmature infants, perhaps we can do something about them. From a physiological point of view we heard from Prof. JONXIS about the change in oxygen consumption and particularly in temperature controle and R.Q. This is terribly important to us in terms of mana ging the infant. We have only touched two other problems, that is the problem of glucose and the problem of bilirubin metabolism. But we barely scraped the surface,

we have not really considered in detail the physiological adjustments, the integrated functions of the cardiovascular system, and
the endocrine system.

Actually I am very much surprised this is a Nutricia sponsored conference. We have been talking for two days about the dysmature infant
which has been defined as an infant suffering from starvation, from
intrauterine growth retardation associated with starvation. We have
not talked at all about postnatal nutrition. We have not said a word
about the caloric requirements, about the type of feeding, about
whether protein in high or low concentrations is better for such an
infant, whether a high fat or low fat intake is better, and what his
mineral intake should be. I am just beginning to touch on those
problems that the paediatrician has been concerned with for the
last fifty years if not longer. I would hope some of my colleagues
will comment in the next few minutes on these aspects of the dysmature infant.

What standards are we going to apply to the abnormal infant in
terms of judging his immediate adjustment in the first few days of
life?

*Dr. Loeb:* I agree completely with Dr. SCHWARTZ. Indeed I was
surprised, maybe a little disappointed that so few things has been
said about the biochemical investigation of the newborn. We leave
now the congress and do not exactly know what to do until the next
meeting in a few years. I would like to stress that it seems to me very
important to go on with the biochemical investigation. Three years
ago, during the first symposium, a lot of things have been said about
biochemical investigation in dysmatures, in infants with respiratory
distress syndrome, hypoglycaemia and so on. It seems that this investigations have not been a very great success in the last year, as we
did not hear a lot of things during the last three days. I think it is
necessary to go on and to study energy metabolism in the newborn.
I know it is very difficult and it is even more difficult to study not
the abnormal but the normal children. When we study the abnormal
children, for instance dysmature infants with the risk of hypoglycaemia,
we have to take as standards probably praemature infants. So we have
to make our own standards for every group in order to better
understanding of energy metabolism. We should think about the

control of energy metabolism and the control is probably partly endocrine. So we have to investigate some endocrine problems like growth hormone, insulin and so on.

*Prof. Visser:* We appreciate your suggestion for the next symposium and we promise to deal with these subjects then.

SUMMING-UP BY PROF. MINKOWSKI

First of all I like to thank again Prof. JONXIS, Prof. VISSER and Nutricia Company for organizing this symposium. Maybe we ware living without having enough biochemical information and the way we should feed babies, but at least I have some ideas and this will stimulate us for a long time until the next symposium.

When we deal with low birthweight babies there is a growing idea now that, 20 years ago we were interested in just survival; I think we move now to another problem, that is *good* survival. This changes not only our investigation, but also our way of thinking. In dealing with the brains of this low birthweight babies, we have to study investigation problems and ethical problems. I should like to summarize the different headings which we are interested in during this symposium.

First is the correlation of growth of the central nervous system in the foetal period versus general body growth. I think it is obvious that from many sides it has been shown that the brain development in those 'small for date' infants does not follow the general line of body growth. According to our criteria a child weighing 1000 g at 39 weeks has a slightly underweight brain, but not too much, but at the same time exhibits a perfect normal behaviour and E.E.G. tracing as a full-term child of 3000 g. This is an interesting phenomenon, which stimulates further research. When this child is normal according to our development criteria this does not mean that the brain has not been damaged. In this line I think, as has been pointed out again, the question of food is of primary importance. As you know if a newborn rat is deprived of food for a few hours, the brain will exhibit damage. This phenomenon will stimulate further investigation about the type and the quantity of food, and also about neurochemistry which we are lacking now.

A second heading is, what shall we do about the biochemical damage to the brain which results from dysmaturity. About hypo-glycaemia we are in need of more investigation to explain why a prae-mature newborn and some infants of diabetic mothers with very low levels of glucose in their blood will not have brain damage as frequently as the dysmature have. I think in this line, and we are studying this, that we should have more information about what is going to the brain and what is coming back from the brain by investigating the circulation through the brain and studying glucose uptake. Not only glucose, but also $pO_2$, $pCO_2$ and pH in the cerebral blood stream should be compared to what happens in the general circulation. There is a chance that it would not be exactly the same. This would be a clue to explain what is going on. Hypernatraemia has also been a matter of concern, it is well known that hypernatraemia can cause convulsions. This should be investigated in a more detailed way.

According to what we have seen from Dr. DRILLIEN and Dr. PRECHTL and others, when we estimate the damage caused by foetal growth retardation to the brains it is obvious now that we should take into account the cause of dysmaturity, namely toxaemia, which probably reduces the blood flow to the brain etc. I would turn to the obstetricians and tell them what our concern is when we have to decide what is the proper time for delivery. We just don't know whether it is better for a baby of a toxaemic mother to be longer in the uterus and then to be not too much praemature. Or if this baby is in distress, the more you wait, the more there is a chance for the brain to be involved. This is a very serious problem, which has not been attacked scientifically and at the moment we lack information. In this line we need of course the help of the experimental workers to know what kind of information we should collect. Otherwise we are just having again the problem of better surviving because longer gestation means more aggression to the brain.

In cases of infertility or difficult conception, we are faced with this problem, that a mother, who has made eight or ten attempts to have children, after a number of either abortions or praemature deliveries with the death of the child, comes to you, and askes 'should I con-tinue'. As you know there is a tendency for these mothers to be very energetic in their attempts to have a child. The problem is there that the more there have been unsuccessful attempts and the more desired is this child, the more there is a risk for the mother to have finally a very praemature or dysmature child with brain damage. I think we are not in a position to give proper advice. The future of this lies in a better basic knowledge of what happens to the brain in those babies.

# INDEX OF AUTHORS

# INDEX OF SUBJECTS